Should this book become sufficiently familiar through usage to earn the title 'Bender's dictionary', it would probably be more correct to call it 'Benders' dictionary', in view of the invaluable assistance of D., D.A., and B.G., guided, if not driven, by A.E.

DICTIONARY OF NUTRITION
AND FOOD TECHNOLOGY

Dictionary of Nutrition and Food Technology

B.Sc., Ph.D., F.R.I.C., F.R.S.H., F.I.F.S.T.

Professor of Nutrition, Queen Elizabeth College,
University of London

NEWNES—BUTTERWORTHS

THE BUTTERWORTH GROUP

ENGLAND: BUTTERWORTH & CO. (PUBLISHERS) LTD.
LONDON : 88 Kingsway, WC2B 6AB

AUSTRALIA: BUTTERWORTH & CO. (AUSTRALIA) LTD.
SYDNEY : 586 Pacific Highway Chatswood, N.S.W. 2067
MELBOURNE : 343 Little Collins Street, 3000
BRISBANE : 240 Queen Street, 4000

CANADA: BUTTERWORTH & CO. (CANADA) LTD.
SCARBOROUGH : 2265 Midland Avenue, Ontario, M1P 4S1

NEW ZEALAND: BUTTERWORTH & CO. (NEW ZEALAND) LTD.
WELLINGTON : 26–28 Waring Taylor Street, 1
AUCKLAND : 35 High Street, 1

SOUTH AFRICA: BUTTERWORTH & CO. (SOUTH AFRICA) (PTY.) LTD.
DURBAN : 152–154 Gale Street

First Edition 1960

Second Edition 1965

Third Edition 1968

Fourth edition published in 1975 by Newnes-Butterworths, an imprint of the Butterworth Group

ISBN 0 408 001437

Printed in Great Britain by
The Whitefriars Press Ltd.,
London and Tonbridge

PREFACE

The study of food as included in the combined subjects of nutrition and food science and technology involves a wide variety of basic sciences ranging from chemistry and biochemistry to microbiology and engineering. Consequently many technical terms and abbreviations are involved.

At the same time the rapidly growing interest in the subject is shared by specialists from many fields such as sociology, medicine, agriculture and commerce. The purpose of this dictionary is to assist the specialist from one field to understand the technical terms used by the variety of specialists in the food fields.

Successive editions have become larger with the broadening scope of the subject matter, changes in policy such as the inclusion of proprietary names, the updating of information, and the introduction by official bodies of defined terminology. In the present edition the energy content of foods is expressed in both joules and calories, and vitamins are expressed, where appropriate, in both micrograms and international units.

ARNOLD E. BENDER

INTRODUCTION

Definitions have been kept simple and brief but in many instances they are followed by a reference indicating where the reader can find further information. The codes refer to the following books.

It should be noted that where the composition of foods is stated, these are average values taken from standard works of reference. It must be borne in mind that different samples of the same food can vary considerably in composition, especially in vitamin content.

Abrams	*Linton's Animal Nutrition and Veterinary Dietetics*, J. T. Abrams. Edinburgh: W. Green & Son Ltd.
AEB	*Nutrition and Dietetic Foods*, A. E. Bender. London: Leonard Hill Books.
Bailey	*Industrial Oil and Fat Products*, A. E. Bailey. New York: Interscience Publishers Inc.
B & R	*The Nation's Food*, A. L. Bacharach and T. Rendle. London: Society of Chemical Industry.
Baum	*Canned Foods, an introduction to their microbiology*, J. G. Baumgartner. London: J. & A. Churchill Ltd.
BDS	*Textbook of Physiology and Biochemistry*, G. H. Bell, J. N. Davidson and Emslie Smith. London: E. & S. Livingstone Ltd.
Bell	*Bell's Sale of Food and Drugs*, J. A. O'Keefe. London: Butterworth & Co. (Publishers) Ltd.
Brav	*Citrus Products*, J. B. S. Braverman. New York: Interscience Publishers Inc.
Clark	*Clark's Applied Pharmacology*, revised by A. Wilson and H. O. Schild. London: J. & A. Churchill Ltd.
Cohen	*Theoretical Organic Chemistry*, Julius B. Cohen. London: Macmillan & Co. Ltd.
Cruess	*The Principles and Practice of Wine Making*, W. V. Cruess. New York: The Avi Publishing Co. Ltd.
Davis	*A Dictionary of Dairying*, J. G. Davis. London: Leonard Hill Ltd.
Davis & Mac	*Richmond's Dairy Chemistry* revised by J. G. Davis and F. J. Macdonald. London: Charles Griffin & Co. Ltd.

1

DP	*Human Nutrition and Dietetics*, Sir Stanley Davidson and R. Passmore. Edinburgh: E. & S. Livingstone Ltd.
FAO	*Food Composition Tables—Minerals and Vitamins*, Food and Agriculture Organisation, United Nations.
FB	*Value of Food*, Patty Fisher and Arnold E. Bender. London: Oxford University Press.
FM	*Food Industries Manual, 21st ed.*, A. H. Woollen, ed. London: Leonard Hill.
GH	*Good Housekeeping's Home Encyclopaedia.*
Gil	*Mineral Nutrition and the Balance of Life*, F. A. Gilbert. University of Oklahoma Press.
GMW	*Trace Elements in Food*, G. W. Monier-Williams. London: Chapman & Hall.
Griswold	*The Experimental Study of Foods*, Ruth M. Griswold. Boston: Houghton, Mifflin Co.
Hawk	*Practical Physiological Chemistry*, B. L. Oser. London: J. & A. Churchill Ltd.
Hilditch	*Industrial Fats and Waxes*, T. P. Hilditch. London: Baillière, Tindall & Cox.
Hutch	*Hutchison's Food and the Principles of Dietetics*, revised by V. H. Mottram and G. Graham. London: Edward Arnold (Publishers) Ltd.
Jacobs	*Food and Food Products*, M. B. Jacobs. New York: Interscience Publishers Inc.
Johnson	*Laboratory Manual in Cookery*. Doris B. Johnson. London: Putnam.
KJ	*Modern Cereal Chemistry*, D. W. Kent Jones and A. J. Amos. Liverpool: The Northern Publishing Co. Ltd.
Loes	*Outlines of Food Technology*, H. W. von Loesecke. New York: Reinhold Publishing Corp.
M & W	*Composition of Foods*, R. A. McCance and E. M. Widdowson. M.R.C. Special Report Series No. 297. London: H.M.S.O.
MP	*Food Science and Technology*, Magnus Pyke. London: John Murray.
Matz	*Food Texture*, S. A. Matz. Westport: The Avi Publishing Co. Inc.

Matz 2 — *The Chemistry and Technology of Cereals as Food and Feed*, S. A. Matz. Westport: The Avi Publishing Co. Inc.

Meat — *The Science of Meat and Meat Products*, American Meat Institute Foundation. San Francisco & London: W. M. Freeman & Co.

Merory — *Food Flavorings, Composition, Manufacture and Use*, J. Merory. Westport: The Avi Publishing Co. Inc.

OF — *The Oxford Book of Food Plants*, S. G. Harrison, G. B. Masefield and M. Wallis. London: Oxford University Press.

Platt — *Tables of Representative Values of Foods Commonly used in Tropical Countries*, B. S. Platt. Medical Research Council Special Report, Series No. 302, 1962.

RJC — *Process Engineering in the Food Industries*, R. J. Clarke. London: Heywood & Company Ltd.

Sebrell — *The Vitamins*, W. H. Sebrell, Jr. and R. S. Harris. New York: Academic Press Inc.

Tanner — *The Microbiology of Foods*, F. W. Tanner. Illinois: Garrard Press.

TND — *Tropical Nutrition and Dietetics*, L. Nicholls, H. M. Sinclair, and D. B. Jelliffe. London: Baillière, Tindall & Cox.

Tressler — *Marine Products of Commerce*, D. K. Tressler and J. McW. Lemon. New York: Reinhold Publishing Corp.

WHSS — *Principles of Biochemistry*, A. White, P. Handler, E. L. Smith, D. Stetten. New York: McGraw-Hill Book Co. Inc.

3

A

Abalone. A shellfish, gastropod mollusc of the genus *Haliotis*; found in the water round Japan, California, Channel Islands and France.
Also called Ormer.

Abbé Refractometer. *See* Refractometer.

Abernethy. Hard biscuit flavoured with carraway seed.

Abomasum. *See* Rumen.

Absinthe. Green liqueur prepared from oils of wormwood, angelica, anise and marjoram. It is toxic and the manufacture has been banned in many countries. The toxic principle is oil of thujol, which is cumulative, and is a cerebral convulsant. (Clark.)

Absorptiometer. Instrument used to measure the absorption of light, and therefore used as a quantitative measure of coloured solutions. Frequently (incorrectly) called colorimeters. Many substances, minerals, vitamins, amino acids, will react with a particular reagent to form a coloured complex. The colour developed is proportional to the amount present and is measured in an absorptiometer or a true colorimeter. (Hawk.)

Acaricide. Chemical that kills acarids, i.e. ticks and mites, e.g. tetraethylpyrophosphate.

Ac'cent. Trade name (International Mineral & Chemical Corpn., U.S.A.) for mono sodium glutamate. *See* Glutamate.

Acerola. West Indian Cherry, *see* Cherry, West Indian.

Acetate. Salt of acetic acid, *which see*.

Acetate, Active. The form in which the acetyl radical CH_3CO-, is transferred from one compound to another, as the acetyl-Coenzyme A complex (*see* Coenzyme A).
The metabolism both of glucose and of fats involves the formation of active acetate. (WHSS.)

Acetate Replacement Factor. *See* Lipoic acid.

Acetic Acid. One of the simplest of the organic acids,—formula CH_3COOH. *See* Vinegar. (Cohen.)

Acetobacter. Genus of bacteria of family *Acetobacteriaceae*, which oxidizes alcohol to acetic acid. *Acetobacter pasteurianus* (also known as *Mycoderma aceti* and *Bacterium aceti* or *pasteurianum*) is one of this type and is used in the manufacture of vinegar. Also grow in film on beer wort, pickle brine and fruit juices. *See also* Vinegar. (Tanner.)

Aceto-glycerides. Differ from the triglycerides in that either one or two of the long chain fatty acids attached to the glycerol molecule are replaced by acetic acid. There are three types, diaceto-triglycerides (e.g. diaceto-monostearin), monoaceto-triglycerides (e.g. monoaceto-distearin) and monoaceto-diglycerides (e.g. monoaceto-monostearin) in which one hydroxyl group of the glycerol is free.
Also known as **Partial glyceride esters.**
They are non-greasy and have lower melting points than the corresponding triglycerides and are used in shortenings and

spreads, as films for coating foods, and as plasticisers for hard fats.

Acetoin. Acetyl methyl carbinol, $CH_3.CO.CHOH.CH_3$, precursor of diacetyl, butter flavour. Produced by bacteria during butter ripening and by yeast during fermentation.

Acetone Bodies. *See* Ketone bodies.

Acetylcholine. Acetyl derivative of choline (*which see*) which is liberated at certain nerve endings (cholinergic nerves) to stimulate the muscle. (BDS.)

ACH Index. Arm, chest, hip index. The arm girth, chest diameter and hip width used as a method of assessing the state of nutrition. (DP.)

Achlorhydria. Deficiency of hydrochloric acid in the gastric secretion.

Achrodextrin. A product formed during the enzymic breakdown of starch to maltose; it is a dextrin that gives no colour with iodine (hence achro).

Achromotrichia. Loss of hair pigment. *See* Para-amino benzoic acid *and* Pantothenic acid.

Acid-base Balance. Body fluids are maintained just on the alkaline side of neutrality, pH $7 \cdot 3$ to $7 \cdot 45$, by buffers in the blood and tissues. Buffers include proteins, and sodium and potassium phosphate and bi-carbonate.

Acidic products of the body's metabolism are excreted in the urine in combination with bases such as sodium and potassium. These bases are thereby lost to the body and the acid-base balance is maintained by replacing them from the diet.

Buffer materials in the blood and tissues are termed the alkaline reserve. (BDS.)

Acid Calcium Phosphate. *See* Calcium acid phosphate.

Acid Foods and Basic Foods. Minerals sodium, potassium, magnesium and calcium are base-forming, and phosphorus, sulphur and chlorine are acid-forming. Which of these predominates in the food determines whether the food itself leaves an acid or alkaline residue. An acid residue is left by meat, fish, eggs, cheese, cereals. An alkaline residue is left by milk, vegetables, some fruits. Fats and sugars are neutral as they contain no minerals at all.

Acid-tasting citrus fruits are actually alkali formers, as, although they contain a mixture of citric acid and sodium citrate, the citric acid and the citrate radical are oxidized to carbon dioxide and water, and the sodium remains as the alkaline residue. *See also* Acid-base balance. (Hutch.)

Acid Number. With reference to fats is a measure of hydrolytic rancidity. Defined as milligrams of caustic potash required to neutralise the free fatty acids in 1 g of the fat.

The acid number, also known as the **acid value,** is an index of the efficiency of refining, during which process the free fatty acids are removed and the acid number falls to very low values; it is also an index of the deterioration in storage. (Bailey.)

Acidophilus Therapy. The consumption of milk containing a high concentration of viable *Lactobacillus acidophilus* (the milk itself being unfermented) as a treatment for constipation. The effect is said to be due to the implantation of these organisms in the intestine. (Tanner.)

Acidosis. Increase in the ratio of acid to base in the blood plasma, or a reduction in its buffering power. Causes may be alteration in carbon dioxide excretion, metabolic overproduction of acid or excessive loss of base. *See also* Acid-base balance. (BDS.)

Acid Rebound. Term used in reference to the secretion of gastric acid to signify the increase in acidity of the stomach that results from the administration of alkalies. There is conflicting evidence as to whether this really occurs.

Acid Value. *See* Acid Number.

Aconitine. Toxic alkaloid of Monkshood *(Aconitum)*, slows the pulse and reduces blood pressure, fatal in small doses.

Acorn Sugar. Quercitol, extracted from acorns; pentahydroxycyclohexane.

A.C.P. Acid calcium phosphate. *See* Calcium acid phosphate.

Acraldehyde. *See* Acrolein.

Acrodynia. A specific type of dermatitis seen in animals fed on diets deficient in vitamin B_6. (Sebrell.)

Acrolein. Acraldehyde, CH_2: CHCHO. Formed when glycerol is heated to a high temperature, and is responsible for the acrid odour and lachrymatory vapour produced when fats are overheated. (Cohen.)

Acronize. Trade name (Cyanamide Co., U.S.A.) for the antibiotic chlortetracycline (used, for example, as "acronized ice").

ACTH. Abbreviation for adrenocorticotropic hormone, *which see.*

Actin. One of the proteins of muscle, about 13% of total, combines with myosin to form the contractile protein, actomyosin.

Activators. With reference to enzymes, substances that increase the activity of the enzyme in a non-specific manner. Those substances that are part of the activating system, and are required before the enzyme can activate its substrate, are activators. Substances that are part of the reaction system but play no part in the activation of the substrate are coenzymes. Many inorganic radicals are activators; thus salivary amylase requires the presence of chloride; others are potassium, calcium, magnesium, phosphate. (WHSS.)

Active Oxygen Method. A method of measuring the stability of fats and oils by bubbling air through the heated material and following the formation of peroxides.

Also known as the **Swift Stability Test.**

Actomyosin. The contractile protein of muscle formed from actin plus myosin. It also appears to be identical with the enzyme that catalyses the decomposition of adenosine triphosphate ("ATP-ase") and liberate its energy. This procedure provides the energy for the work of the muscle. (WHSS.)

Addison's Disease. Destruction of the cortex of the suprarenal glands; symptoms are low blood pressure, anaemia, muscular weakness, fall in metabolic rate. Treatment partly successful by taking sodium chloride, or by implantation of pellets of deoxycorticosterone acetate. (BDS.)

Additives. Include all materials deliberately added to food to help manufacture and preserve food, improve palatability and eye-

7

appeal; such as emulsifiers, flavours, thickeners, curing agents, humectants, colours, vitamins, minerals, and mould, yeast and bacterial inhibitors. Most of these are controlled by law in all countries.

Additives, Baking. *See* Baking additives.

Adenine. *See* Purines *and* Nucleic acids.

Adenosine. Combination of the base, adenine, with the sugar, ribose. Of special importance, as adenosine triphosphate plays a central part in the energy release in muscle.
See also Adenosine diphosphate, Adenosine triphosphate, Phosphate bond, energy-rich *and* Phosphokinase. (WHSS.)

Adenosine Diphosphate (or ADP). Adenine + ribose + phosphate + phosphate. Involved in energy exchange in muscle metabolism as the addition and subtraction of the third phosphate (to form adenosine triphosphate) is the means of trapping and releasing energy respectively.
See also Adenosine triphosphate, Phosphate bond, energy-rich *and* Phosphokinase. (WHSS.)

Adenosine Monophosphate. *See* Adenylic acid.

Adenosine Triphosphate (ATP or adenyl pyrophosphate). A compound of central importance in the liberation of energy from foodstuffs, consisting of adenine linked to ribose and three phosphate molecules. The last two phosphates are linked by what is called "the energy-rich phosphate bonds". On hydrolysis they liberate energy for muscular work, etc. The energy obtained by the

oxidation of carbohydrates, fats and amino acids is trapped as ATP. *See* Phosphate bond, energy-rich *and* Phosphokinase. (WHSS.)

Adenylic Acid. Combination of the base, adenine, with the sugar, ribose, and phosphoric acid. Also known as adenosine monophosphate or AMP; of importance in muscle metabolism. (BDS.)

Adenyl Pyrophosphate. *See* Adenosine triphosphate.

Adermin. *See* Vitamin B_6.

Adipose Tissue. Groups of cells that store and mobilize fat; constitutes a fifth to a quarter of the total body mass—more in fat people. Composed of 82–88% fat, 2–2·6% protein and 10–14% water and contains 8–9 kcal (34–38 kJ) per gram or 3,600–4,000 (15·1–16·8 MJ) per lb. (DP.)

Adlay. A tall grass that grows wild in parts of Asia and Africa. Latin name *Coix lachryma-jobi*,—Job's tears. Used as a cereal to eke out rice supplies in parts of India, China, Siam and Philippines. Belongs to the same tribe (*Tripsaceae*) as maize.
Protein 14%, fat 4%, kcal 363 (1·52 MJ), Ca 20 mg, Fe 4 mg, vitamin B_1 0·3 mg, B_2 0·2 mg, nicotinic acid 3 mg—per 100 g (TND, Platt.)

ADI. Acceptable daily intake: refers to chemical additives used in food processing.

ADP. *See* Adenosine diphosphate.

Adrenal Glands. Also called **suprarenal glands**; situated just above each kidney. Comprise the inner part, or medulla, which secretes adrenaline and nor-drenaline (*which see*), and the

8

outer cortex, which secretes steroid hormones.

Steroid hormones include steroid sex hormones, corticosterone (affects carbohydrate metabolism and is anti-inflammatory) and aldosterone (controls excretion of salt and water through the kidneys.) (BDS.)

Adrenaline. Hormone secreted by the medulla of the adrenal glands; the first hormone to be discovered. It is secreted under conditions of emotional stress and causes an increase in blood pressure, blood sugar levels and metabolic rate, thus mobilising the body's reserves of energy.

Also known as epinephrine, chemically hydroxy, dihydroxyphenyl-ethylmethylamine. (BDS).

Adrenocorticotropic Hormone. Hormone extracted from the anterior part of the pituitary gland of animals and used in the treatment of rheumatoid arthritis. Acts by stimulating the adrenal gland to secrete corticosteroids.

Aequum. Amount of food necessary to maintain body weight under normal or specified conditions of activity (rarely used).

Aerobes. Micro-organisms that need oxygen for growth. Obligate aerobes cannot survive in the absence of oxygen. (Tanner.)

Aesculin. A glycoside (dihydroxycoumarin glycoside) found in chestnuts, with "vitamin P" activity. (WHSS.)

AFD. Accelerated freeze-drying. See Freeze-drying.

Aflatoxins. Toxic metabolites of the mould *Aspergillus flavus.* The cause of an outbreak of a fatal disease among turkeys in United Kingdom in 1960, called **turkey** X disease, arising from groundnuts infected with the mould. Since then found in cottonseed meal and cereals.

Eight forms isolated; chemically related to furocoumarins; carcinogenic to several animal species.

Also formed by other strains of *Aspergillus* and *Penicillium puberulum.*

Agar. Dried, purified stems of a seaweed, *Gelidium algae, Gracilaria* and other genera. Partly soluble and swells with water to form a gel. It has a wide temperature range between gelling and melting points.

Used in soups, jellies, ice-cream, meat and fish pastes, in bacteriological media, for sizing silk, as adhesive and as a stabiliser for emulsions. Also called agar-agar, Macassar gum and vegetable gelatine. (Jacobs.)

Agar is a galactan, i.e. a complex of galactose units but it is not digested by man.

Agene. See Aging.

Ageusia. Lack or impairment of sensitivity to taste stimuli.

Agglutinins. See Haemagglutinins.

Aging. (1) Term applied to treatment of flour with oxidising agents, i.e. aging agents.

When freshly milled flour is stored for several weeks it undergoes an aging effect and produces a stronger and more resilient dough and a bolder loaf, and the flour slowly bleaches. Chemical agents can produce these effects immediately.

Oxidising agents, such as ammonium persulphate (used at 160 ppm) and potassium bromate (20 ppm), are "improvers" but

9

do not bleach. Nitrogen peroxide (5 ppm) and benzoyl peroxide (Novadelox, 20–40 ppm) bleach but do not "improve". Nitrogen trichloride (agene) (60 ppm) and chlorine dioxide (Dyox, 30 ppm) bleach and "improve".

The Bread and Flour Report 1960 recommends the use of only one bleaching agent, benzoyl peroxide at not more than 50 ppm. No specific limit is set on maturing agents such as ascorbic acid, potassium bromate, ammonium and potassium persulphate, chlorine dioxide, chlorine (cake flour only) sulphur dioxide (brown flour only). (KJ.)

(2) In reference to wine "aging" refers to the development of bouquet and smooth mellow flavour, and disappearance of harsh and yeasty taste—due to slow oxidation and formation of esters.

(3) With reference to meat *see* Rigor mortis. (Cruess.)

Aginomoto. *See* Glutamate, sodium.

Aglycon. The non-sugar part of a glycoside.

Agnelloto. Envelope of pasta stuffed with minced meat or vegetables; cut in half-moon shape, so differing from ravioli, which is cut in squares.

A/G Ratio. *See* Albumin/Globulin ratio.

Ajinomoto. Trade name (Hercules Powder Co.) for range of flavour enhancers—Ajinomoto IMP, disodium inosinate; Ajinomoto GMP, disodium guanylate; Ajinomoto, monosodium glutamate.

Akee. *Blighia sapida*; fruit of West African origin, long grown in West Indies; unripe fruits are toxic. (OF.)

Ala. Bulgur, *which see.*

Alanine. A non-essential amino acid, amino propionic acid. The alpha amino acid is found in all proteins; there is also beta-alanine (the amino group attached to the second carbon atom) which is part of the molecule of pantothenic acid, of carnosine and of anserine. (BDS.)

Albedo. White pith of the inner peel of citrus fruits, also known as the mesocarp; 20–60% of the whole fruit. Consists of sugars, cellulose and pectins; used as a source of pectin for commercial manufacture. (Brav.)

Albumen. *Oxford Dictionary* spelling of albumin.

Albumin. Often used as a non-specific name for protein, strictly should refer to one of the albumins, *which see. See also* Egg white, Lactalbumin, *and* Albumin/Globulin ratio.

Albumin/Globulin Ratio. Ratio of the blood albumin to the globulins; in normal human serum $1 \cdot 82$. Change in the A/G ratio is of diagnostic value.

Albumin Index. A measure of the quality of an egg; the ratio of height of the albumin to the width when broken on to a flat surface. As the egg deteriorates the albumin index decreases, i.e. the egg white spreads. (Griswold.)

Albumin milk. *See* Protein milk.

Albuminoids (or scleroproteins). Fibrous proteins that have supporting or protective function in the animal (in plants cellulose fulfils this function). Three types: (1) collagens in skin, tendons and bones, resistant to pepsin and

10

trypsin, converted to water-soluble gelatin by boiling with water; (2) elastins in tendons and arteries, not converted to gelatin; (3) keratins, proteins insoluble in dilute acids and alkalies, not attacked by any animal digestive enzymes, comprise horns, hoofs, feathers, scales, nails. (Hawk.)

Albumins. Simple proteins (i.e. free from other subtances) soluble in water and coagulated by heat, e.g. ovalbumin in egg-white, serum albumin in blood serum, lactalbumin in milk.

The name albumin is often used for any protein, e.g. albuminuria is the presence of protein in the urine, and although this protein is often largely serum albumin it is not necessarily so. (Hawk.)

Albumoses. Old name for proteoses, *which see*.

Alcaptonuria. A rare inborn error of metabolism of the two amino acids phenylalanine and tyrosine. Their metabolism ceases at homogentisic acid, which is excreted in the urine. Homogentisic acid oxidizes to black melanoid pigments, hence the urine of alcaptonurics slowly turns black. The defect appears to be harmless. (BDS.)

Alcohol. The name without further description refers to ethyl alcohol, chemical formula C_2H_5OH. This is the second member of a series of alcohols of the general formula $C_nH_{2n}OH$, the first member being methyl alcohol CH_3OH, and rising to long molecules such as cetyl alcohol, *which see*.

Alcohol is produced by yeast fermentation of carbohydrates and is the basis of a large number of beverages. It has an energy value of 7 kcal (29 kJ) per gram;

the quantity of alcohol contained in various drinks is shown under Alcoholic Beverages. (Cohen.)

Alcohol, denatured. Alcohol to which unpleasant materials have been added to prevent it being drunk, e.g. methylated spirits contains 10% methyl alcohol, a blue dye and unpleasant-smelling pyridine. Denatured alcohol is used for industrial purposes and not subject to Excise Duty.

Alcoholic Beverages. Yeast fermentation of sugar or starchy materials yields a solution of approximately 15% alcohol, (wine) at which strength the alcohol kills off the yeast. If sweet wines are wanted the fermentation is stopped at an earlier stage when there is still some sugar left. If stronger wines are required, such as port, they are fortified by the addition of brandy.

The strong spirits are made by distilling the alcohol from wine.

Alcohol content (per cent by volume):— spirits — gin, whisky, brandy, rum—25 under proof, 43% alcohol; 35 under proof, 37%. Wines, — port, sherry, madeira 20%; burgundy, 14%; champagne, claret, hock, 10%; cider, 4·3%; ale 3·1 to 6·6%; stout, 3·9 to 5·3%; porter 4·0%. Liqueurs; curacao, 55%; benedictine, 52%; absinthe, 59%; anisette, 42%; chartreuse, 43%; kummel, 34%. *See also* Proof spirit. (Hutch.)

Aldehyde. One of a large class of organic substances derived from primary alcohols by oxidation, and containing the grouping —CHO. E.g. formaldehyde, acetaldehyde, benzaldehyde. (Cohen.)

Aldosterone. Hormone secreted by the adrenal cortex which

11

controls the excretion of salt and water through the kidneys. (BDS.)

Ale. *See* Beer.

Aleurone Layer. Single layer of large cells under the bran coat and outside the endosperm of cereal grains; about 3% by weight of the grain, rich in protein. Botanically is part of the endosperm but during milling remains attached to the inner layer of bran.

Contains about 20% of the thiamin, 30% of the riboflavin and 50% of the nicotinic acid of the grain. (KJ.)

Alewives. River herrings, mostly used for canning after salting. (Tressler.)

Algae. Sub-group, mainly aquatic, of the division of plants called *Thallophyta* which show no differentiation into root, stem and leaf. Includes seaweeds, such as Dulse and Irish Moss, which have long been eaten by man.

Unicellular varieties such as *Chlorella, Scenedesmus* and *Spirulina* are being grown experimentally in tanks as a potential source of food. They require only carbon dioxide and mineral salts since they obtain their energy by photosynthesis.

Protein content on dry weight basis: Spirulina 60–70%, Scenedesmus and Chlorella 50–60%; fat, Spirulina 2%, Chlorella 8–20% depending on growing conditions; nutritional value of the proteins is similar to that of casein, i.e. NPU 50–70, per 2·2–2·5. (FM.)

Alginates. Salts of alginic acid found as the free acid and calcium salt in many seaweeds. Alginic acid is a polysaccharide complex built from mannuronic acid units.

Salts such as iron, magnesium and ammonium alginates form viscous solutions. They hold large amounts of water and are useful as thickeners, stabilisers and gelling, binding and emulsifying agents in ice-cream, synthetic cream. The propyl glycol ester is used under the trade name of "mannucol ester". (Tressler.)

Alginic Acid. *See* Alginates.

Alimentary Canal. The digestive tract, comprising, in man, mouth, oesophagus, stomach, duodenum, small and large intestines. (BDS.)

Alimentary Pastes. Shaped dried doughs made from semolina or wheat flour with water, and sometimes egg and milk. The dough is partly dried in hot air, then more slowly.

Macaroni — tubular-shaped, about $\frac{1}{4}$ inch diameter; at $\frac{3}{4}$ inch it is called fovantini or maccaroncelli; at $\frac{1}{2}$ inch, zitoni.

Spaghetti is solid rod about $\frac{3}{32}$ inch diameter; vermicelli is a third of this thickness.

Noodles are shaped into sheets or ribbons.

Farfals are ground, granulated or shredded. (Loes, Matz 2.)

Aliment de Sevrage. Protein-rich baby food, 20% protein. Algerian version made from wheat, chick peas, lentils, skim milk powder and sugar with added vitamin D. Senegal version made from millet flour, peanut flour, skim milk powder and sugar with vitamins A and D and calcium.

Aliphatic. Name given to those organic chemicals that have open-chain structure in distinction to the alicyclic compounds, which contain rings of carbon compounds. (Cohen.)

Alkali Formers. *See* Acid Foods and Basic Foods.

Alkaline Reserve. *See* Acid-base balance.

Alkaloids. Group of organic compounds containing nitrogen, occurring in plants and having powerful effects on animals. Many drugs and poisons are alkaloids, such as strychnine, codeine, morphine, atropine, nicotine, quinine. (Cohen.)

Alkalosis. Decrease in the acid–base ratio in the blood plasma, or an increase in its buffering power. Causes may be excessive loss of carbon dioxide, excessive intake of base as in antacid drugs, loss of gastric secretion by vomiting, high intake of sodium or potassium salts of weak organic acids. *See also* Acid-base balance. (BDS.)

Alkannet (Alkanet, Alkannin, Alkanna). Colouring obtained from root of *Anchusa tinctoria* (*Alkanna tinctoria*); legally permitted in food in most countries; colouring principle is alkannin. Insoluble in water but soluble in alcohol and ether. Blue in alkalies, blue with lead, crimson with tin, violet with iron. Used for colouring fats, cheese, essences (and inferior port wine). Also known as orcanella. (Jacobs.)

All Bran. Trade name (Kellogg's Ltd.) for a breakfast cereal derived from wheat bran.

Composition per 100 g: 14 g protein, 2 g fat, 65 g soluble carbohydrate, 6·3 g fibre, 350 kcal (1·4 MJ), 11 mg iron, 0·6 mg B_1, 2·5 mg B_2, 32 mg nicotinic acid.

Allantoin. Oxidation product of uric acid; end-product of purine metabolism in most mammals except man and the anthropoid apes (where it is uric acid). (BDS.)

Allergen. *See* Allergy.

Allergy. An altered or abnormal tissue reaction which may be caused by contact between a foreign protein, the allergen, and sensitive body tissues.

Food allergies are more common in infants and the usual causes are eggs, milk and wheat, together with fish and various fruits. The reactions may include nettle-rash, hay fever, asthma, and dyspepsia. (DP.)

Allicin. Sulphur compound responsible for the flavour of garlic. (Griswold.)

Alligator Pears. *See* Avocados.

Allinson Bread. A whole wheat bread named after Allinson who advocated its use in England at the end of the nineteenth century, as did Graham in the United States (thus Graham bread).

Allolactose. A sugar, which may be a modification of lactose, which, together with **gynolactose,** has been claimed to be found in human milk. (Davis & Mac.)

Allotriophagy. Unnatural desire for foods, alternative words cissa, cittosis and pica.

Alloxan. Pyrimidine derivative that can induce diabetes when given orally or by injection, by damaging the Islets of Langerhans (that part of the pancreas which secretes insulin). (BDS.)

Alloxan Diabetes. Experimental diabetes caused by alloxan.

Alloxazine. Three-ring structure, the central part of riboflavin. The latter is dimethyl ribityl isoalloxazine. (BDS.)

13

Allspice. Dried fruits of the ever-green *Pimenta officinalis*, also known as **pimento** or **Jamaican pepper** (differs from pimiento). The name allspice derives from the volatile oil, which has an aroma similar to a mixture of cloves, cinnamon and nutmeg. Used to flavour meat products. (Jacobs.)

Almond, Sweet. Ripe seeds of *Prunus amygdalus* var. *dulcis;* yields sweet almond oil.

Almond Oil, Bitter. Essential oil from seeds of almond tree (*Prunus amygdalus*) or apricot tree (*Prunus armeniaca*); mostly manufactured from the apricot. Contains 95% benzaldehyde, with hydrocyanic acid and benzaldehyde cyanhydrin. When freed from hydrocyanic acid is used as flavour, in perfumes and in cosmetics.

Aloe. Dried juice of leaves of *Aloe perryi*; used in medicine. Contains a glycoside, aloe-emodin or rhabarberone, aloe oil, and aloin or barbaloin.

Alpha-Laval Centrifuge. Continuous bowl centrifuge for separating liquids of different densities for clarifying. Widely used for cream separation.

Aluminium. One of the most abundant elements in Nature, as it occurs in rocks and clay. It is found in animal and plant tissues in traces but has not been shown to be essential to either.

There is a popular misconception that aluminium cooking vessels are in some way harmful but the fact that relatively large doses of aluminium hydroxide are often consumed as an antidote to gastric hyperacidity demonstrates the harmlessness of aluminium.

"Alum" baking powders, in which sodium aluminium sulphate was the acid constituent, used to be used. (GMW.)

"Silver" beads used to decorate confectionery may be coated either with silver foil or an aluminium copper alloy.

Alveographe. Measures stretching quality of dough as index of protein quality for baking. A standard disc of dough is blown into a bubble and the pressure curve and bursting pressure measured; gives the stability, extensibility and strength. (FM.)

Amama. Trade name (Glaxo Laboratories) for a protein-rich baby food based on casein (1 part) and groundnut flour (10 parts)—obsolete.

Amaranth. Burgundy red colour, fast to light; trisodium salt of 1-(4-sulpho-1-naphthylazo)-2-naphthol-3:6-disulphonic acid.

Ambergris. Morbid concretion obtained from the intestine of the sperm whale. Contains cholesterol, ambrein, benzoic acid. Appears as a mottled or striped grey-brown or black wax. Used in drugs and perfume. (Tressler.)

Amberlite. Group of polystyrene resins used to absorb specific radicals from solutions. The sulphonic acid derivative, strongly acidic (IR 120), and the carboxylic acid, weakly acidic (IRC 150), are used for cation exchange; basic types used for anion exchange (IR 4B, IR 45, IRA 400). Used for water softening, metal recovery, purification of chemicals, chemical analysis, particularly amino acids. *See also* Ion-exchange resins.

Amino Acid. Characterized by an amino group and an acid group attached to the same carbon atom. Proteins are made of combinations of large numbers of amino acids of twenty different kinds.

Eight of these amino acids must be provided in the diet, i.e. the essential amino acids—namely, lysine, methionine, valine, tryptophan, threonine, leucine, isoleucine and phenylalanine. Possibly arginine and histidine are essential for infants.

The remaining twelve can be synthesized in the body so long as a source of nitrogen is available in the diet. These are the non-essential amino acids—histidine, glycine, arginine, alanine, aspartic acid, glutamic acid, proline, hydroxyproline, serine, cystine, cysteine and tyrosine. (BDS, DP.)

Amino Acid, Limiting. That essential amino acid present in the protein in question in least amount (relative to the dietary needs). The ratio of the amount of the limiting amino acid to the requirements serves as a chemical estimation of the nutritive value of the protein. *See* Chemical score.

Most cereal proteins are limited by lysine and most animal and vegetable proteins by the sulphur amino acids (methionine plus cystine).

In complete diets it is the sulphur amino acids that are usually limiting. *See also* Lysine *and* Methionine. (DP, AEB.)

Amino Acid Oxidase. *See* Flavoproteins.

Amino Acid Profile. Amino acid composition of a protein.

Amino Acids, Antiketogenic. Those which are metabolized to glucose. They are glycine, alanine, serine, cystine, aspartic acid, glutamic acid, arginine, proline and hydroxyproline. (WHSS.)

Amino Acids, Ketogenic. Those which are metabolized to acetoacetic acid (ketone bodies). They are leucine, isoleucine, phenylalanine and tyrosine. (WHSS.)

Aminogram. Amino acid composition of a protein.

Aminopeptidase. Enzyme of the pancreatic juice that splits polypeptides to dipeptides. Removes the terminal unit of the polypeptide chain at the end at which the amino radical is free, hence is an exopeptidase. (WHSS.)

Aminopterin. Aminopteroylglutamic acid, specific antagonist to folic acid.

Ammonotelic. Animals that excrete their waste nitrogen as ammonia, e.g. various worms, leeches, molluscs, sea urchins, fish.

AMP. Adenosine monophosphate or adenylic acid, *which see*.

Amphetamine. *See* Anorectic drugs.

Amphoteric. *See* Iso-electric point.

Amydon. Starchy material made by steeping wheat flour in water and drying the starch sediment in the sun; used for many centuries for thickening broths.

Amygdalin. Glucoside in almonds, apricot and cherry stones, hydrolysed by the enzyme, emulsin, to glucose, hydrocyanic acid and benzaldehyde. The benzaldehyde gives the characteristic odour. (Merory.)

Amylases. Enzymes that hydrolyse starch and glycogen to maltose. Alpha-amylase, or dextrino-

15

genic amylase, breaks starch down to small dextrin-like molecules and does not proceed to maltose.

Beta-amylase, or maltogenic amylase, is specific for the 1:4-alpha-glucosidic linkages of starch and liberates maltose. Complete degradation of starch requires the attack of both these enzymes.

Salivary amylase and pancreatic amylase in animals behave like the alpha-amylase. Also known as diastase. *See also* Z-enzyme. (WHSS.)

Amyloamylose. Old name for amylose, as distinct from erythro-amylose, old name for amylopectin.

Amylodyspepsia. Inability to digest starch.

Amylograph. Measures the viscosity of flour paste as it is heated from 25°C to 90°C (the same temperature rise as in baking) and serves as a measure of the diastatic activity of the flour. (KJ.)

Amyloins. Carbohydrates that are complexes of dextrins with varying proportions of maltose. (KJ.)

Amylolytic. General adjective applied to enzymes that can split starch into soluble products.

Amylopectin. Starch consists of 20–25% amylose and the remainder amylopectin.

Amylose consists of 1:4 alpha-linked glucose units and gives a pure blue with iodine. **Amylopectin** is a branched structure built up of 20–24 glucoside units linked 1:4, and gives a purplish colour with iodine. *See also* Amylases. (WHSS.)

Amylopsin. Pancreatic amylase.

Amylose. *See* Amylopectin.

Anabiosis. Suspended animation

(with stoppage of respiration and the heart-beat), caused by freezing or freezing and drying, as achieved, for example, by Alaskan and Siberian insects during cold spells.

Anabolism. The process of building up or synthesising. *See* Metabolism.

Anaemia. A shortage of red blood cells. May be caused by a deficiency of any of the factors needed to form red cells, namely protein, iron, vitamins C and B_{12} and folic acid, or damage to the bone marrow.

Nutritional anaemia is the commonest form and is due to iron deficiency. Pernicious anaemia is usually due to a failure to absorb vitamin B_{12}. *See also* Intrinsic factor *and* Blood, red cells. (BDS.)

Anaerobes. Micro-organisms that grow in the absence of oxygen. Obligate anaerobes cannot survive in the presence of oxygen. Facultative anaerobes normally grow in oxygen but can also grow in its absence. (Tanner.)

Analysis, Gastric. *See* Fractional test meal.

Analysis, Proximate. An analysis for the major ingredients, usually nitrogen (as a measure of the protein), and fat and ash (as a measure of the mineral salts); these are added together and subtracted from 100 to give what is called "carbohydrate by difference". The latter may be corrected for crude fibre.

See Carbohydrate by difference.

Anchovy. A fish *Engraulis encrasicholus*. Usually prepared semi-preserved with 10–12% salt and sometimes benzoic acid.

Aneurine. Obsolete name for vitamin B_1.

16

Angelica. Bright green crystallized sticks used for decorating and flavouring confectionery goods, prepared from the young stalks of *Angelica archangelica*. This is a tall umbelliferous herb (not to be confused with wild English angelica, *Angelica sylvestris*) and the crystallized material is imported from S. France.

The roots are used with juniper berries for flavouring gin and the seeds are used in vermouth and chartreuse. Essential oils are distilled from the roots, stem and leaves.

Angostura. Essential oil distilled from the bark of *Galipea cusparia*. Contains galipol, cadinene, galipene and pinene; used in preparation of bitters and liqueurs.

Ångström Unit. One ten-millionth part of a millimetre, or one ten-thousandth part of a micron: symbol Å.

Angular Stomatitis. An affection of the skin at the angles of the mouth, characterised by heaping-up of epithelium into ridges, giving the appearance of fissures: a symptom of riboflavin deficiency but also a symptom of other diseases. (DP.)

Anhydrovitamin A. Form of retinol in which the OH group has been removed by treatment with HCl, with a corresponding shift in the double bonds. Once incorrectly called cyclized or spurious vitamin A. Has very slight biological activity. When fed in large doses to rats, a more active material called rehydrovitamin A is obtained.

Animal Protein Factor. Name given to certain growth factor or factors which were found to be present in animal but not vege-table proteins. Vitamin B_{12} was identified as one of these.

Anion. *See* Ionization.

Anise. *See* Aniseed.

Aniseed. Or Anise, is the dried fruit of *Pimpinella anisum* (parsley family). Chief component of the volatile oil is anethole (methoxypropenyl benzene). The seed is used to flavour baked goods, meat products and drinks. (Jacobs, Merory.)

Anisette. Liqueur based on aniseed.

Annatto. Also known as bixin or butter colour; colour from seed-pods of *Bixa orellana*.

Used for colouring butter and cheese (not margarine); legally permitted. Contains orellin, of minor importance, soluble in water, and bixin, the major colour, insoluble in water. Also used to dye cotton and silk and in wood stains. (Jacobs, Davis.)

Anomers. A pair of stereoisomers related to each other in the same way as alpha and beta glucose are related, are termed anomers.

Anorectic or Anorexigenic Drugs. Drugs that depress the appetite and are used as an aid to weight reduction. E.g. amphetamine (or dextro-amphetamine or dexedrine) preludin (phenmetrazine hydrochloride) "Tenuate" (diethylpropion). (AEB.)

Anorexia Nervosa. Psychological disturbance resulting in a refusal to eat; sensations of hunger usually not felt. There may be a restriction of the diet to particular foods. The result is great weight loss, atrophy of tissue and fall in basal metabolic rate. (DP.)

Anosmia. Lack or impairment of sensitivity to odour stimuli.

Anserine. Beta-alanyl methylhistidine; a dipeptide originally isolated from goose muscle; found in muscle of mammals, fishes and birds; function unknown.

Antabuse. Tetra-ethyl thiuramdi-sulphide, drug used in the treatment of alcoholism. The drug alone has no effect, but if alcohol is subsequently taken, it gives rise to headache, palpitation, nausea and vomiting. (Clark.)

Antacids. Bases or buffers that neutralize acid; used generally in relation to the partial neutralization of stomach acidity. Substances like magnesium carbonate, sodium bicarbonate, magnesium hydroxide, glycine, etc., are used.

Anthelminthics. Chemicals used to destroy intestinal worms.

Anthocyanins. Violet, red and blue water-soluble colouring matter of many fruits, flowers and leaves. Consist of glucose plus anthocyanidins (these consist of two 6-membered carbon rings containing one oxygen atom). Examples are delphinin, pelargonidin, cyanidin. Can attack iron and tin and cause trouble in canned foods. (Cohen.)

Anthoxanthins. Alternative name for flavonoids, *which see.*

Antibiotics. Substances produced by living organisms which inhibit the growth of other organisms. Classic example is penicillin, produced by a mould and inhibitory to many bacteria.

When fed to animals in minute doses (a few gm per ton of food) many antibiotics, such as penicillin, aureomycin, terramycin, increase growth rate.

Used in some countries as food preservatives but not permitted in Great Britain with the exception of nisin.

See also individual antibiotics; Nisin, Penicillin, Tetracyclines, Oleandomycin. (Bell.)

Antibodies. *See* Toxins.

Anti-caking Agents. Added to powder foodstuffs to prevent caking, e.g. small amounts of anhydrous disodium hydrogen phosphate added to salt or sugar; aluminium calcium silicate or calcium or magnesium silicate in table salt; calcium silicate in baking powder.

Anticoagulants. With reference to blood, substances that prevent clotting by interfering with the mechanism. Oxalate and citrate are anticoagulants as they combine with the calcium which is needed; dicoumarin and heparin inhibit the formation of prothrombin, needed to release fibrin from fibrinogen; hirudin inactivates the thrombin. (BDS.)

Antidiuretics. Drugs that reduce the rate of formation of urine, i.e. reduce water loss from the body.

Antienzymes. Substances that specifically inhibit enzymes; produced by the lining of the digestive tract to prevent attack by the digestive enzymes, by intestinal parasites, and as antibodies in the blood stream. (BDS.)

Antifoaming Agents. Octanol (capryl alcohol), sulphonated oils, silicones; reduce foaming often caused by the presence of dissolved protein or other stabilizer.

Antigalactics. Substances that suppress the secretion of milk.

Anti-Grey Hair Factor. *See* Para-amino benzoic acid.

Anti-mould Agents. *See* Antimycotics.

DICTIONARY OF NUTRITION AND FOOD TECHNOLOGY

Antimycotics. Substances that inhibit mould growth, such as sodium and calcium propionate, methyl hydroxybenzoate, quaternary ammonium chloride, sodium benzoate, sorbic acid.

Antioxidants. Substances that retard the oxidative rancidity of fats. E.g. propyl gallate, octyl gallate, dodecyl gallate, butylated hydroxyanisole (BHA) and butylated hydroxytoluene (BHT). Many fats, particularly vegetable oils, contain naturally-occurring antioxidants, such as tocopherol, which protect the oils from rancidity for a limited period. *See* Induction period.

Antisialagogues. Substances that arrest the flow of saliva.

Anti-spattering Agents. Added to fats used in frying, e.g. lecithin, sucrose esters (laurates and stearates), and sodium sulphoacetate derivatives of mono- and diglycerides. They function by preventing the coalescence of water droplets. (Bailey.)

Anti-staling Agents. Substances that retard the staling of baked products, and also soften the crumb, e.g. Sucrose stearate, polyoxyethylene monostearate, glyceryl monostearate, stearoyl tartrate.

A.O.M. *See* Active Oxygen Method.

Apastia. Refusal to take food as an expression of mental disorder.

Aphagosis. Inability to eat.

Apo-carotenal. *See* Carotenal.

Apoerythein. Name suggested for the Intrinsic factor, *which see.*

Apoferritin. The protein part of ferritin, the iron storage complex in the intestinal mucosal cells.

Apollinaris Water. An alkaline, highly aerated water, containing sodium chloride and calcium, sodium and magnesium carbonates; obtained from a spring in the valley of the Ahr (Prussia). (Hutch.)

Aporinosis. Term for any disease due to deficiency of an element in diet. (Greek aporos—scarce.)

Aporrhegma. Ptomaine or other toxic substance split off from an amino acid during the bacterial decomposition of a protein.

Aposia. Absence of feeling of thirst.

Apositia. Aversion for food.

Apparent Digestibility. *See* Digestibility, apparent.

Appertization. Term applied by the French to the process of destroying all the micro-organisms of significance in food, i.e. "commercial sterility"; a few organisms remain alive but are quiescent. (Named after Nicholas Appert.)

Apple. Fruit of many species of *Malus sylvestris.* Water 84%, protein 0·3%, fat 0·3%, sugar 9%, kcal 49 (210 kJ), Ca 5 mg, Fe 0·3 mg, vitamin A 23 μg, B₁ 0·03 mg, nicotinic acid 0·2 mg, vitamin C, 4 mg—per 100 g. It contains 0·7% malic acid, 3% pectin and the aromatic constituents are largely amyl esters of formic, caproic and caprylic acids and geraniol. (FAO, OF.)

Apple Butter. Apple that has been boiled in an open kettle to a thick consistency. Similar to apple sauce but darker in colour due to the prolonged boiling.

Apples, Dried. Composition, protein 3·1%, fat 0·6%, kcal 280 (1·2 MJ), Ca 54 mg, Fe 2·3 mg, vitamin A 300 μg, B₁ 0·06

19

mg, B_2 0·12 mg, nicotinic acid 1·5 mg, vitamin C 10 mg—per 100 g. (FAO.)

Apple Jack. American name for apple brandy; distilled cider, also known as Calvàdos.

Apple, Liquid. American preparation of apple juice plus pulverised apple pulp in suspension.

Apple Nuggets. Crisp granules of apple of low moisture content. Dehydrated apples of 24% moisture content are cut into small cubes and dried down to 2% moisture; used to make applesauce.

Apricot. Fruit of *Prunus armeniaca*. Analysis, raw—protein 0·6%, fat trace, carbohydrate 7%, kcal 28 (120 kJ), Fe 0·2 mg, vitamin A 830 μg, B_1 0·04 mg, B_2 0·05 mg, nicotinic acid 0·6 mg, vitamin C 7 mg—per 100 g.

Apricot kernel sometimes used (plus oil of almonds) in place of almond to make marzipan substitute. (M&W.)

Arachidonic Acid. Straight-chain fatty acid containing 20 carbon atoms and four double bonds (a tetraene). Found only in animal fats, e.g. brain, liver, egg yolk. *See* Essential fatty acids.

Arachin. One of the globulin proteins from the peanut. Precipitated by 40% saturated ammonium sulphate from a salt extract of peanut. Conarachin can be precipitated from the residue by 85% saturated ammonium sulphate.

Arachis Oil. *See* Peanuts.

Arginase. Enzyme that hydrolyses arginine to urea and ornithine, the last stage of urea synthesis from the amino groups of the amino acids. Present in most animal cells. (WHSS.)

Arginine. Chemically amino-guanido valeric acid. Dibasic amino acid that is non-essential to adult man. Since it is partly essential to growing rats (growth only 80% of optimum in its absence) it may similarly be partly essential to children. It is essential to the chick. (BDS.)

Argol. Crust of crude cream of tartar (potassium acid tartrate) that forms on the sides of wine vats (also called Wine Stone). White argol from white grapes, red argol from red. 50–85% potassium hydrogen tartrate and 6–12% calcium tartrate. Used in vinegar fermentation, as mordant in dyeing, and in the manufacture of tartaric acid. (Cruess.)

Ariboflavinosis. Name given to set of symptoms caused by deficiency of riboflavin (vitamin B_2). Characterized by swollen, cracked, bright red lips (cheilosis), enlarged tender, magenta-red tongue (glossitis), cracking at the corners of the mouth (angular stomatitis), congestion of the blood vessels of the conjunctiva. (Sebrell.)

Arlac. Protein-rich baby food (42% protein), made in Nigeria by Cow & Gate Ltd., from peanut flour and skim milk powder with added vitamins B_1, B_2, B_{12} and D and minerals.

Armenian Bole. Or ferric oxide; occurs naturally as haematite or prepared by heating ferrous sulphate, etc. Used in metallurgy, polishing compounds, paint pigment and as a food colour.

Arogel. Trade name, Arogel 909 P (Morningstar-Paisley, U.S.A.) for a potato starch preparation used as thickener in gravies, sauces and canned foods; it is stable to heat.

20

Arrowroot. Tuber of the West Indian plant, *Maranta arundinacea*, mainly used to prepare arrowroot starch, the most refined of all feculas. The starch contains only a trace of protein (0·2%) and is free from vitamins. It is used in bland, low-salt and protein-restricted diets and, unfortunately, as an infant food in some West Indian islands. (TND.)

Arsanilic Acid. Used to stimulate growth in poultry.

Arsenic. One of the few elements not essential in traces to either plants or animals, it is toxic to both, even in small amounts. There is a legal limit to the amount permitted to be present in foodstuffs. (GMW.)

Ascorbic Acid. Vitamin C, also called L-xyloascorbic acid in distinction from D-araboascorbic acid (isoascorbic acid or erythorbic acid) which has only slight vitamin C activity.

Erythorbic acid has strong reducing properties and is used as an antioxidant in foods and to preserve the red colour of fresh or preserved meats.

Physiological properties of ascorbic acid are described under Vitamin C.

Ascorbic Acid Oxidase. Plant enzyme that oxidizes ascorbic acid to the dehydro form. In the living tissue it appears to be separated from the vitamin, but in the wilting leaf, or, for example, in shredded cabbage, the enzyme comes into contact with its substrate and there is a rapid destruction of the vitamin. For preservation of the vitamin in greens on cooking it is recommended that the vegetables be plunged into boiling water, when the enzyme is destroyed. (FB.)

Ascorbin Stearate. Ester of ascorbic acid (vitamin C) and stearic acid; a fat-soluble form of the vitamin which is used as an antioxidant at concentrations around 0·1%.

Ascorbyl Palmitate. Ester of ascorbic acid and palmitic acid used as an anti-staling agent in bakery products. Amounts of 0·1–0·4% by weight of the flour retard staling for 2–4 days.

Aseptic Filling. When food, solid or liquid, is sterilised in the can it is subjected to heat treatment that can affect the quality of the food. Instead it can be sterilised in thin films or in narrow tubes by shorter treatment that inflicts less damage, and must then be filled into cans under strictly aseptic conditions. (FM.)

Ash. Residue left behind after all the organic matter has been burned off. Serves as a measure of the inorganic salts that were present in the original material.

Asparagine. Amide of the amino acid, aspartic acid; serves in plants as a store of ammonia. During the growth of seedlings ketonic acids are formed during photosynthesis, and these are aminated to amino acids at the expense of the ammonia in asparagine. (WHSS.)

Asparagus. Young shoot of *Asparagus officinalis*. Protein 1·4%, fat 0·1%, Ca 14 mg, Fe 0·6 mg, kcal 14 (60 kJ), vitamin A 220 μg, B₁ 0·11 mg, B₂ 0·13 mg, nicotinic acid 0·9 mg, vitamin C 22 mg—per 100 g. (FAO.)

Aspartic Acid. A non-essential amino acid; amino succinic acid (dibasic). Its amide is asparagine. (BDS.)

21

Aspartyl-phenylalanine Methyl Ester. Dipeptide ester which is 100–200 times as sweet as sucrose.

Aspergillus. *See* Moulds *and* Taka-diastase.

Aspic Jelly. A jelly flavoured with lemon, tarragon vinegar, sherry, peppercorns and vegetables used as a garnish.

Astaxanthin. A carotenoid pigment; the pink colour of salmon muscle.

Atherosclerosis. The deposition of a fatty material, called atheroma, on the inner lining of the arteries. If atheroma is laid down in the coronary arteries the formation of a thrombus or clot may be encouraged—coronary thrombosis. Several dietary factors have been implicated in causation of atherosclerosis. (AEB.)

Atmungsferment. Name given by Warburg to the respiratory enzyme, later called cytochrome oxidase. (WHSS.)

ATP. Adenosine triphosphate, *which see.*

Atwater Factors. Factors used to calculate the energy content of foods in kilocalories after allowing for losses in digestion and urinary nitrogen: Protein 4, fat 9, carbohydrates 4, derived by Atwater from the heats of combustion, namely, protein $5 \cdot 7$, fat $9 \cdot 4$, carbohydrates $4 \cdot 1$. *See also* Energy *and* Rubner Factors. (DP.)

AT–10. *See* Tachysterol.

Aubergine. Also known as egg plant, *Solanum melongena*, native of South East Asia; 3–5 inches in diameter and up to 12 inches long, purple in colour.

Carbohydrate 6%, protein $1 \cdot 4\%$, vitamin B_1 $0 \cdot 06$ mg, B_2 $0 \cdot 05$ mg, nicotinic acid $0 \cdot 8$ mg, vitamin C 5 mg—per 100 g. (TND.)

Aurantiamarin. Glucoside present in the albedo of the bitter orange; partly responsible for the flavour. (Brav.)

Aureomycin. *See* Tetracyclines.

Autoclave. A vessel in which high temperatures can be reached by using high pressure. The domestic pressure cooker is an example.

At atmospheric pressure water boils at 100°C; at 10 lb extra pressure the boiling point is 115°C; at 15 lb, 121°C and at 20 lb, 126°C.

Autoclaves have two major purposes. As in the domestic pressure cooker, the higher temperature permits cooking in a shorter time. The second major use is in sterilization. Bacteria are destroyed more readily at these elevated temperatures, and autoclaves are used to sterilize food, for example in cans, and for sterilizing instruments and dressings in surgery. *See also* Cooking, losses of vitamins.

Autolysis. Process of self-digestion effected by the enzymes naturally present in the tissue. E.g. tenderizing of game while hanging is autolytic breakdown of connective tissue.

Autotrophes. Organisms that can synthesize their own tissues from simple inorganic salts, as distinct from heterotrophes that must be supplied with complex ready-made foods. Thus plants are autotrophes, animals heterotrophes. Bacteria can be of either type. Autotrophes are not involved in food spoilage; hetero-

22

trophic bacteria include pathogens and food-spoilage organisms. (Baum.)

Auxins. Plant hormones produced in the growing buds, embryos and young leaves of plants, as well as many fungi and bacteria. They are organic acids, e.g. indolyl acetic acid, indolyl butyric acid and naphthalene acetic acid. Used to stimulate root formation and control growth.

Available Carbon Dioxide. *See* Baking powder, *and* Flour, self-raising.

Available Nutrients. In some foodstuffs nutrients shown to be present by chemical tests may not be available, or only partly available, to the animal. For example, the calcium combined in phytin, and lysine that is combined with sugar in the Maillard complex, are not available as they cannot be liberated by the digestive enzymes.

Avenalin. The globulin protein present in oats.

Avenin. The glutelin protein present in oats.

Avicel. Trade name (American Viscose Co.) for microcrystalline alpha-cellulose—natural cellulose partly hydrolysed with acid and reduced to a fine powder. Disperses in water and has the properties of a gum; used to make oily foods such as cheese, peanut butter, as well as syrups and honey, into dry granular powders; also used in sauces and dressings. (AEB.)

Avidin. Protein in white of egg which combines with vitamin H (biotin), and renders it unavailable to the body. It is inactivated in cooked eggs. *See* Biotin.

Avitaminosis. Absence of a vitamin; may be used specifically, as avitaminosis A.

Avocado. Or Alligator pears, *Persea americana*, grown mostly in tropical America and in many Asiatic and African countries. Unusual as a fruit in its high fat content.

Composition: carbohydrate 5%, protein $2 \cdot 0\%$, fat 17–27%; Fe 1 mg, vitamin A 70 μg, B_1 $0 \cdot 1$ mg, B_2 $0 \cdot 15$ mg, nicotinic acid $1 \cdot 1$ mg, vitamin C 16 mg— per 100 g. (TND.)

Axerol. Axerophthol. Suggested names for vitamin A but not used.

Azaserine. Diazoacetyl derivative of the non-essential amino acid serine. Appears to interfere with the metabolism of serine and acts as an anti-cancer agent.

Azeotrope. A mixture of water and organic solvent that distils at a temperature below the boiling point of either. Use is made of this property in azeotropic drying, when the addition of the solvent allows the water to be distilled off at a reduced temperature.

Azlon. Name given to textile fibres produced from proteins, such as casein, zein.

Azo Dyes. A group of compounds formed by combining a diazonium salt to an aromatic amino- or hydroxy-compound; they contain two nitrogen atoms combined together and are all strongly coloured. Some are permitted in foods. (Cohen.)

Azotobacter. Genus of bacteria of family *Azotobacteriaceae* which can use atmospheric nitrogen and synthesize nitrogenous tissue from it.

23

B

Babassu Oil. Edible oil from the Brazilian palm nut; similar to coconut oil and used in food, soap and cosmetics.

Babcock Test. Test for fat in milk. Sample is mixed with sulphuric acid in a Babcock bottle, centrifuged, diluted and recentrifuged. The level of the fat in the neck of the bottle is read off. (Davis.)

Bacalao. South American name for Klipfish, *which see.*

Bacitracin. Antibiotic isolated from an organism of the *B. subtilis* group; a polypeptide.

Bacon. Cured and smoked flesh of pigs raised with less subcutaneous fat than pigs for pork and with long backs.

Streaky, fried. Protein 24%, fat 45%, carbohydrate nil; kcal 500 (2·1 MJ) vitamin B_1 0·6 mg, B_2 0·24 mg, nicotinic acid 2 mg—per 100 g.

Gammon, fried. Protein 31%, fat 33%, carbohydrate nil; kcal 420 (1·8 MJ), vitamin B_1 0·6 mg, B_2 0·24 mg, nicotinic acid 2 mg—per 100 g.

Pig meat is rich in vitamin B_1, containing twice as much as other meat.

Green bacon—cured but not smoked; mild cure—less salt.

Bacteria. Microscopic, unicellular plants which do not contain chlorophyll; mostly 0·5—3 microns in size. They are responsible for much food spoilage and for disease but are also made use of as in biological oxidation, and fermentation such as the pickling process and the souring of milk.

Some bacteria, the so-called pathogens, produce toxins which cause disease. Some are sporeformers and in this form they are more resistant to heat and sterilising agents. Bacteria contain 45–85% protein and are grown on a large scale as a potential source of food for animals, using petroleum residues, methane or methanol as a source of energy. (Baum, FM.)

Bacterial Count. *See* Plate count.

Bacteriophage. Group of viruses that attack bacteria; composed of nucleoprotein and capable of multiplying in host cells. They are smaller than bacteria and can pass through ordinary bacterial filters.

Cause of considerable trouble in culture suspensions, e.g. in milk starter cultures, as these readily become infected with phages.

Bacterium aceti. See Acetobacter.

Bactofugation. A Belgian process for removing bacteria from milk by high-speed centrifuging.

Bagasse. Mill residues from sugar cane consisting of the crushed stalks from which the juice has been expressed; 50% cellulose, 25% hemicelluloses, 25% lignin. Sometimes also applied to residues from other plants such as beet.

Used as fuel, cattle feed, preparation of paper and fibre board, and in the manufacture of furfural. (Jacobs.)

Bain Marie. Double saucepan (French for water-bath).

Baker's cheese. *See* Cheese, cottage.

Baking Additives. Materials added to baked products to improve them. For example in bread-making yeast-stimulating preparations may be used, and bleaching and improving agents (ascorbic acid, potassium bromate, ammonium persulphate, chlorine dioxide, benzoyl peroxide).

Cakes may contain added sodium lactate to improve the texture of the sponge and biscuits may contain the same substance to prevent "checking".

Baking Powder. A mixture that liberates carbon dioxide when moistened or heated. Sodium bicarbonate is the source of CO_2 and an acidic substance is required, such as tartaric acid or acid salt, calcium acid phosphate, sodium pyrophosphate or sodium aluminium sulphate. Quick-acting powders contain tartrate and liberate CO_2 in the dough before heating; slow-acting contain phosphate and liberate most of the CO_2 during heating.

Legally must contain not less than 8% available, and not more than 1·5% residual, CO_2. Golden raising powder (similar but coloured yellow; formerly called egg-substitute) must contain not less than 6% available, and not more than 1·5% residual, CO_2. (KJ.)

Bal-ahar. Protein-rich baby food (22–26% protein) made in India from wheat flour, oil-seed flour and vegetables with added vitamins and calcium.

Balance. With reference to diet means equilibrium between intake and output, e.g. nitrogen balance, calcium balance, etc. Negative and positive balance respectively refer to net loss from, or gain to the body.

Balling. A table of Specific Gravity published by von Balling in 1843, giving the weight of cane sugar in 100 g of solution corresponding with S.G. determined at 17.5°C.

It is used in calculating the percentage extract in beer worts. It was corrected for slight inaccuracies by **Plato,** 1900. Extracts are referred to as per cent Plato.

For S.G. greater than unity S.G.=200 divided by (200 minus scale reading); for S.G. less than unity=200 divided by (200 plus scale reading).

Ball Mill. Vessel in which material is ground by rolling heavy balls; used for hard materials.

Bambarra Groundnut. *Voandzeia subterranea.* Resembles true groundnut but seeds are low in oil content. Seeds are hard and need soaking or pounding before cooking.

Composition per 100 g: 18 g protein, 6 g fat, 60 g carbohydrate, 367 kcal (1·5 MJ), 65 mg calcium, 6 mg iron, 0·3 mg B_1, 0·1 mg B_2, 2 mg nicotinic acid. (OF, Platt.)

Bamboo Shoots. Thick, pointed shoots of *Bambusa vulgaris* and *Phyllostachys pubescens* eaten in eastern Asia.

Composition per 100 g: 2·3 g protein, 0·2 g fat, 6 g carbohydrate, 35 kcal (0·15 MJ), 0·15 mg B_1, 0·07 mg B_2, 0·6 mg nicotinic acid, 4 mg C. (OF, Platt.)

Bamies. *See* Okra.

Banana. Fruit of genus Musa, but since the cultivated kinds are sterile hybrid forms they cannot be given exact species names.

Dessert bananas have a high sugar content (17–19%) and are eaten raw (*see also* Plantains).

Composition per 100 g: 1 g protein, 0·3 g fat, 27 g carbohydrate, 116 kcal (0·49 MJ), 0·5 mg iron, 30 μg vitamin A, 0·05 mg B_1, 0·05 mg B_2, 0·7 mg nicotinic acid, 10 mg C. Sodium content is low, 1·2 mg per 100 g, so used in low-sodium diets. (OF, Platt.)

Banana, False. *Ensete ventricosum*, closely related to the banana; fruits are small and contain seeds (bananas are sterile and have no seeds); the rhizome and inner tissues of the stem are eaten after cooking (major food in S. Ethiopia).

Composition of rhizome per 100 g: 1·5 g protein, 45 g carbohydrate, 190 kcal (0·8 MJ), 5 mg iron, 0·02 mg B_1, 0·05 mg B_2, 0·2 mg nicotinic acid, 0·5 mg C. (OF, Platt.)

Banana Figs. Bananas are split longitudinally and sun-dried without treating with sulphur dioxide. The product is dark in colour and sticky.

Bannock. Flat round cake made of oat, rye or barley meal; baked on a hearth or griddle.

Pitcaithly bannock is a type of almond shortbread containing caraway seeds and chopped peel.

Bap. A soft, white, flat, floury-coated Scottish breakfast roll.

Barbados Cherry. *See* Cherry, West Indian.

Barding. *See* Larding.

Barfoed's Test. For all mono-saccharides. Barfoed's solution is copper acetate in acetic acid, which gives a red precipitate of cuprous oxide with monosaccharides. (Hawk.)

Barium Meal. A meal containing barium sulphate, which is opaque to X-rays, and allows examination of the shape and movements of the stomach for diagnostic purposes. (BDS.)

Barley. Grain of *Hordeum vulgare*, of considerable importance as human and animal food and in brewing; one of the hardiest of cereals.

The whole grain with only the outer husk removed is called **Pot, Scotch** or **Hulled Barley** (this requires several hours cooking).

Pearl Barley—most of the bran and germ removed, ash reduced from 2·5 to 1%, vitamin B_1 to one tenth. Analysis: protein 9%, fat 1·4%; calcium 20, iron 0·7, vitamin B_1 0·15, B_2 0·08, nicotinic acid 2·5—mg per 100 g. (FAO.)

Barley Meal is ground hulled barley; **Barley flour** is ground pearl barley; **Barley flakes** are the flattened grain. (GH.)

Barley, Malted. *See* Malt.

Barm. Another name for yeast or leaven, or the froth on fermenting malt liquor.

Spon or virgin barm (short for spontaneous) is made by allowing wild yeast to fall into a sugar medium and multiply there.

Barmene. Trade name (English Grains Ltd.) for yeast extract—prepared from autolysed brewer's yeast—plus vegetable juices, used for flavouring. Composition; 38% protein, 13% carbohydrate; 6 mg thiamin, 6 mg riboflavin, 60 mg nicotinic acid, 3 mg pantothenic acid, 1·5 mg pyridoxine, 1 mg folic acid per 100 g.

Basal Metabolic Rate. When the body is at complete rest, free from draughts, at moderate room temperature and 12–14 hours after a meal, energy is being used at the basal rate—the basal metabolism. This energy is needed to maintain the heart beat, respiration, &c. but largely to maintain body temperature and the tension of the muscles. BMR is therefore related to muscle mass and the surface area of the body.

It may be calculated from surface area, the output per sq m varies with age and sex.

For male infants BMR is 50–70 kcal per m^2 per hour, falling steadily with age to 30–40 kcal at the age of 70, about 10% less for women.

Average BMR about 1,500 kcal (6 MJ) per day. It is, under control of the thyroid gland, increased in fever and hyperthyroidism and by administration of thyroxine or dried thyroid, and reduced when the thyroid is underactive. *See also* Surface Area *and* Energy. (BDS.)

Base Formers. *See* Acid foods and basic foods.

Basic Foods. *See* Acid foods and basic foods.

Basic 7 Foods Plan. Division of foods into seven groups, with the recommendation that some food from each group should be eaten every day, so ensuring a well-mixed diet.

Group 1—Green and yellow vegetables. Group 2—Oranges, tomato, grapefruit and raw salads. Group 3—Potatoes and other vegetables and fruits. Group 4— Milk and cheese. Group 5—Meat, poultry, fish and eggs. Group 6— Bread, flour, cereals. Group 7— Butter, margarine. (Johnson.)

Basil. May be one of four different types of herb but the main one is the European sweet basil, *Ocimum basilicum.* Used in seasoning.

Batata. *See* Sweet potato.

Bath Chap. Cheek and jawbones of the pig, salted and smoked. Originated at Bath.

Baumé. A table of Specific Gravity used for salt solutions. For S.G. greater than unity S.G. = 145 divided by (145 minus degrees Baumé): for S.G. less than unity = 140 divided by (130 plus degrees Baumé).

Baycovin. Trade name (Bayer Co.) for diethyl pyrocarbonate.

Bdelygmia. Extreme loathing for food.

Bé. Abbreviation for degrees Baumé.

Beans. A wide variety of leguminous seeds rich in protein (20–30%) moderate sources of iron (2–10 mg per 100 g) and of vitamins B_1, B_2 and nicotinic acid. When soaked in water and allowed to germinate they become a good source of vitamin C.

Many have different names in different countries, e.g. Lima bean (U.S.A.), butter bean (U.K.), curry bean, madagascar bean, sugar bean (*Phaseolus lunatus*).

Navy, pinto, or snap bean (U.S.A.), haricot (U.K.), kidney, French—the pods sometimes called string beans (*Phaseolus vulgaris*).

Broad bean, horse bean (*Vicia faba*). Scarlet runner bean (*Phaseolus multiflorus*).

Mung bean, black gram, woolly pyrol (*Phaseolus mungo*). Field bean, hyacinth bean, Egyptian

27

kidney bean, tonga bean (*Dolichos lablab*). *See also* Pulses, *and* Peas. (TND, Platt, FB.)

Beans, Baked. Usually mature haricot beans *Phaseolus vulgaris*, (*see* Beans); cooked by autoclaving.

Beans, Broad. *Vicia faba.* Analysis after cooking, whole beans without pod, water 84%, protein 4%, carbohydrate 7%; kcal 43 (176 kJ), Fe 1 mg, nicotinic acid 3 mg, vitamin C 15 mg—per 100 g. Also known as horse bean. (M&W.)

Beans, Butter. *Phaseolus lunatus.* Analysis after cooking:—water 70·5%, fat trace, protein 7%, carbohydrate 17%; kcal 93 (390 kJ), Fe 1·7 mg—per 100 g. Also known as lima beans, (U.S.A.) curry beans, madagascar beans and sugar beans. (M&W, Platt.)

Beans, French. *Phaseolus vulgaris*, eaten unripe in the pod, analysis of cooked pod and beans: water 95·5%, fat trace, protein 0·8%, carbohydrate 1·1%; kcal 7 (30 kJ), Fe 0·6 mg, carotene 800 i.u., vitamin C 5 mg—per 100 g. Mature bean is the haricot bean. (M&W.)

Beans, Haricot. Ripe seeds of *Phaseolus vulgaris* (unripe seed is the French bean).

Analysis of cooked bean:— water 70%, fat trace, protein 6·6%, carbohydrate 16·6%; kcal 89 (370 kJ), Ca 65 mg, Fe 2·5 mg—per 100 g.

Also known as Navy, pinto, or snap beans (U.S.A.). (M&W, Platt.)

Beans, Runner. *Phaseolus multiflorus*, eaten unripe with pod, total analysis after cooking:—water 93·6%, protein 0·8%, carbo-

hydrate 0·9%; kcal 7 (30 kJ). 0·6 mg, carotene 500 i.u., nicotinic acid 0·5 mg, vitamin C 5 mg —per 100 g. (M&W.)

Bêche-de-mer. Sea slug, *Stichopus japonicus*, also called trepang; an occasional food in most parts of the world.

Composition, protein 22%, carbohydrate 1%, fat trace; Ca 120 mg, Fe 1·4%; kcal 94 (394 kJ)—per 100 g. (Platt.)

Beechwood Sugar. Xylose.

Beef. Composition varies with the amount of fat present; usually classified as fat, medium and lean with the following composition per 100 g.

Fat: 22 g fat, 14·2 g protein, 259 kcal (1·1 MJ), 1·7 mg iron, 1·2 μg vitamin A, 0·05 mg B_1, 0·13 mg B_2, 3 mg nicotinic acid.

Medium: 17 g fat, 14·9 g protein, 217 kcal (0·9 MJ), 1·8 mg iron, 9 μg vitamin A, 0·05 mg B_1, 0·13 mg B_2, 3·1 mg nicotinic acid.

Lean: 10 g fat, 1·54 g protein, 156 kcal (0·66 MJ), 1·8 mg iron, 6 μg vitamin A, 0·05 mg B_1, 0·14 mg B_2, 3·2 mg nicotinic acid. (FAO.)

Beef Tea. An extract of stewing beef prepared by simmering for 2–3 hours. Used to be used for invalids as the meat extractives stimulate the appetite. *See also* Meat extract *and* Bovril.

Beer. Alcoholic beverage produced be fermentation of cereals. The first step in manufacture is **malting** of the barley. It is allowed to sprout when the enzyme amylase develops and hydrolyses the starch to dextrins and maltose. The sprouted barley is dried and extracted with hot water (the process is called **mashing**) to produce **wort**. After the addition of hops for flavour the wort is allowed to ferment.

Ale is a light-coloured beer made by top fermentation and containing more alcohol and hops.

Porter is made from partly charred malt and is darker in colour; it is also a top fermentation.

Stout is similar to porter but contains more extract and a higher alcohol content.

Lager is made by bottom fermentation, is low in alcohol content, rich in extract and aged after fermentation.

Most beers, ale and stout contain 3–7% alcohol and 30–60 kcal per 100 ml. (Loes.)

Beestings. The first milk given by the cow after calving.

Beet, Common Red. Root of *Beta vulgaris*. Boiled, water 83%, protein 1·8%, fat trace, carbohydrate 10%; kcal 44 (185 kJ), Fe 0·7 mg, Ca 30 mg, vitamin A trace, B_1 0·02 mg, B_2 0·04 mg, nicotinic acid 0·06 mg, vitamin C 5 mg—per 100 g. (M&W.)

Beet Sugar. Sucrose extracted from the sugar beet. It is identical with sucrose extracted from any other source.

Beeturia. Red pigmented urine after eating beetroot; occurs only in one person in eight and not consistently.

The colour is due to the pigment betanin.

Bee Wine. Wine produced by the usual alcoholic fermentation of sugar, but using yeast in the form of a clump of yeast and lactic bacteria. The clump rises and falls with bubbles of carbon dioxide produced, hence the "bee".

Bemax. Trade name (Vitamins Ltd.) of a wheat germ preparation. Composition, protein 27·8%, fat 9·3%, carbohydrate 44·7%; Ca 54 mg, Fe 7·7 mg, kcal 368 (1·55 MJ), vitamin B_1 1·6 mg, B_2 0·7 mg, nicotinic acid 7 mg—per 100 g. (M&W.)

Benedictine. French liqueur, invented, and made, by the Benedictine monks at the Abbey of Fécamp. Approximately 75% of proof spirit.

Benedict-Roth Spirometer. *See* Spirometer.

Benedict's Test. For reducing sugars; solution of copper sulphate, sodium citrate and sodium carbonate which gives a green, yellow or red precipitate on heating with a reducing agent, depending on the amount present. Benedict's quantitative reagent also includes potassium thiocyanate and potassium ferrocyanide. (Hawk.)

Benniseed. *See* Sesame.

Benzidine Test. Very sensitive test for blood. The substance under test is added to a saturated solution of benzidine in glacial acetic acid, followed by hydrogen peroxide. A blue or green colour is positive. *See also* Peroxidase. (Hawk.)

Benzoate. *See* Benzoic acid.

Benzoic Acid. Carboxylic acid derived from benzene. The free acid and the sodium and potassium salts are effective preservatives, but in U.K. permitted only in coffee extracts, pickles, sauces and soft drinks.

Has antimicrobial activity, especially in acid solution (little effective at pH above 5), half as effective as SO_2. Permitted level

29

in concentrated soft drinks 600 ppm.

Benzoic acid appears to be harmless as it is excreted in the urine in combination with glycine as hippuric acid; up to 4 g per day can be consumed and excreted in this way.

Esters of the acid are more potent preservatives than the salts. (Cohen.)

Bergamot. An orange, *Citrus bergamia*, confined almost entirely to the province of Calabria in southern Italy. Used only for extraction of the peel oil for perfumery. (Brav.)

Beriberi. Result of a severe vitamin B_1 deficiency; common in the Far East where white (polished) rice forms the bulk of the diet and vitamin B_1 is poorly supplied.

There are two forms of beriberi; the wet form—where oedema is present—and dry beriberi—where there is extreme emaciation. In both forms there is a degeneration of the nerves affecting the lower limbs first, gastro-intestinal disorders, mental symptoms, an enlarged heart with an increased rate of beat, and death ultimately results from cardiac failure. (DP.)

Berries. Botanical name for fruits in which seeds are embedded in pulpy tissue, e.g. strawberry, currant, tomato.

Berries, Golden. The berries of the Cape Gooseberry or Chinese Lantern, (*Physalis peruviana*).

Water 85%, fat 0·5%, protein 2%, fibre 2·8%, carbohydrate 9%; kcal 48 (0·2 MJ), Fe 1·5 mg, vitamin A 600 μg, B_1 0·1 mg, B_2 0·04 mg, nicotinic acid 2·8 mg, vitamin C 30 mg—100 g. (Platt.)

Betaine. Trimethyl glycine. Occurs in beetroot and cottonseed; also known as lycine and oxyneurine (obsolete names).

Related to choline; possesses labile methyl groups. (BDS.)

Beta-oxidation. One of the routes of fatty acid metabolism. Oxidation at the carbon atom beta to the carboxyl group of the fatty acid, i.e. next but one, with the formation of the beta-ketonic acid. Acetic acid then splits off, leaving a fatty acid two carbon atoms shorter than the original. (WHSS.)

Betel. Leaf of the creeper *Piper betel* or *betle*, which is chewed in some parts of the world for its stimulating effect (due to the presence of the alkaloids arecoline and guvacoline). The leaves are chewed with nuts of the areca palm, *Areca catechu*, which is therefore often called the betel palm and the nut is called the betel nut.

Bezoar. A hard ball of undigested food that forms in the stomach and can cause intestinal obstruction. Foods with a high content of indigestible pectin such as orange pith can form bezoars if swallowed without chewing. (DP.)

BHA Butylated hydroxyanisole.

BHT Butylated hydroxytoluene.

B.I.B.R.A. British Industrial Biological Research Association.

Bicarnesine. Trade name for synthetic carnitine.

Bifidus factor. Name given to factor present in human milk— now known to be lactulose—that stimulates growth of *Lactobacillus bifidus* and makes faeces of breast-fed infants slightly more acid

30

than those of babies fed on cow's milk (AEB.)

Biffins. Apples that have been peeled, partly baked, then pressed and dried.

Bigaradier. French term for the bitter orange, *see* Orange, bitter.

Bilberry. Berry of shrub of species *Vaccinium.* Variously named whortleberry, blaeberry (Iceland) windberry, huckleberry. Not cultivated but grows wild.

Composition: water 76·6–87%, protein 0·7%, free acid 1·1–1·7%, sugar 3·8–6·8%, pentosans, etc., 0·6–1·4%, fibre 3·7–12·0%, ash 0·3–1·0%.

Bile. A liquid produced by the liver and stored in the gall bladder which is embedded in the liver. It consists of bile salts (sodium glycocholate and sodium taurocholate) bile pigments (bilirubin and biliverdin) and cholesterol. The bile salts play a part in the digestion of fats as they lower the surface tension and aid the formation of a fine emulsion of fat. The bile pigments are waste products formed from the breakdown of haemoglobin and they are excreted in the faeces.

The bile travels from the gall bladder to the duodenum via the bile duct. (BDS.)

Bile Salts. *See* Bile.

Bilirubin. One of the bile pigments; formed by the degradation of haemoglobin; a reduction product of biliverdin.

Biliverdin. One of the bile pigments; formed by the degradation of haemoglobin.

Biltong. Dried meat strips (South Africa). The meat is cut in 2 inch strips, 2–3 feet long, along the muscle fibres, salted, spiced and dried in air for 10–14 days.

Composition per 100 g: 11·5 g water, 1·9 g fat, 12·5 g ash, 65 g protein, 308 kcal (1·3 MJ).

Biocytin. One of the bound forms of biotin that occurs naturally, the lysine derivative; not fully usable by all organisms until it has been hydrolysed to free biotin. (Sebrell.)

Bioflavonoids. Alternative name for flavonoids. *See* Vitamin P.

Biological Oxygen Demand (B.O.D.). Micro-organisms consume oxygen for their respiration and the uptake of oxygen by a contaminated material, e.g. sewage, water, milk, etc., is a measure of microbial activity. Also termed biochemical oxygen demand.

Biological Value. A quantitative measure of the nutritive value of a protein food carried out under conditions where quality of the protein is the limiting factor. Defined as the amount of absorbed protein that is retained in the body (expressed as a ratio), i.e. digestibility is not taken into account. If digestibility is included, i.e. the amount retained is expressed as a fraction of the amount in the diet, the measure is net protein utilisation. NPU = BV × Digestibility.

Previously expressed as a percentage scale, now as a ratio; thus the perfect protein has BV = 1·0 (100% retained). Examples are egg and human milk protein, 0·9–1·0; meat, fish and cow's milk, 0·75–0·8; wheat bread, 0·5; peanut, 0·4–0·45; gelatin, zero. When fed as mixtures these proteins complement one another. *See* Complementation. (AEB.)

Bios. During the early investigations into the factors necessary for

31

yeast growth it was found that a substance derived from yeast had to be added to the medium. This was called bios. It was later fractionated into Bios I, identified as inositol, and Bios II, identified as biotin. (Sebrell.)

Biostat. Trade name (Pfizer Ltd., U.S.A.) for ice containing the antibiotic oxytetracycline.

Biosterol. Obsolete name for vitamin A.

Biotin. Also known as vitamin H, identical with bios II and with coenzyme R (growth factor and respiratory stimulant for the organism Rhizobium, present in the root nodules of legumes).

Essential to a wide variety of animals, including man, but synthesized in the intestines. Is inactivated by combination with avidin, a protein in raw egg-white, and deficiency symptoms can be produced by feeding raw egg-white (not cooked). Deficiency causes dermatitis, loss of fur, and disturbances of the nervous system in experimental animals.

Present in liver, kidney, egg yolk, yeast, vegetables, grains, nuts. (Sebrell.)

Biotoprotein. A soluble biotin-protein complex that occurs naturally. (Sebrell.)

Birch Beer. Non-alcoholic carbonated beverage flavoured with oil of wintergreen or oil of sweet birch and oil of sassafras.

Biscuit. Essentially bakery confectionery dried down to low moisture content, name derived from Latin for twice-cooked. Made from soft flour; mostly rich in fat and sugar and consequently of high energy content 420–510 kcal (1·7–2·1 MJ), per 100 g.

Termed cookie in the U.S.A. where the word biscuit means a small cake-like bun. (KJ.)

Biscuit Check. The development of splitting and cracks in biscuits immediately after baking. (KJ.)

Biskoids. Trade name (Andomia Products) for saccharine.

Bitot's Spots. Foam-like irregular plaques on the surface of the eye due to vitamin A deficiency. (Sebrell.)

Bitters. Gentian, quassia and calumba, and, in small doses, quinine and strychnine. Used to stimulate gustatory nerves in the mouth and thus stimulate appetite. (Clark.)

Biuret Test. For proteins (actually for peptide bonds). Violet colour is developed when a drop of copper sulphate solution is added to a solution of protein in caustic soda. (Hawk.)

Bixin. A carotenoid pigment found in the seeds of the tropical plant *Bixa orellana*, the crude extract is the colouring agent annatto, *which see.*

Blackberry. Berry of bramble, *Rubus fruticosus*. Protein 1·2%, fat 1·0%; kcal 57 (0·24 MJ), Fe 1·0 mg, vitamin A 50 μg, B_1 0·03 mg, B_2 0·05 mg, nicotinic acid 0·4 mg, vitamin C 24 mg—per 100 g. (FAO.)

Blackcurrant. Fruit of the bush, *Ribes nigra*. Of special interest as a fruit because of its high vitamin C content. Protein 0·9%, fat trace, carbohydrate 6·6%; water 77%; kcal 29 (0·12 MJ), Fe 1·3 mg, vitamin A 90 μg, B_1 0·03 mg, B_2 0·06 mg, nicotinic acid 0·25 mg, vitamin C 200 mg—per 100 g. (M&W.)

Black Jack. *See* Caramel.

Black PN. Food colour, tetra sodium salt of 8-acetamido-2-(7 - sulpho - 4 - p - sulphophenyl-azo - 1 - naphthylazo) - 1 - naphthol-3:5-disulphonic acid. Also called Brilliant black BN. Not very stable.

Black Tongue. A symptom of nicotinic acid deficiency in dogs that was used in the isolation of the vitamin. (DP.)

Blaeberry. *See* Bilberry.

Blanching. A partial pre-cooking. Fruits and vegetables are blanched before canning, dehydrating, or freezing, for a variety of reasons: softening of texture, shrinkage, removal of air, destruction of enzymes, removal of undesirable flavours. Consists of dipping in hot water, 82–93°C, for half to five minutes.

Also done to remove excess salt from preserved meat and to aid removal of skin, e.g. from almonds. Can result in losses of 10–20% of sugars, salts, and protein, some of the vitamins B_1, B_2 and nicotinic acid, and up to one-third of the vitamin C.

Blanching, Infra-red. Superior to steam blanching for apples, celery, peas and potatoes as it reduces the amount of water left in the product, does not leach out flavour and nutrients, and improves the texture, flavour and appearance. In potatoes the process reduces fat absorption during frying.

Blancmange Powders. Usually a cornflour base with added flavour and colour.

Bland Diet. One that contains the minimum of crude fibre or roughage and is therefore non-irritating and soothing to the intestine. (AEB.)

Bleaching. In the context of food usually refers to the bleaching of flour. (*See* Aging.) Also refers to the bleaching of oils, a stage in the purification by which colloidally dispersed impurities and natural colouring matters are removed by activated earth or Fuller's earth.

Bleaching Agents. *See* Aging.

Bleeding Bread. A bacterial infection with *B. prodigiosus* that stains the bread bright red. Under optimal conditions of warmth and damp the infection can appear overnight and contamination of shewbread with this organism in churches has led to accusations and riots against religious minorities over the centuries.

Bloaters. *See* Red herring.

Blood Cells, White. *See* Leucocytes.

Blood, Citrated. Blood that has been prevented from clotting by the addition of citrate, which combines with the calcium. (*See* Coagulation, blood.) 600 mg of sodium citrate will prevent coagulation of 100 ml blood. (BDS.)

Blood, Defibrinated. Blood clots rapidly after it has been shed when the soluble protein fibrinogen is converted into insoluble fibrin. If the blood is stirred with a rod the fibrin can be removed as it forms and the blood, still containing the cells, will remain fluid. This is defibrinated blood. (BDS.)

Blood, Oxalated. Blood that has been prevented from clotting by the addition of oxalate, which combines with the calcium. (*See* Coagulation, blood.) 160 mg of sodium oxalate will prevent the clotting of 100 ml blood. (BDS.)

33

Blood, Red Cells. Carry the red colouring matter, haemoglobin, which is the means of transporting oxygen and carbon dioxide in the blood stream. The cell, or erythrocyte, is $8 \cdot 8$ microns in diameter, $1 \cdot 9$ microns at its greatest thickness; 5 million per cubic millimetre of blood; exists for 120 days then destroyed in the body and the iron re-used. (BDS).

Blood Sugar. The blood sugar is glucose, normally present (before breakfast) at 80–100 mg per 100 ml. The level rises after a meal (to around 150 mg per 100 ml) but rapidly returns to normal as glucose is taken up by the tissues (except in cases of diabetes mellitus, *which see*).

Glucose provides the energy for muscular activity and it is stored in the liver and muscles after conversion to glycogen. (BDS.)

Blood Sugar Test. *See* Glucose tolerance.

Blood Volume. Average: males—$5 \cdot 3$ litres, females—$3 \cdot 8$ litres; 78 and 66 ml per kg body weight, respectively. Can be calculated from Wilson's formula: vol. in ml $= 43 \times$ wt in kg $+ 131 \times$ height in inches $- 6250$. Determined by injecting known amount of a dye, such as Evans Blue, and determining the degree of dilution in a sample of the blood. (BDS.)

Blood, White Cells. *See* Leucocytes.

Bloom. Fat bloom is the whitish appearance on the surface of chocolate that sometimes occurs on storage. It is due to a change in the form of the fat at the surface or to fat diffusing outward and being deposited on the surface.

Bloom Gelometer. Instrument used for measuring the strength of jellies, and also for any test of firmness, e.g. staleness of bread. For jelly strength the jelly is prepared at $6 \cdot 66\%$ concentration and chilled at $10°C$ for 16–18 hours. The instrument measures the load in grams needed to produce a 4 mm depression in the gel with a ½-inch diameter plunger.

Gelatin at 250 bloom grams is used in jellied meat, 200 in marshmallows.

Blueberry. Highbush blueberry (*Vaccinium corymbosum*) and lowbush (*V. augustifolium*) grown in North America.

Blue Cheese. *See* Cheese, Blue.

Blue Value. (1) Of vitamin A—refers to the transient blue colour produced by reaction with antimony trichloride, the depth of colour being proportional to the amount of the vitamin present. (2) Referring to starch—it is an index of the free soluble starch, i.e. the amylose, in a food, e.g. potatoes.

Blue VRS. Sodium salt of 4:4′-di (diethylamino)-4″:6″-disulphotriphenylmethanolanhydride.

B.M.R. Basal Metabolic Rate, *which see.*

B.O.D. *See* Biological oxygen demand.

Body-building Food. A term indiscriminately used, usually refers to proteins. The Code of Practice suggests that no claim should be made for the body-building properties of a food unless a reasonable amount of protein (not specified) is present in a normal portion. (AEB.)

Body Fluid. *See* Water balance.

Body Surface. *See* Surface area.

Bog Butter. Norsemen, Finns, Scots and Irish used to bury firkins of butter in bogs to ripen it for the strong flavour that developed. (Davis.)

Boiled Sweets. Sugar and water boiled at such a high temperature, 149–166°C, that practically no water remains and a vitreous mass is formed on cooling. Actually a supersaturated solution of sugar.

Boiling or Stewing. For meat of second quality, i.e. containing much connective tissue, boiling or stewing is the preferred method of cooking since it slowly breaks down the connective tissue to water-soluble gelatin and improves the tenderness.

The meat extractives expressed into the water through shrinkage, are not lost since the water is normally used.

Destruction of vitamin B_1 approx. 75%, B_2 30%, and nicotinic acid 50%, according to Johnson. Fish loses 20% B_1. *See also* Autoclave.

Bole. *See* Armenian bole.

Bombay Duck. Fish found in Indian waters; eaten fresh or after salting and curing.

Bomb Calorimeter. *See* Calorimeter.

Bone. Organic matrix of collagen, osseoalbumoid and osseomucoid with an inorganic mixture of 85% calcium phosphate, 10% calcium carbonate and 1·5% magnesium phosphate. The inorganic mixture has the crystal structure of the mineral hydroxyapatite which is composed of one molecule of calcium hydroxide to three of calcium phosphate.

Fluoride and sulphate are also present in bone. (Hawk.)

Bone Broth. Prepared by prolonged boiling of chopped bones. Of little nutritive value, consisting of 2–4% gelatin, with very little calcium.

Bone Charcoal. Bones degreased, broken to required size and heated in closed retorts. The organic matter is carbonized leaving about 10% carbon deposited on a framework of calcium phosphate.

Used to purify solutions by virtue of its properties of absorbing colouring matter and impurities.

Bone Meal. Prepared from degreased animal bones and used as a supplement both to animal feed and human food as a source of both calcium and phosphate; also used as plant fertiliser as a source of phosphate. (AEB.)

Bontrae. Trade name (General Mills, Inc., U.S.A.) for textured vegetable protein preparation made by spinning or extrusion. (FM.)

Borage. A herb, *Borage officinalis*, not grown on a commercial scale. The flowers and leaves are sometimes used to flavour beverages and have a flavour resembling that of cucumber.

Borax. Sodium salt of boric acid.

Boric acid. Derived from boron; has, in the past, been used as a food preservative (in bacon and margarine) but accumulates in the body.

Boron. Element essential to plants but not to animals.

Boston Brown Bread. In the United States, a spiced pudding steamed in the can.

Bottles. The customary wine bottle holds 26⅔ fluid oz, or one sixth of a gallon, which is the "reputed quart".

2 bottles = magnum; 4 bottles = Jeroboam; 6 bottles = Rehoboam, 8 bottles = Methuselah; 12 bottles = Salamanzar; 16 bottles = Balthazar; 20 bottles = Nebuchadnezzar.

Botulism. Rare form of food poisoning due to the endotoxin botulinum produced by *Clostridium botulinus;* extremely minute quantities are fatal. The organism is anaerobic, and the spores can withstand boiling for 3 hours. They require a temperature of 120°C and a pH below 4·5 for destruction. Hence cooked foods, especially meat and non-acid canned vegetables, can still contain these spores. The toxin itself is destroyed at 65°C. (Tanner.)

Bouillabaisse. Fish stew common in Southern France, made from several kinds of fish and shellfish, cooked with oil, spices and herbs. So named since it is repeatedly boiled.

Bouillon. Plain, unclarified beef or veal broth.

Bouquet Garni. *See* Faggot.

Bourbonal. Ethylvanillin, *see under* Vanilla.

Bournvita. Trade name (Cadbury Schweppes, Ltd.) for a preparation of malt, milk, sugar, cocoa, eggs and flavouring, for consumption as a beverage when added to milk.
Protein 11·4%, fat 7·5%, carbohydrate 67·6%; Ca 89 mg. Fe 3 mg, kcal 370 (1·6 MJ)—per 100 g. (M&W.)

Bovril. Trade name (Bovril Ltd.) for a preparation of meat extract, hydrolysed beef, beef powder and yeast extract used as a beverage, breadspread and flavouring agent.
Protein 28%, vitamin B_2 3·5

mg, nicotinic acid 24 mg, Fe 12 mg—per 100 g.

Boysenberry. Similar to loganberry.

Bradycardia. An unusually slow heart-beat; a symptom, among other causes, of certain vitamin deficiencies.

Bradyphagia. Eating very slowly.

Braising. Brief frying in shallow fat followed by stewing. Proteins coagulate very rapidly during frying and may become tougher. Loss of vitamin B_1 may be up to 50%, B_2 25%, nicotinic acid 35%. (Johnson.)

Bran. *See* Wheatfeed.

Bran Plus. Trade name (Allinson's Ltd.) for untreated wheat bran with germ.
Composition per 100 g: 13·7 g protein, 57·4 g carbohydrate, 13 g water, 3·6 g fat, 4·5 g ash, 7·8 g fibre.

Brandy. A spirit distilled from wine. Name derived from the German Brantwein (burnt wine) corrupted to brandywine.
There are two types, (1) of high alcohol content, 80–94·5%, used to fortify dessert wines, and (2) beverage brandies of 50% alcohol.
The age of brandies used to be designated by stars (one for 3 years, two for 4 years, three for 5 years) and the initials V.S.O. (very special old, 12–17 years) V.S.O.P. (very special old pale, 18–25 years), V.V.S.O.P. (very, very, special old pale, up to 40 years old)—but these designations have largely lost their meaning through indiscriminate use.

Brawn. Made from meat, ears and tongue of the pig; boiled with peppercorns and herbs, minced and pressed into a mould. Mock brawn differs in that other meat by-products are used.

Bread. Usually refers to loaf made from wheat or rye. Composition depends on extraction rate of flour and on enrichment with vitamins and minerals; may also be enriched with milk powder, fish protein concentrate or other sources of protein.

Composition of white bread in U.K. (enriched with iron, calcium, thiamin and nicotinic acid) per 100 g: 38 g water, 53 g starch, 8 g protein, 1·4 g fat, 240 kcal (1·0 MJ), 0·18 mg B_1, 0·04 mg B_2, 1·7 mg nicotinic acid, 1·8 mg iron, 90 mg calcium. *See also* Flour, Flour Enrichment *and* Gluten. (KJ, FB.)

Bread, Aerated. The dough is made with water saturated with carbon dioxide under pressure. The object is to produce an aerated loaf without the loss of carbohydrate involved in a yeast fermentation (7% of the total ingredients). The result was insipid in flavour and the method went out of use, *but see* Glucono-delta-lactone. (Hutch.)

Bread, Allinson's. Trade name for a wholemeal loaf.

Protein 8·2%, fat 2%, carbohydrate 47·1%; Ca 26 mg, Fe 3 mg, kcal 228 (0·97 MJ), per 100 g. (M&W.)

Bread, Black. Coarse wholemeal wheat or rye bread leavened with "sauerteig," that is a mixture of fermenting micro-organisms. These include: (1) peptonizing bacteria that turn the dough to a more plastic state, (2) yeast, (3) lactic or acetic bacteria that produce the sour flavour. (Tanner.)

Bread, Brown. A loaf may not legally be described as brown (or wholemeal) unless it contains not less than 0·6% fibre (on dry weight), i.e. a high rate of extraction. (Bell.)

Bread, Cornell. Loaf of increased nutritional value by addition of 6% soya flour and 8% skim milk solids. So-called because of participation of staff of Cornell University in its development.

Breadfruit. The starchy fruit of the tree *Artocarpus communis* or *incisa*. Staple though seasonal food of the West Indies; eaten roasted whole when ripe or boiled in pieces when green.

Water 70%, carbohydrate 26%, protein 1·5%, fat 0·4%; kcal 113 (0·47 MJ), Fe 1 mg, vitamin B_1 0·1 mg, B_2 0·06 mg, nicotinic acid 1·2 mg, vitamin C 20 mg—per 100 g. (TND, Platt, OF.)

Bread, Gluten. Loaf with added wheat gluten to increase the protein content. The name may legally be applied only to loaves containing not less than 16% protein (calculated on dry weight).

When the protein level is not less than 22% the loaf may be designated protein bread. *See also* Bread, starch reduced. (Bell, KJ.)

Bread, Lactein. Milk bread. (*See* Bread, milk).

Bread, Malt. Contains 6–13% ground malt or malt extract which produces a sweeter, stickier and darker loaf.

Bread, Milk. A loaf cannot legally be described as milk bread unless it contains not less than 6% whole milk solids or skim milk solids. (Bell.)

Bread, Protein. Loaf containing not less than 22% protein (calculated on dry weight). High protein bread is an alternative designation. (Bell.)

Bread, Soda. Bread leavened with sodium bicarbonate and an acidic substance instead of yeast, although legally it may contain yeast as well.

Breads, Quick. *See* Quick breads.

Bread, Starch-reduced. Bread is normally 9–10% protein and about 50% starch; if the starch is reduced either by washing some part of it out of the dough or by adding extra protein, the bread is referred to as starch-reduced and is often claimed of value in slimming and diabetic diets.

Legally the term starch-reduced bread may be applied only to bread containing less than 50% carbohydrate and the wording claiming its value as a slimming aid is legally controlled. *See also* Bread, gluten *and* Bread, protein (Bell.)

Bread, Wheat Germ. A loaf which must contain not less than 10% added processed wheat germ. (Bell.)

Breakfast Food, Cereal. Legally defined as any food obtained by the swelling, roasting, grinding, rolling or flaking of any cereal. Described under individual names (e.g. All-Bran, Bemax, Cornflakes, Wheat, puffed, Wheat, shredded, Force).

Break Rolls. Special type of rollers used in flour mills. Consist of a pair of corrugated chilled-iron rolls that rotate at a differential speed of $2\frac{1}{2}:1$ so shearing the grain and scraping out some of the endosperm.

Bredsoy. Trade name (British Soya Products Ltd. for unheated (enzyme-active) full-fat soya flour.

Brewers' Grains. Cereal residue from brewing, contains about 25% protein; used as animal feed and also a source of unidentified growth factors.

Brewers' Pounds. Before specific gravity was used in breweries the strength of wort was expressed as the difference between the weight of a barrel of wort and that of a barrel of water (360 lb.). The excess weight over 360 lb. is denoted by Brewers' pounds.

Brewing. *See* Beer.

Brislings. Young sprats, *Clupea sprattus*. Canned brislings contain 1,000 i.u. vitamin A and 1–2,000 i.u. vitamin D per 100 g.

British Industrial Biological Research Association. Joint Government–Industry sponsored body that investigates food additives.

Brix. A table of Specific Gravity based on the Balling tables (*which see*) calculated in grams of cane sugar in 100 g solution at 20°C, i.e. degree Brix = per cent sugar.

Used to refer to concentration of sugar syrups used in canned fruits.

Brodie's Solution. Fluid used in the Warburg manometer (*which see*) with specific gravity of $1 \cdot 033$ so that 10,000 mm equals 1 atmosphere pressure. 23 g sodium chloride, 5 g bile salts in 500 ml water, coloured with crystal violet or gentian violet, and preserved with thymol. (Hawk.)

Broiler. Chicken 10–12 weeks old weighing about 3 lb. Alternative definition—chicken 70–76 days old weighing 2–2½ lb of a rapidly growing strain.

At this stage the chicken is at its most rapid, and therefore economically most profitable, growth.

Broiling. *See* Grilling.

Bromatology. Science of foods (from the Greek *broma*—food).

Bromelin. Proteolytic enzyme in pineapple juice, used for tenderizing meat and sausage skin casings.

Brominated Oils. Brominated olive, peach, apricot kernel, soya oils, etc., used to help to stabilize emulsions of flavouring substances in soft drinks; also described as weighting oils.

Brose. A Scottish dish made by pouring boiling water on oatmeal or barley meal; fish, meat or vegetables may be added.

Broth. A soup made from meat or bone extractives, with vegetables, meat, farinaceous material, spices, and herbs. Legally, in the case of canned soups, the "meat nitrogen" content must be equivalent to not less than 1% protein.

Brown Colours. *Brown FK*, a mixture of the disodium salt of 1:3-diamino-4:6-di - (p-sulphophenylazo)benzene and the sodium salt of 2:4-diamino-5-(p-sulphophenylazo) toluene—"kipper brown".

Chocolate brown FB. The product of coupling diazotised naphthionic acid with a mixture of morin and maclurin (*see* Fustic).

Chocolate brown HT. Disodium salt of 2:4- dihydroxy - 3:5 - di- (4-sulpho-1-naphthylazo) benzyl alcohol. Both these colours are "baking browns".

Browning Reaction. *See* Maillard reaction *and* Phenol oxidases.

Brussels Sprouts. Leaf buds of *Brassica oleracea gemmifera.* Protein 3·6%, fat 0·4%; Ca 26 mg, Fe 1·0 mg, kcal 36 (0·15 MJ), vitamin A 90 μg, B_1 0·06 mg, B_2 0·12 mg, nicotinic acid 0·5 mg, vitamin C 71 mg—per 100 g. (FAO.)

Buckling. Hot-smoked herring. (The kipper is cold-smoked).

Buckwheat. A cereal, *Fagopyrum esculentum*, also known as Saracen corn and, when cooked, as Kasha (Russian). Unsuitable for bread-making, eaten as the cooked grain, porridge or pancakes.

Protein 11%, fat 2%, carbohydrate 70%; 350 kcal (1·5 MJ), Fe 3 mg, vitamin B_1 0·3 mg, B_2 0·3 mg, nicotinic acid 3 mg—per 100 g. (Platt.)

Budde's Process. For preserving milk, *see* Milk, Buddeized.

Buffers. Substances that resist change in acidity or alkalinity. Salts of weak acids and weak bases are buffers, also proteins and amino acids by virtue of their content of both acidic and basic groups. *See also* Acid-base Balance.

Bulgur. Prepared, precooked wheat originating in the Near East. Wheat is soaked, cooked and dried; it is lightly milled to remove the outer bran and cracked. Eaten with soups, cooked with meat, etc.

Bulgur is the oldest processed food known; also called **ala** and **American rice**; cooked with meat it is called Kibbe.

Bullace. Wild damson.

Bullock's Heart. *See* Custard Apple.

Bunt. *See* Smut.

Burghul. Alternative name for bulgur.

Burning Feet Syndrome. Aching and throbbing in the feet later spreading upwards to the knees; results from long periods on a diet poor in protein and B vitamins.
Claimed to be cured by pantothenic acid but not confirmed and the whole vitamin B complex appears to be necessary. (DP.)

Busa. *See* Milks, Fermented.

Bushel. A dry measure of capacity equivalent to 80 lb of distilled water at 17°C with barometer reading 30 inches, i.e. 8 gallons or 4 pecks. Used as a measure of corn, potatoes, etc.
The weight of a bushel varies with the product, e.g. wheat—60 lb, maize—56 lb, rye—56 lb, barley—48 lb, oats—32 lb, paddy rice—45 lb.
The American measure is the Winchester bushel which is 3% greater.

Butane 1:3 diol. Of possible use in food manufacture; energy content kcal 6 (24 kJ) per g.

Butt. Cask for beer or wine containing 108 imperial gallons.

Butter. Prepared from cream by souring naturally or with bacterial culture (starter) and churning. Legally in U.K. must contain not less than 80% fat (may be 78% if salt added), not more than 2% other milk solids and not more than 16% water; usually contains 1% protein, 0·4% lactose, 1·5–4·5% salt and coloured with annatto. Vitamin A content varies between 500 μg per 100 g in winter and 1350 μg in summer; 1 mg vitamin D. (FM.)

Butter, Black. Butter that has been browned by heating then vinegar, salt, pepper or other seasoning added, and used as a sauce.

Butterine. *See* Margarine.

Buttermilk. Residue left after churning butter, 0·1–2·0% fat, with the other milk constituents proportionately increased. Has a slightly acid flavour together with a distinctive flavour due to diacetyl and related substances. (Davis & Mac.)

Buttermilk, Cultured. The modern equivalent of sour buttermilk, produced by acid-producing streptococci in skim milk.

Butter, Mowrah. *See* Vegetable butters.

Butter, Process or Renovated. Butter that has been melted and rechurned with the addition of milk, cream or water.

Butter, Vegetable. *See* Vegetable butters.

Butter, Whey. Or **serum butter;** made from the small amount of fat left in whey. It has a fatty acid composition slightly different from that of ordinary butter.

Butylated Hydroxyanisole. Or BHA. An antioxidant, used for fats and fatty foods, derived chemically from phenol, not destroyed by heat and therefore useful in baked products: active at concentration of 0·01–0·1%.

Butylated Hydroxytoluene. Or BHT, an antioxidant used for fats and fatty foods.

Butyric Acid. A short chain fatty acid, with the formula $CH_3CH_2CH_2COOH$. Occurs as the triglyceride as 5–6% of butter fat, and small amounts in other fats.

Butyrine. Alternative name for alpha-amino-n-butyric acid; found in the blood stream, derived from threonine and not present in the diet.

BV. Biological Value.

Bynin. Name given (by Osborne and Campbell 1896) to an alcohol-soluble protein of malt; later shown to be identical with the alcohol-soluble protein of barley and the name was abandoned.

C

Cabbage. Leaves of *Brassica oleracea capitata.* Protein 1·1%, fat 0·1%; Ca 35 mg, Fe 0·3 mg, kcal 17 (0·07 MJ), vitamin A 20 μg, B_1 0·04 mg, B_2 0·03 mg, nicotinic acid 0·2 mg, vitamin C 35 mg—per 100 g. (FAO.)

Cachexia. An extreme state of general ill-health, with malnutrition, wasting, anaemia, and circulatory and muscular weakness.

Cadaverine. *See* Ptomaines.

Cadmium. A mineral considered to be of no biological interest until the recent isolation of metallothionein from horse kidney cortex. This is a protein complex including 2·9% cadmium and 0·6% zinc per gram of protein; significance unknown.

Cadmium is highly toxic and there have been many cases reported of poisoning arising from cadmium derived from cadmium-plated vessels. (GMW.)

Caecum. First part of the large intestine, separated from the small intestine by the ileo-colic sphincter. It is small in carnivorous animals, very large in herbivores as it is involved in cellulose digestion, intermediate size in man. (BDS.)

Caeruloplasmin. A blue copper-protein complex present in traces in the blood.

Caffeine. Alkaloid drug (trimethylxanthine) found in coffee and tea. Raises blood pressure, stimulates kidneys and averts fatigue temporarily.

Coffee beans contain 1% caffeine, hence the beverage contains about 18 mg per oz or 100 mg per cup; tea contains 1·5–2·5% caffeine, about 12–15 mg per oz of beverage: cola drinks contain 3–4·5 mg per oz.

Also called theine.

Caffeol. Volatile oil giving characteristic flavour and aroma to coffee.

Calabash. *See* Gourds.

Calamondin. A citrus fruit resembling a small tangerine, with

41

a delicate pulp and a lime-like flavour.

Calciferol. Old name for ergocalciferol or vitamin D_2, made by irradiation of ergosterol. *See* Vitamin D.

Calcium. A dietary essential needed for the formation of bones and teeth, which are composed largely of calcium phosphate. It is present in the body in larger amounts than any other mineral (1·0–1·5 kg).

The small amount circulating in the blood (9–11 mg per 100 ml) and in the soft tissues plays a vital part in the metabolic processes, controls the heart beat and the excitability of muscle and nerve, plays a part in blood clotting and in the maintenance of acid-base equilibrium. A fall in the level of blood calcium results in increased sensitivity of the motor nerves to stimuli, i.e. tetany.

Its absorption from food is aided by vitamin D and protein and hindered by excess fat, phosphate, oxalate and phytate; the result is that only 15–35% of dietary calcium is absorbed.

Daily requirements 0·4–0·5 g increased to 0·4–0·7 g in growing children, and 1·0–1·2 g in pregnancy and lactation.

Richest sources are milk and cheese; calcium is added to flour as *creta praeparata* at the rate of 14 oz per 280 lb sack: eggs and vegetables are moderate sources.

The chemical form in which calcium is added to foods for enrichment does not appear to be important, e.g. carbonate, phosphate, chloride, etc., appear to be equally well absorbed. *See also* Phytic acid, Parathyroid glands *and* Hypercalcaemia. (DP, FB.)

Calcium Acid Phosphate. Also known as monocalcium phosphate, and acid calcium phosphate or A.C.P., $Ca(H_2PO_4)_2$.

Used as the acid ingredient of baking powder and self-raising flour since it reacts with bicarbonate to liberate carbon dioxide.

Chemically similar to "superphosphate" fertiliser but purer. (KJ.)

Calcium Gluconate. Water-soluble salt of calcium and gluconic acid useful for intravenous administration (e.g. in the relief of tetany).

Calcium-phosphorus Ratio. Earlier work suggested that a high ratio of phosphate to calcium in the diet hindered the absorption of calcium from the intestine into the blood stream and gave rise to rickets. It was thought that a Ca:P ratio of between 1:2 and 2:1 was essential for maximum absorption but this belief has been discarded.

Calculus. Stone formed in tissues such as kidney and gall bladder. Kidney stones consist of uric acid, urates, and calcium oxalate, carbonate and phosphate. Possibly of dietary causation.

Renal calculus—stones in kidney or ureter.

Vesical calculus — prostatic gland obstruction.

Biliary calculus — gallstone, *which see.* (DP.)

Calfos. Trade name (Croda Food Ingredients Ltd.) for a prepared bone meal, i.e. calcium phosphate used as a source of calcium and of phosphate in foods. Similarly Calphos is a trade name (Joseph Crosfield & Sons Ltd.). (AEB.)

Calorie. The unit of heat used in nutrition is the kilocalorie—the amount of heat required to raise

42

the temperature of 1 kg of water from 15° to 16°C—abbreviated to kcal or written with a capital C to distinguish it from the small calorie. (DP.)

Calorie Conversion Factors. *See* Atwater factors *and* Rubner factors *and* Energy Conversion Factors.

Calorie Expenditure. *See* Energy expenditure.

Calorie Values. *See* Energy, available.

Calories, Empty. Refers to foods that supply only energy with little, if any, of the nutrients.

Calorimeter (or bomb calorimeter). Instrument for measuring the amount of oxidizable energy present in a substance by burning it in oxygen and measuring the heat released. The heat liberated by burning a food in this way will coincide with the metabolizable energy in that food only if it can be completely metabolized. E.g. proteins liberate 5·65 kcal/g in the bomb calorimeter in which the nitrogen is oxidized to the dioxide, but only 4·4 kcal/g in the body where the nitrogen is excreted as urea and uric acid, etc. (containing 1·25 kcal/g). (DP.)

Calorimetry, Direct. Direct measurement of heat production. It is measured in man in a respiration calorimeter (Atwater-Benedict type); the subject is placed inside the calorimeter, which is a small room with insulated walls. The heat produced is measured by the rise in temperature of water flowing round the walls. This type of apparatus was used in the early days of research into energy metabolism. (BDS.)

Calorimetry, Indirect. Measurement of energy output by calculation from the oxygen consumption and carbon dioxide output. *See* Spirometer. (BDS.)

Caltrops. *See* Chestnut, Water.

Calvados. *See* Apple Jack.

Campbell's Process. A method of drying milk by first concentrating by blowing hot air through, followed by drum-drying; patented in England 1901. (Davis & Mac.)

Campden Process. The preservation of food by the addition of sodium bisulphite which liberates sulphur dioxide. Also known as cold preservation since it replaces heat sterilization.

Campden Tablets. Tablets of sodium bisulphite.

Camu-camu. A Peruvian fruit from the bush *Myrciaria paraensis*; burgundy red in colour, 6–14 g wt, 3 cm diameter: 3,000 mg vitamin C per 100 g pulp.

Canapés. Small open sandwiches.

Canbra Oil. Oil extracted from genetically selected variety of rapeseed with not more than 2% erucic acid. (*See* Erucic Acid).

Candida. *See* Yeast.

Candied Peel. Used in confectionery; prepared by softening the peel, often of citrus fruits, and boiling for prolonged period with sugar syrup.

Candy. United States term for sugar confectionery. (Griswold.)

Candy Doctor. *See* Sugar doctor.

Cane Sugar. Sucrose extracted from the sugar cane; identical

43

with sucrose prepared from any other source, such as sugar beet.

Canner's Alkali. Mixture of sodium hydroxide and sodium carbonate used to remove skin from fruit before canning (sodium hydroxide alone more frequently used). (Jacobs.)

Canning, Aseptic. Foods are pre-sterilised at very high temperatures, 150–175°C, for a few seconds and then sealed into cans under aseptic conditions. The flavour, colour and vitamin retention are superior with this short time–high temperature process compared with conventional canning.

The rate of bacterial spore destruction is approximately multiplied tenfold for every 10°C rise in temperature while the chemical reactions responsible for loss of quality are doubled for every 10°C rise in temperature. (Baum.)

Canthaxanthin. A red carotenoid pigment, chemically related to beta-carotene but without any vitamin-A activity. Suggested use as addition to the diet of broiler chickens to impart a pigmented skin and shanks, and to the diet of trout to produce the bright colours of wild trout; these colours are normally derived from natural foodstuffs which may be variable or in short supply.

Similarly beta-apo-8'-carotenal which is four-fifths of the beta-carotene molecule, can be used in chick–diets to increase the colour of the egg yolks.

Capers. Buds of unopened flowers of *Capparis spinosa* (Europe and North Africa): flavour for pickles and sauces. (Merory.)

Capillary Fragility. Refers to the resistance to rupture of the walls of a blood vessel, which would result in the leakage of red blood cells into the tissue spaces. There is some evidence that the flavonoids (*see* Vitamin P) increase the resistance to rupture and this has given rise to unverified suggestions that this group of compounds will protect against the common cold by increasing the resistance of the capillaries to infection.

Capon. Castrated cockerel; slightly increased growth with more tender flesh than the cockerel. Surgery mostly replaced by "chemical caponization", i.e. implantation of pellets of female sex hormone.

Capric Acid. One of the fatty acids, $C_9H_{19}COOH$. occurs as triglyceride in coconut, goat and cow butter, and in the fat of the spice bush.

Caproic Acid. One of the fatty acids, $C_5H_{11}COOH$.
Found as triglyceride in goat and cow butter and coconut fat.

Caprylic Acid. One of the fatty acids, $C_7H_{15}COOH$. Occurs as triglyceride in goat and cow butter, coconut oil and human fat.

Capsicum. *See* Pepper.

Carageenan. Extract of red seaweed, *Chondrus crispus* (Irish Moss) and *Gigartina stellata;* the name is also given to extracts of other red seaweeds (*Eucheuma* and *Iridea* varieties).
Used in low-calorie jams and jellies, chocolate milk drinks, ice-cream, instant milk puddings, oil emulsions, toothpastes and processed cheese. Increases viscosity, binds water and emulsifies and stabilises by reacting with the

proteins present. Its setting properties depend on temperature only, not time and temperature as, for example, with pectin gels. (Tressler.)

Caramel. Brown colour prepared by heating sugar above its melting point; permitted additive to foods. Also known as Black Jack.

Caramelization. The brown colour produced when sugars are heated or treated with acid. Sweetened fruit juices turn brown on storing at elevated temperatures through caramelization. The effect is distinct from the Maillard reaction between sugar and proteins which also occurs on storage.

Caramels. *See* Toffee.

Caraway. Dried ripe fruit of *Carum carvi*. Main component of the volatile oil is carvone, with smaller amounts of limonene. Used for the liqueur kümmel, and on bread and rolls.

Carbohydrate by Difference. In the analysis of foods it is difficult to determine the various carbohydrates and they are usually approximated by subtracting the measured protein plus ash plus fat from 100. The figure can be corrected by subtracting crude fibre which is non-available carbohydrate.

Carbohydrate by difference is the sum of:—
(a) unavailable carbohydrate—pentosans, pectins, hemicelluloses and celluloses;
(b) available carbohydrate—dextrins, starch and sugars;
(c) non-carbohydrates, such as organic acids and crude fibre.

Carbohydrate Metabolism. *See* Glucose metabolism.

Carbohydrates. Substances composed of carbon, hydrogen and oxygen with 2 atoms of hydrogen for every oxygen. They include polysaccharides such as starch, dextrins and glycogen which are digested to glucose, and sugars such as lactose, fructose and glucose, as well as undigestible materials (*see* Carbohydrates, Unavailable).

They form the major part of the diet of man in the form of starch and sucrose in particular, and provide energy at the rate of 4 kcal or 16 kJ per g. The loss of water in the formation of disaccharides and polysaccharides from the monosaccharides results in slight differences in energy content—monosaccharides 3·74 kcal or 15·6 kJ, disaccharides 3·95 kcal or 16·5 kJ, starch 4·18 kcal or 17·5 kJ and glycerol 4·32 kcal or 18·0 kJ per g. (DP, AEB.)

Carbohydrates, Unavailable. The term includes pentosans, pectins, hemicellulose, cellulose, lignin and gums which are not digested and therefore unavailable to monogastric animals, but some are available to ruminants.

Carbon Dioxide, Available. *See* Baking powder *and* Flour, self-raising.

Carbon Dioxide Storage. *See* Gas storage.

Carbonic Anhydrase. Enzyme that converts carbon dioxide and water into carbonic acid. This is normally a slow process and its acceleration by the enzyme is an essential part of respiration (transfer of carbon dioxide from the tissues to the lungs). Present in red blood cells, plays part in gastric secretion of hydrochloric acid; contains zinc. (WHSS.)

45

Carboxymethylcellulose. Prepared from the pure cellulose of cotton or wood. Absorbs up to 50 times its weight of water to form a stable colloidal mass and used (in combination with stabilisers) as a whipping agent, in ice-cream, confectionery, jellies, etc., and as an inert food filler in slimming aids.

Methyl cellulose is another cellulose derivative but differs from the above (and other gums) since its viscosity increases with rise in temperature instead of decreasing, hence it is soluble in cold water and gels on heating. Used as thickener, emulsifier, in foods low in gluten, etc.

Other cellulose derivatives with similar properties are ethyl methyl cellulose, and hydroxyethyl-cellulose.

Carboxypeptidase. Enzyme of the pancreatic juice which splits polypeptides to dipeptides. Removes the terminal unit of the chain in which the carboxyl radical is free, hence it is an exopeptidase. (WHSS.)

Cardamom. Dried, nearly ripe, fruit, and the seed of *Elettaria cardamomum* (ginger family). The volatile oil contains cineol and terpineol. Used as flavouring in sausages, bakery goods and in curry powder and used in whole, mixed pickling spice. (Merory.)

Carenol. Name once suggested for vitamin A but not accepted.

Carmine-Fibrin. Chopped blood fibrin that has been soaked in ammoniacal carmine solution. It is used as a test for proteolytic activity, since, when digestion takes place, the liberation of the carmine into the solution acts as an indicator. (Hawk.)

Carmoisine. Red colour permitted in food in U.K. and many other countries, also called Azorubin; disodium salt of 2-(4-sulpho-1-naphthylazo) - 1 - naphthol-4-sulphonic acid.

Carnitine. Plays a role in transferring the acetyl group from inside the mitochondrion to the outside where fat synthesis takes place.

Occurs in animal muscle and is particularly rich in meat extract but is not a dietary essential for man and the higher animals. The only organisms that have been shown to require carnitine as a dietary essential are the mealworm and a few related species; it was originally called vitamin B_T.

Carnosine. Beta-alanyl histidine; dipeptide found in muscle of most animals; function unknown.

Carob Seed. Seeds and pod of *Ceratonia siliqua*, also known as **locust bean** and **St. John's bread**. Contains a sweet pulp rich in sugar and gums used for fodder and for the preparation of carob-seed gum used for emulsifiers, cosmetics and textile sizes.

Carophyll. Trade name (Hoffman La Roche) for apo-8-carotenal, *see* Carotenal.

Carotenal. Or apo-8-carotenal; a modified form of beta-carotene found in the intestine and is possibly the first intermediate in the conversion of carotene to retinol. Also found in nettles, spinach and citrus fruits. When fed to laying chickens it is deposited in the egg yolk and so it is added to chick diets to produce deeply coloured yolks. (AEB.)

46

Carotene. Red pigment in plants, obvious in carrots, red palm oil and yellow maize, masked by chlorophyll in leaves.

It is converted into retinol in the body. About one-third of the vitamin A of western diets is supplied as carotene. Present to only a limited extent in animal tissues, for example there is some caretone as well as retinol in milk.

Occurs in three forms, alpha, beta and gamma carotenes, and lends name to a range of pigments of similar structure—the, carotenoids—only a few of which are vitamin A-active.

Before the preparation of pure retinol, beta-carotene was used as the vitamin A standard—$0 \cdot 6$ microgram of beta-carotene = 1 i.u. of vitamin A. Alpha and gamma carotenes have only half the vitamin A potency of beta-carotene.

Since carotene is poorly absorbed from foods (about 33%) and the efficiency of conversion to vitamin A in the body is one-half of the available β-carotene, the utilisation efficiency is taken as one-sixth. Thus 1 microgram of β-carotene in the diet is equivalent to $0 \cdot 167$ microgram retinol.

Used as a colouring material in foods and as a source of vitamin A in vegetarian and kosher margarines. (DP, AEB.)

Carotenoids. A group of yellow to red pigments occurring widely in plants and animals and structurally related to carotene. Some are converted into retinol in the body, the carotenes, cryptoxanthin, echinenone, torularhodin, and apocarotenal, others are not—canthaxanthin, lycopene, zeaxanthin, bixin.

Carotenols. Carotenoid pigments carrying the hydroxyl group. The term xanthophylls is often used collectively for these hydroxylated carotenoids, apart from the substance xanthophyll itself.

Carotin. Obsolete spelling of carotene.

Caroto-albumin. Carotene-protein complex in the blood serum, presumed to be the mode of transport of carotene in the body. (Sebrell.)

Carrot. Root of *Daucus carota*. An outstanding source of vitamin A, present as its precursor, carotene. Not all the carotene is absorbed, the amount depends on the fineness of mincing of the vegetable.

Protein $1 \cdot 0\%$, fat $0 \cdot 2\%$; Ca 31 mg, Fe $0 \cdot 7$ mg, 37 kcal ($0 \cdot 16$ MJ), vitamin A 500 μg, B_1 $0 \cdot 06$ mg, B_2 $0 \cdot 04$ mg, nicotinic acid $0 \cdot 6$ mg, vitamin C 6 mg— per 100 g. (FAO.)

Carr-Price Reaction. A test for vitamin A which gives a blue colour with a solution of antimony trichloride in chloroform (the Carr-Price reagent). (Hawk.)

Carter's Spread. Name given to a mixture of butter (68%) with hydrogenated oil ($12 \cdot 4\%$) plus salt, preservative and lecithin, used as a breadspread. (Loes.)

Cartilage. Consists mainly of collagen, chondromucoid (protein plus chondroitin sulphuric acid) and chondroalbumoid (a protein similar to elastin). New bone growth consists of cartilage on which calcium salts are deposited at a later stage to form the bone. (Hawk.)

47

Cartose. Trade name (Winthrop Laboratories, USA) for a steam hydrolysate of maize starch used as a carbohydrate modifier in milk preparations for infant feeding. Consists of a mixture of dextrin, maltose and glucose.

Casein. The main protein of milk, about 3%; lactalbumin and lactoglobulin comprise about 1% of milk. Casein is precipitated under acid conditions, when the other two are not, thus cheese contains the casein, and the lactalbumin and lactoglobulin are left in the whey.

Casein is one of the most easily prepared proteins and is therefore used as a dietary supplement. Its biological value is 70.

Casein may be precipitated by acid or by rennet. Acid casein contains 2% ash, 0·1% calcium, and is used as a binder for chinese clay in coating paper, for glue and in casein-bound water paints as well as for food. Rennet casein contains 8% ash, 3·5% calcium and is used in plastics.

Casein, Hammarsten's. *See* Hammarsten's casein.

Casein, Iodinated. When iodine is introduced into the casein molecule it has thyroactive properties similar to those of the thyroid hormone, but without some of the hypermetabolic effects of, for example, thyroxine.

Caseinogen. According to the older nomenclature, caseinogen is the form present in milk, and when precipitated with rennin it becomes casein. In the American nomenclature the two forms are casein and paracasein, which is now the accepted usage.

Casilan. Trade name (Glaxo Laboratories) for a casein preparation—protein 90%, fat 1·8%, mineral salts 3·8%, calcium 340 mg per oz.

Cassareep. The juice of the bitter cassava or manioc. It is boiled to a thick syrup and used as a base for sauces.

Cassava. Or **Manioc.** Tuber of the plant *Manihot utilissima*. Staple article of diet in many tropical countries although an extremely poor source of protein.

One of the most productive crops, yielding (e.g. in Nigeria) 13 million kcal per acre compared with yam, 9 million, sorghum, 1 million and maize 1 million.

Composition, protein 0·9%, fat 0·2%; Ca 25 mg, Fe 0·5 mg, kcal 109 (0·46 MJ), vitamins B_1 0·04 mg, B_2 0·02 mg, nicotinic acid 0·4 mg, vitamin C 27 mg—per 100 g. (FAO.)

The juice from the roots is **Cassareep,** used in sauces and fermented with molasses. The leaves are eaten as a vegetable. The tuber is a source of **Tapioca,** *which see*. (TND.)

Cassia. Inner bark of a tree grown in the Far East—used as a seasoning; similar in appearance and flavour to cinnamon.

Cassina. Beverage (tea substitute) made from cured leaves of a holly bush, *Ilex cassine*; contains 1–1·6% caffeine and 8% tannin. (Jacobs.)

Castor Oil. From the castor oil bean, *Ricinus*. The oil itself is non-irritating, but in the small intestine is hydrolysed by lipase to liberate ricinoleic acid which is an irritant to the gastro-intestinal mucosa and therefore acts as a purgative. (Clark.)

48

Catabolism. *See* Metabolism.

Catalase. Enzyme in plants and animals that splits hydrogen peroxide into water and gaseous oxygen. It is a conjugated protein containing haem (identical with the haem of haemoglobin) as its prosthetic group. (WHSS.)

Catalyst. Substance that alters the rate of a chemical reaction; mostly of use when it accelerates the reaction. Metallic platinum is a catalyst in the manufacture of sulphuric acid, metallic nickel is a catalyst for the hardening of oils with hydrogen.

Enzymes are defined as organic catalysts produced by living cells.

Catchup. Alternative spelling of catsup or ketchup, *see* Tomato Ketchup.

Cathepsins. Group of intracellular proteolytic enzymes in animal tissues. Probably function in the normal breakdown and resynthesis of tissue proteins. Are responsible for the autolytic softening of the flesh when game is "hung".

There are four enzymes in the group, cathepsins I, II, III and IV, respectively similar to pepsin, trypsin, aminopeptidase and carboxypeptidase. (WHSS.)

Cation. *See* Ionization.

Catsup. *See* Tomato Ketchup.

Cauliflower. White edible flower of *Brassica oleracea botrytis*. Protein 1·3%, fat 0·1%; Ca 12 mg, Fe 0·6 mg, kcal 13 (0·05 MJ), vitamin A 15 μg, B_1 0·06 mg, B_2 0·05 mg, nicotinic acid 0·03 mg, vitamin C 37 mg—per 100 g. (FAO.)

Caviar(e). Salted hard roe of the sturgeon. 30% protein, 20% fat, nil carbohydrate, 340 kcal (1·42 MJ)—per 100 g. (Hutch.)

Celacol. Trade name (British Celanese Ltd.) for derivatives of cellulose, methyl, hydroxyethyl, etc.

Celery. (*Apium graveolens*). Protein 0·7%, fat 0·1%; Ca 31 mg, Fe 0·3 mg, kcal 12 (0·05 MJ), vitamin A nil, B_1 0·03 mg, B_2 0·02 mg, nicotinic acid 0·2 mg, vitamin C 4 mg—per 100 g. (FAO.)

Cellobiose. Two molecules of glucose joined together in the 1·4′-beta position (as distinct from the 1·4′-alpha bond in maltose). Cellobiose is the basic structural unit of cellulose and does not exist in the free state in nature. (WHSS.)

Cellofas. Trade name (Imperial Chemical Industries Ltd.) for derivatives of cellulose, e.g. cellofas A, methyl ethyl, cellofas B, sodium carboxymethyl.

Celluflour. Powdered cellulose; used in experimental diets to provide indigestible bulk.

Cellulase. Enzyme that attacks cellulose; present in the digestive juices of various snails, wood-boring insects, and micro-organisms. The cellulase present in the intestinal micro-organisms of ruminants is responsible for the ability of these animals to obtain energy from straw, for their own digestives juices do not contain cellulase. (WHSS.)

Cellulose. Polysaccharide that forms the supporting cell structure in plants, does not occur in animals. Consists of long chain of glucose units.

49

Is not digested in man or other monogastric animals, but serves a useful purpose in providing bulk for intestinal functioning. It is digested by the bacteria in the rumen of ruminating animals, which can therefore subsist on grass and hay.

Paper and wood are essentially cellulose. Commercial sources are cotton and wood pulp. (BDS.)

Cellulose Derivatives. *See* Carboxymethylcellulose.

Centrifuge. Machine that exerts a pull many times stronger than gravity by spinning. Used to clarify liquids by settling the heavier solid in a few minutes, a process that might take several days under gravity. Also used to separate two liquids of different densities, e.g. cream from milk.

Cephalins. Alternative spelling to kephalins, *which see*.

Ceplapro. Protein-rich baby food (18–20% protein) made in granular form from degerminated maize flour, wheat, defatted soya flour and skim milk powder with added calcium and vitamins. Made in United States.

Cereal Coffee. Prepared from roasted cereal grains.

Cereals. Any grain or edible fruit of the grass family that may be used as food. Include wheat, rice, oats, rye, barley, maize and millet.

Provide the largest single type of foodstuffs. In the Far East cereal often constitutes 90% of the diet; even in Gt. Britain bread and flour provide one-third of the calories and at the same time one-third of the protein of the average diet.

Cerebrosides. Part of the structural matter of brain and the myelin sheath of nerves. Contain phrenosin, kerasin, fatty acid, sphingosine and galactose. This is the only structure of the body that contains the sugar galactose. (BDS.)

Cerelose. Commercial glucose with about 9% water. (Loes.)

Cervelat. *See* Sausage.

Cetavlon. Trade name for detergent and bacteriostat, cetyltrimethylammonium bromide.

Cetyl Alcohol. A solid, waxy, straight chain alcohol of sixteen carbon atoms, found in spermaceti (from the sperm whale) and waxes. Can be spread as a thin (monomolecular) film on the surface of water in reservoirs where it reduces evaporation of the water. (Cohen.)

CF. *See* Citrovorum factor.

Challah. *See* Cholla.

Chalva. *See* Halva.

Chamomile. Can be two herbs, *Anthemis nobilis* and *Matricaria recutica*. Essential oil used for flavouring liqueurs; chamomile tea made by infusing dried flower heads, used as old-fashioned tonic; whole herb used to make herb beers. (OF.)

Chapati. Flat, pancake-like baked product made from wheat flour, commonly eaten in India and Pakistan.

The standard chapati is made from 95% extraction wheat flour and water only; other types are leavened or may be made with white flour (Nan) or have added fats, milk, sugar, baking powder.

Chappati. *See* Chapati.

Charcoal. *See* Bone charcoal.

50

Charqui. Dried meat of Brazil, chiefly from beef but also from sheep, llama and alpaca in Peru. Strips of meat cut lengthways and pressed after salting then air dried; finished form is in flat, thin sheets, rather flaky, so differing from the long strips of biltong.

Chartreuse. Liqueur made by monks of Chartreux, using, it is said, more than 200 ingredients. There are 3 varieties:—green, 96% of proof spirit, yellow 74·5% and white 52·5%.

Chastek Paralysis. Acute dietary disease of foxes caused by the inclusion of 10% of raw fish in the diet. It is due to a deficiency of vitamin B_1 caused by the presence of the enzyme, thiaminase, in the fish that destroys the vitamin. It is cured by adding vitamin B_1 to the diet. (Hawk.)

Cheddaring. In the manufacture of cheese, after coagulation of the milk, heating of the curd and draining, the curds are piled along the floor of the vat when, in the case of Cheddar cheese, they consolidate to a rubbery sheet of curd. This stage is the Cheddaring process. (In the case of Cheshire cheese it is not allowed to settle so densely and has a more crumbly texture.) (Davis.)

Cheese. Prepared from the curd precipitated from milk by rennin or lactic acid. Cheeses other than cottage or cream are cured by being left to mature with salt, under various conditions that produce the characteristic flavour of the particular type of cheese.
Analysis (hard cheese) Protein 25%, fat 31%; kcal 387 (1·62 MJ), Ca 700 mg, Fe 1 mg, vitamin A 420 μg, B_1 0·01 mg, B_2 0·45 mg, nicotinic acid 0·1 mg—per 100 g.

Most of the lactose of the milk is lost with the whey.
Legally must contain not less than 40% fat on a dry weight basis and the fat must be milk fat. (Davis, FAO.)

Cheese, Blue. Cheese that contains an internal growth of the mould, *Penicillium roqueforti*; e.g. Blue Vinney, Stilton and Roquefort. (Tanner.)

Cheese, Cottage, Pot, Dutch or **Schmierkase.** A soft, uncured white cheese made from pasteurised skim milk (or milk powder) by lactic acid starter (with or without added rennet) heated, washed and drained (salt may be added). Contains more than 80% water.
Farm cheese is as above but the curd is pressed.
Baker's cheese or **hoop cheese** is as cottage cheese but not washed and is drained in bags so giving a finer grain and contains more water and acid than cottage cheese.

Cheese, Processed. Natural cheese passes its peak of flavour rapidly and processing temporarily arrests the deterioration. Processed cheese is loaf cheese, melted, pasteurized, flavourings added (pimento, caraway, etc.), plus emulsifiers, and repacked.
Nutritive value identical with original cheese.

Cheese, Whey. Made from whey by heat-coagulation of the proteins (lactalbumin and lactoglobulin).

Cheilosis. *See* Ariboflavinosis.

Chemical Caponization. *See* Capon.

Chemical Ice. Ice containing chemicals used as preservative, e.g. a solution of antibiotics or other chemicals frozen and used to preserve fish.

Chemical Score. A chemical method of defining the nutritional value of proteins, proposed by Block and Mitchell (1946). The limiting amino acid in the protein under consideration is expressed as the percentage of the same amino acid present in egg (taken as the standard). Chemical score numerically equals biological value.

A later modification is Protein Score, in which a standard amino acid reference mixture is used instead of egg protein. (AEB.)

Chemotherapy. Treatment of disease by chemicals that have toxic effect on the micro-organisms.

Cherry. Fruit of *Prunus* species. Protein 1·0%, fat 0·4%; kcal 54 (0·23 MJ), Fe 0·4 mg, vitamin A 170 μg, B₁ 0·05 mg, B₂ 0·05 mg, nicotinic acid 0·4 mg, vitamin C 7 mg—per 100 g. (FAO.)

Cherry, West Indian. Fruit of a small bushy tree native to tropical and semi-tropical regions of America — *Malpighia punicifolia*. The richest known source of vitamin C; the edible portion of the fruit contains 1000 mg of vitamin C per 100 g when ripe, and the green fruit 3000 mg.

Also known as **Barbados cherry** and **Acerola** (Spanish), and Antilles cherry. (FAO.)

Chervil. A herb, *Anthriscus cerefolium*, used in the fresh green state for flavouring salads and soups, and as a garnish.

Chest Sweetbread. *See* Pancreas.

Chestnut, Water. *Trapa natans*, also known as **Caltrops** and

Singharanut. Seed is eaten raw or roasted.

Composition per 100 g: 3 g protein, 15 g carbohydrate, 75 kcal (0·32 MJ), 0·8 mg iron, 0·05 mg B₁, 0·6 mg nicotinic acid, 16 mg C.

Chinese water chestnut is the tuber of the sedge *Eleocharis tuberosa*, imported in cans from Hong Kong. (OF, Platt.)

Chewing Gum. *See* Gum, chewing.

Chick Anti-pellagra Factor. Obsolete name for pantothenic acid.

Chicken. Protein 12·3%, fat 7·7%; Ca 7 mg, Fe 0·9 mg, kcal 122 (0·5 MJ), vitamin A 75 μg, B₁ 0·06 mg, B₂ 0·1 mg, nicotinic acid 4·9 mg—per 100 g. (FAO.)

Chicle. Basis of chewing gums, the partially evaporated latex of the evergreen sapodilla tree (*Achras sapota*); contains gutta (with elastic properties, consists of polymers of isoprene) and resins (triterpenes and sterols) together with carbohydrates, waxes and tannins.

The same tree produces the sapodilla plum.

Chicory. *Cichorium intybus*. The leaves are eaten as a salad and the root, dried and partly caramelised is often added to coffee as a diluent to cheapen the product.

The leaves are grown in the dark to prevent the development of the bitter flavour and so are very pale in colour. Also called succory and (in Belgium) witloof. The French call chicory "Endive Belge" and endive is called "Chicorée": in U.S. chicory is called endive.

Analysis of leaf and stem, water 96%, protein 0·8%, fat trace, carbohydrate 1·5% (some of which is inulin); Fe 0·7 mg per 100 g.

Chili Sauce. Sauce made from tomatoes with spices, onions, garlic, sugar, vinegar and salt—similar to tomato catsup but containing more cayenne, onions and garlic.

Chilli. *See* Pepper.

Chillproofing. A term used in reference to beer; treatment to prevent the appearance of haze when the beer is chilled. Chillproofs include tannic acid to precipitate the proteins, materials such as bentonite to adsorb them, and proteolytic enzymes to hydrolyse them. (Matz.)

Chimche. Basic Korean dish (in addition to fish and rice) consisting of fermented cabbage with garlic, red peppers and pimientos. Vitamin C content 126 mg per 100 g—led to the suggestion that the Koreans have the highest intake of vitamin C.

Chinese Eggs. Known as Pidan, Houeidan and Dsaoudan according to variations in the method of preparation. Prepared by covering fresh duck eggs with a mixture of caustic soda, burnt straw ash, salt and slaked lime, and storing for several months. The white and yolk coagulate and become discoloured with partial decomposition of the protein and phospholipids. (Tanner.)

Chinese Restaurant Disease Syndrome. Headache, sweating, nausea, weakness, thirst, flushing of face, abdominal pain, lachrimation—occurs occasionally when Chinese food rich in mono-sodium glutamate is eaten. Mild symptoms can result from 25 mg/kg body weight taken on an empty stomach; results follow 25–35 min. after ingestion and pass off after a few hours.

Chitin. The organic base of the hard parts of insects and crustacea and present also in small amounts in mushrooms. Similar in composition to cellulose but contains glucosamine instead of glucose; insoluble and indigestible. (DP.)

Chitterlings. Intestine of ox, calf or pig.

Chive. *Allium schoenoprasum*, a plant grown for its bulbs and its long thin leaves, both with a mild onion flavour used in salads, soups and omelettes.

Chlorella. *See* Algae.

Chlorine. An element that is found in biological tissues as the chloride ion. The body contains about 100 g of chloride and the average diet contains 6–7 g, mainly as sodium chloride.

Free chlorine is used as a sterilising agent e.g. in drinking water.

Chlorine Dioxide. A bread "improver", *see* Aging.

Chlorocruorin. The copper-containing protein that carries oxygen in the bloodstream of the Annelid worms—analogous to haemoglobin in mammals.

Chlorophyll. Green colouring matter of all plant materials, by the aid of which plants manufacture foodstuffs from simple salts and carbon dioxide with energy derived from sunlight, i.e. photosynthesis. This is the true distinction between plants and animals, the latter must be supplied with complex foods ready made. Bacteria are on the border-line between the plant and animal kingdoms. Chlorophyll is a mixture of chlorophyll alpha and beta, and two other pigments, xanthophyll and carotene.

Chlorophyllase. Enzyme present in all green plants, which hydrolyses chlorophyll to phytol and chlorophyllide. Reversible in action and can catalyse the synthesis of chlorophyll.

Chlorophyllide. The green colour found in the water after cooking certain vegetables. The fat-soluble chlorophyll is converted to water-soluble chlorophyllide by removal of the phytyl side-chain by alkali or enzyme. (Griswold.)

Chlortetracycline. *See* Tetracyclines.

Chocolate. Chocolate nibs (*see* Cocoa), refined and mixed with sugar, cocoa butter, lecithin, and, if milk chocolate, milk solids.

Analysis (plain unsweetened): protein 5%, fat 50%; kcal 517 (2·2 MJ), Ca 98 mg, Fe 4·4 mg, vitamin A 20 μg, B_1 0·07 mg, B_2 0·24 mg, nicotinic acid 1·1 mg —per 100 g. (FAPO.)

Cholagogue. A substance that promotes the flow of bile from the gall bladder into the duodenum. (Clark.)

Cholecalciferol. *See* Vitamin D.

Cholecystokinin. A hormone secreted by the mucosa of the duodenum and jejunum and carried in the blood to the gallbladder which is thus stimulated to contract and secrete bile. (BDS.)

Cholelithiasis. Gallstones, *which see.*

Choleretics. Substances that stimulate the secretion of bile; e.g. bile salts themselves taken by mouth, or cholic acid by intravenous injection. (BDS.)

Cholesterol. *See* Sterols.

Choline. Essential dietary factor, trimethyl hydroxyethylammonium hydroxide, usually classed as a vitamin, although the quantities involved are far from catalytic. Functions as a source of methyl groups and in fat transport; deficiency gives rise to fatty infiltration of the liver; is part of the structure of the phospholipids of animal and plant tissues. Specific dietary deficiency does not occur; daily requirements not established but the daily intake is 0·25–0·5 g. *See also* Acetylcholine. (Sebrell.)

Choline Esterase. An enzyme that hydrolyses acetyl choline (which is liberated by the nerve ending to stimulate muscle) so that the muscle can recover and become prepared for the next stimulus.

A number of substances, anticholinesterases, that inhibit the enzyme paralyse muscle. Examples are war gases of the nerve group, certain insecticides and eserine, which is used clinically in cases of excess choline esterase (the disease myasthenia gravis). (BDS.)

Cholla. Loaf of white bread made in twist form (or Biblical beehive coil) from one large and one small piece of dough plaited together.

The dough is made from white flour, enriched with eggs and a pinch of saffron, and the loaf is decorated with maw or poppy seed.

Mentioned in the Bible and translated as loaves; used for

benediction on the Jewish Sabbath and Festivals.

Chondroitin. A polysaccharide containing galactosamine and glucuronic acid. The sulphuric acid ester, chondroitin sulphate, is found in cartilage and the organic matrix of bone. Classed as a mucopolysaccharide. (DP.)

Chondrus Crispus. *See* Carageenan.

Chorleywood Bread Process. A method of preparing dough for bread-making in which the dough is submitted to intense mechanical working (5 watt-hours or $0 \cdot 4$ H.P. min per lb) so that, together with the aid of oxidising agents, the need for bulk fermentation of the dough is eliminated. This is a "no-time" dough process and saves $1\frac{1}{2}$–2 hours.

Named after the British Baking Industries Research Association at Chorleywood. The process permits the use of an increased proportion (20–25% replacement) of weaker flour, and produces a softer, finer bread which stales more slowly.

Choux Pastry. A light, airy pastry as used in éclairs and cream buns. The batter is pre-cooked in the saucepan, then baked.

The name choux is the French for cabbage—the characteristic shape for cream puffs.

Chowder. An American term for a seafood soup; often made with clams or shrimps.

Chromatography. A method of separating substances by their different degrees of absorption or partition on a stationary phase. The most easily observed procedure is when a mixture of plant pigments is passed down a column of chalk and the various pigments can be seen to separate (column chromatography).

Paper chromatography is the application of the process on strips of filter paper, when extremely small quantities can be examined.

Ion-exchange resin chromatography is used to separate substances like amino acids by virtue of their acidic and basic groups.

Gas-liquid chromatography is the latest development in which the substance is volatilized along a column of a liquid held on an inert solid.

Chromoproteins. Proteins conjugated with a metal-containing prosthetic group, e.g. vertebrate haemoglobins contain iron, invertebrate haemocyanins contain copper, chlorophyll contains magnesium. (Hawk.)

Chyle. Lymph rich in fat. *See* Lymph.

Chylomicrons. Droplets of unhydrolysed fat in the lymph or bloodstream. *See* Lymph.

Chymase. Alternative name for rennin.

Chyme. Partly digested mass of food as it exists in the stomach. (BDS.)

Chymosin. Obsolete name for rennin, also chymase.

Chymotrypsin. Proteolytic enzyme of the pancreatic juice; attacks parts of the protein molecule different from those attacked by pepsin and by trypsin. Secreted as the inactive precursor, chymotrypsinogen, activated by trypsin. (WHSS.)

Cibophobia. Dislike of food.

Cider, Cyder. An alcoholic beverage made by fermenting apple juice; contains 5–6% alcohol (by volume) and $0 \cdot 7$–$2 \cdot 0$% sugar.

In the United States cider or fresh cider are names given to fresh (unfermented) apple juice, and the fermented material is called hard or fermented cider.

Cieddu. *See* Milks, fermented.

Ciguatera. Poisoning from eating fish feeding in the region of coral reefs in the Caribbean Sea and the Indian and Pacific Oceans. The species of fish are normally edible and appear to derive the toxins, ciguatoxins, from their diet. Reported in seafarer's tales in 16th century.

Cinnamon. The bark, of various species of the genus *Cinnamomum*; it is split off the shoots, cured and dried. During drying the bark shrinks and curls into a cylinder or "quill".

Ceylon or true cinnamon differs from other types (*Cinnamomum zeylanicum*) and the oil contains mostly cinnamic aldehyde, together with some eugenol. Saigon cinnamon contains also cineol; Chinese cinnamon has no eugenol. Used as flavour in meat products, bakery goods and confectionery. (Jacobs, Merory.)

Cissa. Unnatural desire for foods, alternative words cittosis, allotriophagy and pica.

Cis-trans Isomerism. Compounds with same molecular and structural formulae but which can exist in two geometric forms exhibit cis-trans isomerism. When the chemical groups in the molecule are paired on the same side the form is cis, on opposite sides it is trans. They have different chemical and physical properties. (Cohen.)

Citral. Important constituent of many essential oils, especially lemon. Occurs in beta and alpha form (*cis*- and *trans*-isomers); $C_{10}H_{16}O$.

Used as the starting material for the synthesis of ionone (the synthetic perfume with the odour of violets), a stage in the synthesis of retinol. (Brav.)

Citrated Blood. *See* Blood, citrated.

Citric Acid. A tribasic acid, $C_6H_8O_7$. Occurs widely in nature in fruits, especially citrus fruits. Is a normal metabolite in the body, therefore when consumed is completely metabolised.

Widely used as flavouring in beverages and confectionery. Commercially produced by moulds or extracted from lemons. (Cohen.)

Citric Acid Cycle. The oxidation stage in the metabolism of foodstuffs. Carbohydrates and fats are broken down to acetate (active acetate or acetyl coenzyme A) and the first step in the cycle is the combination of the acetyl with oxaloacetate to form citrate. This passes through a series of reactions in which energy is released and carbon dioxide and water produced; the end-product is oxaloacetate.

Since many of the amino acids can be converted into substances that lie on this pathway, the citric acid cycle is the common metabolic pathway for all three major foodstuffs. Also known as the **Krebs' cycle.** (WHSS.)

Citrin. A mixture of two flavanones found in citrus pith, namely hesperidin and eriodictin (demethylated hesperidin). *See also* Vitamin P. (Brav.)

Citron. First of the citrus fruits to become known to Europeans; *Citrus medica.* Very sensitive to cold and can be grown only in warm regions. Very thick peel, solid, sweet and acid-free pulp with practically no juice; used for preparing candied peel. (Brav.)

Citronin. Flavanone glycoside from the peel of immature Ponderosa lemons—methoxy dihydroxy rhamnoglucoside.

Citrovorum Factor. Name given to a growth factor for the organism *Leuconostoc citrovorum.* Now known to be tetrahydro formyl pteroyl glutamic acid, which is believed to be the active form of the vitamin, folic acid.

Citroxanthin. Also known as mutachrome. Yellow carotenoid pigment in orange peel; has vitamin A activity.

Citroze. Trade name (J. Lyons Ltd.) for a lemon flavoured glucose drink.

Citrulline. Amino acid formed as an intermediate in the metabolism of urea in the body. Not of nutritional importance since it is not found in food proteins.

Citrus. Genus including *C. limonum* (lemon), *C. aurantifolia* (lime), *C. aurantium* (sour orange), *C. sinensis* (sweet orange), *C. medica* (citron), *C. nobolis* (tangerine), *C. maxima* (grapefruit), *C. bergamia* (bergamot), and *C. grandis* (pomelo). (Brav.)

Clarification. The process of clearing a liquid of suspended particles; may be carried out by filtration, centrifugation, addition of particular enzymes (proteolytic or pectolytic), or the addition of flocculating agents. (*See* Isinglass.)

Clarifixation. A method of homogenising milk in which the cream is separated, homogenised and re-mixed with the milk in one machine—the clarifixator.

Clarke Degrees. *See* Water hardness.

Clostridia. Genus of bacteria of family *Bacillaceae;* sporeformers. *Clostridium botulinum* is the most heat-resistant of the food-poisoning organisms; its destruction is generally accepted as the minimum standard of processing for low-acid and medium-acid canned foods, although other clostridia are more heat-resistant. (Baum.)

Clotting of Blood. *See* Coagulation, blood.

Cloudberry. *Rumus chamaemorus.* Golden-fruited berry growing in northern latitudes; used in similar fashion to blackberries. Extremely rich in natural benzoic acid and the soft fruit will keep for long periods. (OF.)

Clove. Dried flower buds of *Caryophyllus aromaticus;* mother of clove is the ripened fruit, inferior in flavour. Contains 10% fixed oil and a volatile oil mostly eugenol, with small amounts of caryophyllene, vanillin and other substances. Used as flavour in meat products and bakery goods. (Jacobs, Merory.)

CMC. Carboxymethylcellulose.

CoA. Abbreviation for Coenzyme A, *which see.*

Coacervation. Heat-reversible aggregation of amylopectin—suggested as one explanation of the staling of bread. (KJ.)

Coagulase. Name given to an enzyme said to be present in milk and to account for the ability of

57

milk to clot a solution of fibrinogen. (Davis & Mac.)

Coagulation. A process whereby proteins become insoluble; effected by heat, strong acids and alkalies, metals and various other chemicals.

Denaturation is the rupture of hydrogen bonds within and between the peptide chains of the protein. If the process reaches an advanced state it becomes irreversible, there is extreme unfolding and agglomeration of the side chains, and the aggregates of protein reach such a size that they precipitate, i.e. coagulate.

Coagulation occurs when, for example, an egg is cooked or a flour dough is baked.

Coagulation, Blood. The final stage is the precipitation of fibrils of insoluble fibrin from the soluble plasma protein, fibrinogen. The mechanism is as follows: prothrombin in the plasma is converted by thromboplastin (released from blood platelets and damaged tissue) to thrombin, in the presence of calcium. The thrombin then reacts with the fibrinogen to form the fibrin clot.

Hence the addition of oxalate or citrate, which combine with the calcium, will prevent clotting as effectively as heparin, hirudin and coumarin, which interfere with the prothrombin. (BDS.)

Cobalamin. Vitamin B_{12}.

Cobalt. A mineral that is believed to be a dietary essential in trace amounts although a simple cobalt deficiency has never been observed in man. It is part of the molecule of vitamin B_{12} but no other function is known.

Cobalt is not essential to plants but "pining disease" in cattle is due to cobalt deficiency. It is a growth factor for chicks, turkeys, pigs and rats, although large doses are toxic. (Hawk, Gil.)

Coca Leaves. From the S. American plant, *Erythroxylon coca*; contain cocaine, and chewed by the natives of Peru as a stimulant. (Clark.)

Cocarboxylase. Coenzyme that assists the enzyme carboxylase to remove carbon dioxide from various compounds, i.e. decarboxylation.

Cocarboxylase is the diphosphate of vitamin B_1, alternatively known as thiamin pyrophosphate or **diphosphothiamin.** In deficiency of vitamin B_1 the body is unable to oxidize pyruvic acid, an intermediate stage in carbohydrate metabolism, which therefore accumulates in the blood. (BDS.)

Cochineal. Red colour obtained from the female Conchilla, *Coccus cacti*, found in Mexico, Central America and the West Indies; 70,000 insects produce 1 lb of colour. Legally permitted in food in most countries. Slightly soluble in water and alcohol but not ether. (Jacobs.)

Cock-a-leekie. Scottish soup made from leeks and chicken.

Cocoa. Prepared from the cocoa bean—*Theobroma cacao*. The bean is left to ferment before roasting; it is then cracked and the shell removed. The remainder constitutes the nib, which, when ground, is cocoa: 54% fat, 11% protein, 9% carbohydrate, 2% water, together with alkaloids, fibre, tannins, organic acids. (Merory.)

Cocoa, Dutch. Cocoa treated with dilute solution of alkali (carbonate or bicarbonate) to improve colour,

58

flavour and solubility. The process is known as "Dutching".

Cocolait. A form of coconut "milk" made by pressing coconut under high pressure and homogenising the oil and water emulsion plus coconut water (coconut milk) obtained. Bottled and used (e.g. in Philippines) in place of cow's milk.

Coconut. Tropical palm, *Cocos nucifera*. The dried nut is copra, which contains 60–65% coconut oil. The residue after oil extraction is used for animal feed.

The hollow unripe nut contains a watery liquid known as coconut milk—which is gradually absorbed as the nut ripens. Composition of milk from the ripe nut—1·4% solids, 0·2% protein, 3% carbohydrate (largely sucrose).

Composition of mature kernel per 100 g: 48–80 g solids, 4 g protein, 35 g fat, 11 g carbohydrate, 4 g fibre, 375 kcal (1·57 MJ), 2 mg iron, traces of vitamins B_1, B_2 and nicotinic acid. (OF, Platt.)

Cocoyam, New. W. African name for Tannia.

Cocoyam, Old. W. African name for Taro.

Coddle. To cook slowly in water kept just below the boiling point.

Code of Practice. In the context of foods this refers to agreements e.g. in Advertising and labelling Foods published by the U.K. Ministry of Food in 1945. It is here that, for example, it is suggested that claims for vitamin content should not be made unless one sixth of the daily requirement is contained in the amount ordinarily consumed in a day. (AEB.)

Codex Alimentarius. Originally Codex Alimentarius Europaeus; since 1961 part of the FAO/WHO Commission on Food Standards to simplify and integrate food standards for adoption internationally.

Codfish. The composition of all non-fatty fish, such as cod, hake, haddock, flatfish, is similar.

Cod fillet: protein 16·4%, fat 0·5%; kcal 75 (0·31 MJ), Ca 25 mg, Fe 0·7 mg, vitamin A nil, B_1 0·05 mg, B_2 0·08 mg, nicotinic acid 2·2 mg, vitamin C nil—per 100 g.

Cod, round: protein 7·4%, fat 0·2%; Calories 33, Ca 11 mg, Fe 0·3 mg, vitamin A nil, B_1 0·02 mg, B_2 0·04 mg, nicotinic acid 1·0 mg, vitamin C nil—per 100 g. (FAO.)

Cod Liver Oil. Oil from codfish liver; classical source of vitamins A and D, used for its medicinal properties long before the vitamins were discovered.

Average sample contains 120–1,200 μg vitamin A and 1–10 μg vitamin D per gram.

British Pharmacopoeia standard, minimum 180 μg vitamin A and 2 μg vitamin D per g. Ministry of Health "Welfare" cod liver oil, 270 μg vitamin A and 2·2 μg vitamin D per g.

Coeliac Disease (idiopathic steatorrhoea or non-tropical sprue). A disease of unknown origin, usually beginning in early childhood, due to an idiosyncracy to wheat gluten. Characterized by fatty stools, diarrhoea, loss of appetite and failure to grow. The lining of the intestine is severely damaged by the wheat gluten and removal of this from the diet leads to recovery. Hence the use of "gluten-free bread" and "gluten-

59

free biscuits". As well as wheat gluten the subject cannot tolerate rye protein but maize and rice gluten are thought to be harmless. (DP, AEB.)

Coenzyme A. Coenzyme for the transfer of acetyl groups; contains the vitamin, pantothenic acid. Functions by its ability to combine with acetyl, forming acetyl CoA, and to transfer this to another compound.

Important in the oxidation of glucose at the stage between pyruvic acid and the citric acid cycle, and in fat metabolism. (WHSS.)

Coenzyme Q. A group of substances that function in certain respiratory enzyme systems, found in the sub-cellular particles: identical with the ubiquinones.

Also known as Q 275 and mitoquinone.

Coenzyme R. Obsolete name for biotin.

Coenzyme I (and II). *See* Nicotinamide adenine dinucleotide (and nicotinamide adenine dinucleotide phosphate).

Coenzymes. Substances needed to assist certain enzymes. They are part of the enzyme system and differ from activators in that they play no part in the activation of the substrate.

Coenzymes react first with one enzyme then with another during the course of catalysis and so differ from prosthetic groups, which remain bound to the one enzyme during the course of the reaction.

Those enzymes that do require a coenzyme have an absolute specificity for that particular coenzyme, but the same coenzyme can partner a range of enzymes. Most coenzymes contain one of the B vitamins as part of the

molecule, thus Coenzyme I contains nicotinic acid, Coenzyme A contains pantothenic acid, cocarboxylase is vitamin B_1 pyrophosphate. (WHSS.)

Coffee. Berries of the evergreen plant *Coffea arabica*. The beans are roasted at 234–248°C to drive the aromatic oils to the surface. Three types differing in shape and size, Moka, Bourbon and Martinique.

Average composition after roasting: moisture 8%, protein 8·5%, fat 10·1%, carbohydrate 50%, fibre 18%, caffeine 1·3%, together with coffeol oil which supplies the flavour, caffeic acid, chlorogenic acid and trigonelline.

The hot water extract from 100 g of coffee contains 27 mg nicotinic acid, 1 mg Fe, 30 mg Ca, 8 g protein and 56 kcal. The average cup of coffee contains 18 mg caffeine per fl. oz.

Originated from Arabia, introduced into Turkey 16th century, Europe and U.S.A. 17th century. (Merory.)

Coffee, Decaffeinated. The drug caffeine is removed from the coffee by treating the aqueous extract of the coffee with boiling ethylene dichloride or methylene dichloride, and then drying.

Coffee Essence. Not less than 4 lb of roasted coffee must be used to prepare 1 gallon, and no other vegetable extractives are permitted. Must contain not less than 0·5% w/v caffeine derived from coffee.

Coffee and chicory extract must contain not less than 0·25% caffeine, and not less than 2 lb of coffee must be used to prepare 1 gallon. (Bell.)

Cognac. Brandy produced in a limited area of S. France from special varieties of grape grown on shallow soil and claimed to be distilled only in pot not continuous stills. (Cruess.)

Cola Drinks. Carbonated drinks containing extract of cola bean, the seed of the cola tree. The seed contains caffeine. The drinks contain 3–4·5 mg caffeine per fl. oz.

Colchicine. Alkaloid isolated from the meadow saffron, or Autumn crocus (*Colchicum*). Old remedy for gout. Inhibits cell division and used in experimental horticulture to produce plants with abnormal numbers of genes.

Cold Preservation. *See* Campden process.

Cold Sterilization. *See* Sterilization, cold, *and* Irradiation.

"Cold Store" Bacteria. *See* Psychrophilic bacteria.

Cole. *See* Rape.

Coleman Diet. High calorie, largely liquid diet introduced by Coleman for the treatment of typhoid fever.

Coley. *See* Saithe.

Coliform Bacteria. Group of aerobic, lactose-fermenters, of which *Escherichia coli* is the most important member.

Many coliforms are not harmful, but since they arise from faeces they are useful as a test of faecal contamination, particularly as a test for water pollution. (Tanner.)

Collagen. Insoluble protein in bone, tendons, skin and connective tissue of animals and fish, that is converted to soluble gelatin by moist heat. (*See* Connective Tissue *and* Albuminoids.) (Hawk.)

Collagen Sugar. Glycine.

Colloid. Fine particles (the disperse phase) suspended in a second medium (the dispersion medium); can be solid, liquid or gas suspended in solid, liquid or gas.

Examples of gas-in-liquid colloidal systems: beaten egg white, whipped cream; liquid-liquid colloids: emulsions such as milk, salad cream. *See also* Emulsifying agents *and* Stabilizers. (Jacobs.)

Colloids, Lyophilic. Or emulsoids. Colloids in which there is a high affinity between the particles of the disperse phase and the dispersion medium. Include proteins and higher carbohydrates, very viscous, electrically charged, require large amounts of electrolytes for precipitation which is reversible. (Hawk.)

Colloids, Lyophobic. Colloids in which there is no affinity between the particles of the disperse phase and the dispersion medium. The particles carry an electric charge and are flocculated irreversibly by electrolytes. Also called suspensoids. E.g. colloids of metals and inorganic salts. (Hawk.)

Colocasia. *See* Taro.

Colombo Plan. A co-operative effort to develop the resources and living standards of the peoples of South and South-east Asia, started at a meeting held in Colombo in 1950.

Colon. Last part of the intestine; consists of three parts, the ascending, the transverse, and the descending colon, and finishes at the rectum. (BDS.)

Colorimeter. *See* Absorptiometer, *and also* Lovibond comparator.

61

Colostrum. Secretion of the mammary gland shortly before parturition and during the early stages of lactation. Yellowish in colour, contains a higher concentration of solids than does the later milk, especially the globulin fraction. This contains the protective antibodies, hence the colostrum is of special importance to the young mammal.

In farming practice where animals are weaned as early as possible on to artificial mixtures, weaning takes place only after all the colostrum has been given to the young animal.

Colours. As used in foods colours fall into three groups; natural pigments derived mostly from plant materials, inorganic pigments and lakes (combination of organic colouring matters with metals), and synthetic coal-tar dyes. Most of those in the first two groups are legally permitted in most countries, but only specifically named coal-tar dyes are allowed.

Greece and Iceland do not permit any synthetic dyes in foods with specific exceptions; the list of permitted colours varies so much from one country to another that there is not a single dye that is permitted in every country. *See* under individual colours. (Bell.)

Comminuted. Finely divided. Commonly used with reference to orange drink made from crushed whole fruit, including the peel, and called comminuted orange drink. *See also* Soft drinks.

Comparator Block. Method of comparing colours (often used to estimate pH). *See also* Lovibond Comparator.

Comparator, Lovibond. *See* Lovibond comparator.

Complan. Trade name (Glaxo Laboratories) for a mixture of dried skim milk, arachis oil, casein, maltodextrins, sugar, salts and vitamins. Protein 31%, fat 16%, carbohydrate 44%; Ca 825 mg, Fe 8 mg per 100 g, and vitamins A, B_1, B_2, nicotinic acid, B_{12}, C, D, E, K, pantothenic acid and folic acid.

Complementation. This term is used with respect to proteins when a relative deficiency of one amino acid is compensated by a relative surplus of another consumed at the same time. The nutritive value, i.e. biological value or NPU, is then not the mean of the separate values but higher. E.g. maize with BV 35 is limited by the amino acid lysine, but has a relative surplus of methionine; pea flour with a BV 43 is limited by methionine, but has a relative surplus of lysine; the two complement one another so that a mixture of equal parts of the two proteins has BV 70. (AEB.)

Conalbumin. One of the proteins of egg-white comprising 12% of the total solids. Has the property of binding iron in an iron-protein complex that is pink. Accounts for the pinkish colour resulting when eggs are stored in rusty containers.

Condiment. A seasoning added to flavour foods, such as salt, mustard, ginger, curry, pepper, etc. Although some of these are relatively rich in nutrients they are generally used in such small quantities that they make a negligible contribution to the diet.

Conditioning of Meat. After killing, the muscle glycogen is broken down to lactic acid, and this acidity gradually improves the texture and keeping qualities of the meat. When all these changes have occurred the meat is "conditioned". *See also* Rigor mortis.

Confectioners' Glucose. *See* Glucose syrup.

Conge Machine. Used, in the manufacture of chocolate blend, for coating, to obtain smoothness by kneading the material.

Congies. The water from cooking rice which contains much of the thiamin and nicotinic acid from the rice; used as a drink. (DP.)

Conidendrin. A substance isolated from a number of coniferous woods whose derivatives, **nor-conidendrin** and alpha and beta conidendrol, are antioxidants. Chemically similar to the phenolic substance, nordihydroguaiaretic acid.

Connective Tissue. In fish, connective tissue is found between the muscle segments (myotomes) and consists of the protein collagen. In meat it is spread through the muscle, uniting the muscle fibres into bundles and supporting the blood vessels (a kind of soft skeleton), and consists of both collagen and elastin. A higher content of connective tissue results in tougher meat. (Collagen is also present in bones and skin.)

On cooking, the insoluble collagen is converted into water-soluble gelatin, so making the material more tender, but elastin is unchanged on heating. Thus tough meat is softened to some extent by stewing, but roasting or frying has little effect. (Griswold.)

Consommé. A clear soup made from meat or meat extract.

Convenience Foods. Processed foods in which a considerable amount of the preparation has already been carried out by the manufacturer, e.g. cooked meats, canned foods, baked foods, breakfast cereals, frozen foods.

Cookie. American term for biscuit.

Cooking. Required to make food more palatable and more digestible. There is breakdown of the connective tissue in meat and softening of the cellulose in plant tissues.

Broiling: cooking by direct heat over flame.

Pan broiling: cooking through hot dry metal over direct heat.

Sautéing: cooking with small amount of fat.

Simmering: cooking in water slightly below boiling point.

Stewing: prolonged simmering. (*See* Boiling.)

Fricassée: combination of sautéing and stewing.

Devilled: grilled or fried after coating with condiments or breadcrumbs.

Steaming: cooking by heat conveyed by steam either directly or through steam jacket as in double boiler. Steaming also carried out above 100°C by means of pressure cookers. *See also* Connective tissue, Roasting, Boiling, Braising, Grilling, Frying. (Griswold.)

Cooking, Loss of Nutrients. In general the water-soluble vitamins and minerals are leached into the cooking water, the fat-soluble vitamins are unaffected except at frying temperatures, and the proteins are not damaged except under extreme conditions.

Vegetables lose much of their vitamin C, mostly by leaching into the water, but also by oxidation. Losses are minimised by steaming or greatly reducing the volume of the cooking water, and maximised by storing hot after cooking.

The B vitamins show some destruction, B_1 being more sensitive, on heating, and the loss depends on temperature and time. E.g. frying destroys 10% B_1, 10% B_2 and 15% nicotinic acid, braising destroys 55%, 25% and 35% respectively and stewing destroys 75%, 30%, and 50% respectively. (Johnson, Griswold, FB.)

Copper. Copper is part of the enzyme tyrosinase (and in plants, laccase and ascorbic acid oxidase) and is needed to assist the incorporation of iron into haemoglobin. It is therefore thought to be a dietary essential in amounts of about 2 mg per day, but there is no evidence that a dietary deficiency ever occurs in man. Traces of copper are normally present in the blood in combination with an alpha globulin as caeruloplasmin.

Deficiency in cattle gives rise to "swayback." Traces are also essential for plant growth.

Toxic in high concentrations and there is a legal limit to the amount permitted in foodstuffs. (Gil, GMW.)

Copra. Dried coconut meat; used for production of coconut oil for margarine and soap.

Coprophagy. Eating of faeces. As B vitamins are synthesized by intestinal bacteria, animals that eat their faeces can make use of these vitamins.

Cordial, Fruit. *See* Soft drinks.

Coriander. Dried ripe fruit of *Coriandrum sativum* (parsley family). Contains 20% fixed oil and 1% essential oil—largely linool or coriandrol (an isomer of geraniol). Used as flavour in meat products, bakery goods, tobacco, gin and in curry powder. (Jacobs, Merory.)

Cori cycle. The sequence of reactions through which the liver converts lactic acid back to glycogen, namely, liver glycogen —blood glucose—muscle glycogen —blood lactate—liver glycogen. (DP.)

Cori Ester. Name given to glucose-1-phosphate, one of the intermediates of glucose metabolism, *which see.*

Corm. Thickened, underground base of stem of plants, often called bulbs as, for example, taro and onion.

Corn. In Great Britain a generic term for cereals. In U.S.A. means maize.

Corn, Dent. *See* Maize.

Corned Beef. In the U.S. this is **salt beef.** In the U.K. it is a relatively cheap canned product made from lower quality beef; the chopped meat is partially cooked in boiling water when the water-soluble fraction is partly removed to produce, after evaporation, **meat extract.** The scalded meat is cured in brine, together with sugar and preservatives, and canned. The name is derived from grains or 'corns' of salt.

Composition per 100 g: 25 g protein, 14 g fat, 233 kcal (1·0 MJ), 3 mg iron, 10 μg vitamin A, 0·4 mg B_1, 00·2 mg B_2, 3·5 mg nicotinic acid. (FAO.)

Cornflakes. Breakfast cereal made from maize grain. Typical analysis:—Protein 6·6%, fat 0·8%, carbohydrate 88%; Ca 7 mg, Fe 3 mg—per 100 g.

Phytic acid phosphorus 25% of the total P (58 mg/100 g). (M&W.)

Corn, Flint. *See* Maize.

Cornflour. Purified starch from maize; in U.S.A. called corn starch; used in custard, blancmange and baking powders.

Protein 0·5%, fat 0·3%, carbohydrate 87%, fibre 0·2%, no vitamins present. (Platt.)

Corn, Flour. Flour corn is a variety of maize with large, soft grains and very friable endosperm, making it easy to grind the grain to flour. (Matz 2.)

Corn Grits. *See* Hominy.

Corn Starch. *See* Cornflour.

Corn Steep Liquor. The first stage in the preparation of starch from maize is to soak the maize in water containing sulphur dioxide for 24 hours. The liquor is termed corn steep liquor. It was found to be an excellent medium for growing mould to produce penicillin; the yield was greatly enhanced beyond that obtained with synthetic media since the liquor contained a "biochemical precursor" of penicillin.

Corn Sugar. Glucose.

Corn Syrup. *See* Glucose syrup.

Corn, Waxy. *See* Maize.

Coronary Thrombosis. *See* Atherosclerosis.

Cossettes. Thin chips of sugar beet into which it is shredded for hot-water extraction of the sugar.

Cottonseed. Of double use in the food field; the oil is valuable as a cooking oil, or for margarine when hardened, and the protein residue is a valuable animal feedingstuff.

Courgettes. Italian marrows, Italian Squash or Zucchini (U.S.A.), a variety of gourd with small fruits. *See* Gourds.

Courlose. Trade name (British Celanese Ltd.) for sodium carboxymethylcellulose.

Cow Manure Factor. Vitamin B_{12}.

Cozymase. *See* nicotinamide adenine dinucleotide.

Co I and Co II. Abbreviations of Coenzymes I and II, officially named nicotinamide adenine dinucleotide and nicotinamide adenine dinucleotide phosphate, respectively.

Crabs. Shellfish of the suborder *Brachyura* of the Order *Decapoda*.

Large spider crab, *Maia squinado*, common on the south coast of England, 6 inches across, occasionally used as food.

Edible crab, *Cancer pagurus*, found in shallow water among rocks; can grow up to 12 lb weight.

Analysis of edible portion: hydrate 0; kcal 127 (0·53 MJ), Fe 1·3 mg, vitamin B_1 0·1 mg, B_2 0·15 mg, nicotinic acid 2·5 mg —per 100 g.

Cran. Measure for herrings containing 37½ gallons or about 800 herrings.

Cranberry. Fleshy, acid fruit of *Vaccinium oxycoccus* resembling cherry; commonly used for cranberry sauce.

Composition per 100 g: 3·5 g carbohydrate, 15 kcal (0·06 MJ), 1 mg iron, 12 mg vitamin C. (OF, M&W.)

Crawfish. *See* Lobster.

Crayfish. The English crayfish, *Astacus torrentium*, was almost entirely wiped out by disease in 1887 and crayfish for food are all imported, *Astacus fluviatilis. See* Lobster.

Cream. Legally contains (in U.K.) not less than 18% fat; sterilised cream, 23%, double cream or thick cream, 48%; clotted cream, not less than 48% fat; whipping or whipped cream, not less than 35% fat. (Bell.)

Cream, Clotted. This usually has a higher fat content than double cream which legally is 48% fat. Double cream is floated in a shallow layer on a layer of skim milk and scalded. The clotted cream at 63% fat is then skimmed off. This is **Devonshire cream** and contains 29·5% water, 4% protein, 2·8% lactose, 0·67% ash. **Cornish cream** is similar but is prepared by scalding the double cream alone, not floated on a layer of milk. *See also* Cream.

Cream, Cornish. *See* Cream, clotted.

Cream, Devonshire. *See* Cream, clotted.

Creaming quality. As applied to fats is the ability to absorb air during mixing.

Cream Line Index. The cream line or layer usually forms about 6% of total depth of the milk. The cream line index is the ratio of the percentage cream layer to the percentage fat in the milk. It is used as a test of the milk and in ordinary bulk pasteurised milk is about 1·7. (Davis.)

Cream of Tartar. Potassium hydrogen tartrate, used with sodium bicarbonate as baking powder because it acts more slowly than tartaric acid and gives a more prolonged evolution of carbon dioxide. This is tartrate baking powder; similarly phosphate baking powder contains calcium acid phosphate or sodium hydrogen pyrophosphate.

Also used to "invert" sugar in making boiled sweets (*which see*).

Cream, Plastic. Term used for a cream containing as much fat as butter (80–83%) but as a dispersal of fat in water, whereas butter is water in fat. Prepared by intense centrifugal treatment of cream; crumbly not greasy in texture; used for preparation of cream cheese and whipped cream.

Cream, Sleepy. Cream that will not churn to butter in the normal time. (Davis.)

Cream, Synthetic. Name given to (*a*) emulsion of vegetable oil, milk or milk powder, egg yolk and sugar, and to (*b*) emulsion of water with methyl cellulose, monoglycerides, and other synthetic materials. (Davis & Mac.)

Creatine. Methyl guanidine derivative of acetic acid. Essential part of the energy release system of muscle, as creatine phosphate, or phosphagen, possesses an energy-rich bond which is released when energy is required for muscular contraction.

The anhydride of creatine is creatinine, in which form it is found in urine. Meat extract contains a mixture of the two, derived from the creatine that was present in the fresh muscle. Creatine plus creatinine is used as an index of quality of commercial meat extract, and as a measure of extract present in manufactured products, such as soups. (AEB.)

Creatinine. Anhydride of creatine, *which see.*

Cress. *Lepidium sativum.* Seed leaves eaten raw with mustard leaves (mustard and cress, *see* Mustard).

Winter or Land Cress, *Barbarea verna,* is a rarely grown salad plant. (OF.)

Creta Praeparata. Official British Pharmacopoeia name for prepared chalk, made by washing and drying naturally occurring calcium carbonate. The form in which calcium is added to flour (14 oz. per 280-lb sack). (AEB.)

Cretinism. Underactivity of the thyroid gland (hypothyroidism) in children resulting in poor growth and mental retardation. Hypothyroidism in adults is myxoedema. Can result from a dietary deficiency of iodine. *See also* Goitre *and* Thyroid gland. (BDS.)

Crispbreads. Name given to a flour and water wafer, originally Swedish and made from rye flour, but may be made from wheat flour. They have a much lower water content than bread and some brands are richer in protein because of added wheat gluten.

Although popularly believed to be an aid in slimming they provide more energy than the same weight of ordinary bread since they contain less water.

Cristal Height. A measure of leg length taken from the floor to the summit of the iliac crest. Cristal height as a proportion of total height increases with age in children and a reduced rate of increase is an indication of undernourishment. (DP.)

Crowdies. *See* Milks, fermented.

Croûtons. Small diced or shaped pieces of bread fried in fat.

Crude Protein. *See* Protein, crude.

Crumb-softener. *See* Superglycerinated fats *and* Polyoxyethylene.

Crumpets. *See* Dough Cakes.

Cryovac. Trade name of rubber latex wrapping film. Can be heat shrunk on to foods to form a continuous film.

Cryptoxanthin. Yellow colouring matter in certain vegetables such as yellow maize, and in the seeds of *Physalis,* the Chinese Lantern. A hydroxy derivative of carotene; converted into retinol in the body.

Crystallin. Protein of the lens of the eye.

CSM. Corn-soya-milk; protein-rich baby food (20% protein) made in the United States from 68% precooked maize (corn), 25% defatted soya flour and 5% skim milk powder with added vitamins B_1, B_2, B_6, B_{12}, nicotinic acid, pantothenic acid, folic acid, A, D, and E and calcium carbonate.

Cubs. Trade name (Nabisco Foods Ltd.) for a breakfast cereal made from wheat.

Cucumber. Fruit of *Cucumis sativus,* a member of the gourd family.

Composition: protein 0·6%, fat 0·1%; kcal 10 (0·04 MJ), Ca 7 mg, Fe 0·2 mg, vitamin B_1 0·02 mg, B_2 0·03 mg, nicotinic acid 0·1 mg, vitamin C 6 mg—per 100 g. (FAO.)

Cucurbits. Term used for vegetables of the Cucurbitaceae, *see* Gourds.

Cumin Seed. Dried fruit of *Cuminum cyminum* (parsley family); contains about 10% fixed oil and 2–4% essential oil, largely cuminal. Used in curry powder and for flavouring cordials. (Jacobs, Merory.)

Curaçao. A liqueur made from the rind of Seville oranges and brandy or gin; 60% of proof spirit.

Curds. Clotted protein formed when fresh milk is treated with rennet; the fluid left is whey, *which see.*

Curd Tension. A measure of the toughness of the curd formed from milk by the digestive enzymes and used as an index of the digestibility of the milk. The sample is coagulated with rennin and the force needed to pull a knife-blade through the curd is measured in grams under standardised conditions. Ideal score is zero, below 20 satisfactory; cow's milk 46, diluted with equal volume of water 20, reconstituted spray-dried milk 10, reconstituted roller-dried milk 5, evaporated milk 3, human milk 1.

Curing of Meat. Aids colour, flavour and keeping properties. Saturated salt, sodium nitrate (and some nitrite) and sugar, preferably at 5·5°C (42°F). Only salt-tolerant bacteria develop, and convert nitrate to nitrite which combines with muscle pigment, myoglobin, to give the red colour, nitrosomyoglobin. (Baum.)

Currants. Fruit of Ribes species; white, red and black (*see also* Blackcurrants).

Redcurrants: Protein 1·1%, carbohydrate 4·4%, water 83%, kcal 21 (0·09 MJ), Fe 1·2 mg, vitamin C, 40 mg—per 100 g.

White currants: Protein 1·3%, carbohydrate 5·6%, water 83%, kcal 26 (0·11 MJ), Fe 1 mg, vitamin C 40 mg—per 100 g. (M&W.)

Currants, Dried. Made by drying the small seedless black grape grown in and around Greece and in Australia; usually dried in bunches on the vine or after removal from the vine on supports.

Name derived from Raisins of Corauntz (Corinth).

For analysis *see* Fruit, dried; *see also* Raisins, Sultanas *and* Muscatels.

Curry. Mixture of several spices such as turmeric, coriander, mustard, black pepper, caraway, ginger, cumin, cinnamon, cloves, mace, nutmeg, cayenne and cardamom.

Contains 22 mg iron per ounce.

Custard. May refer to custard powder, *which see*, or to egg custard. Egg custard is composed of milk and egg cooked together.

Custard Apple. One of a number of species of tropical American trees of the family Anonaceae; Sour sop, *Anona muricata*, white fibrous flesh, less sweet than the others, fruit may weigh up to 8 lb; sweet sop (*A. squamosa*) also known as 'true' custard apple, popular in West Indies; bullock's heart (*A. reticulata*) buff-coloured flesh.

Composition per 100 g: 22 g carbohydrate, 1 g protein, 93 kcal (0·45 MJ), 0·5 mg iron, 0·1 mg B_1, 0·08 mg B_2, 0·8 mg nicotinic acid, 30 mg C. (OF, Platt.)

Custard Powder. Usually maize starch, coloured and flavoured.

Cyanocobalamin. Vitamin B_{12}.

Cyclamate. *See* Cyclo hexyl sulphamate.

Cyclitols. Cyclic sugars such as inositols, quercitols and tetritols.

Cyclo Hexyl Sulphamate, Sodium. A non-nutritive sweetener, 30 times as sweet as sugar, also used as the calcium salt; synthesised 1937.

Useful in low-calorie foods. Also called cyclamate and sucaryl (trade name). Unlike saccharine it is stable to heat. (AEB.)

Cymogran. Trade name (Allen & Hanbury's Ltd.) for protein-rich food low in phenylalanine for feeding patients with phenyl-ketonuria. (AEB.)

Cysteine. A non-essential amino acid, aminothiol propionic acid. Sometimes used as a dough improver. *See* Cystine.

Cystic Fibrosis. An inborn error of metabolism which causes a disturbance of the exocrine glands with failure to secrete pancreatic enzymes so that food is incompletely digested and absorbed. Treated by feeding predigested protein or adding dried pancreatin to the diet.

Cystine. One of the three sulphur-containing amino acids (cystine, cysteine and methionine).

Chemically consists of two molecules of cysteine joined via the —S—S— link. Methionine is the essential sulphur amino acid and cystine is non-essential, but can replace part of the methionine of the diet. Hence the S amino acids are always considered together. *See* Methionine. (BDS, DP.)

Cytochrome. Pigment present in every type of living cell (except the strictly anaerobic bacteria); acts as an intermediate hydrogen acceptor in passing hydrogen along the chain from the substrate to oxygen, the ultimate hydrogen acceptor. When it accepts the hydrogen it changes to the reduced form, and is re-oxidized by the enzyme cytochrome oxidase, which passes the hydrogen farther along the chain. (WHSS.)

Cytochrome Oxidase. *See* Cytochrome.

Cytochrome Reductase. *See* Flavoproteins.

Cytosine. *See* Pyrimidines *and* Nucleic acids.

D

d-. Obsolete prefix indicating dextrorotatory, now replaced by (+), *see* Optical activity.

D-. A prefix to chemical names, especially sugars and amino acids, indicating their structure. When the first hydroxyl group of a sugar is on the same side as the alcohol group it is the D- form, on opposite sides it is the L- form. Both L- and D- glucose exist.

In the case of amino acids L-alanine is related to the sugar L-glyceraldehyde and follows the same nomenclature. The other amino acids follow alanine. All the naturally occurring amino acids are L-, synthetic are DL, few D- amino acids are found in nature.

Capital L- and D- are not to be confused with l- and d- which are the old terms for $(+)$ and $(-)$, *see* Optical activity.

D-Araboascorbic Acid. *See* Ascorbic Acid.

Dadhi. *See* Milks, fermented.

Daltose. Trade name (Cow & Gate Ltd.) of a carbohydrate preparation consisting of maltose, glucose and dextrin for infant feeding.

Damson. Small dark-blue plum. Protein 0·5%, water 70%, carbohydrate 8·6%; kcal 34 (0·14 MJ), Fe 0·4 mg, vitamin B_1 0·1 mg, nicotinic acid 0·25 mg— per 100 g. (M&W.)

Dandelion Greens. The leaves of the weed, *Leontodon taraxacum*, used sometimes as a salad. Protein 2·4%, fat 0·6%; Ca 135 mg, Fe 2·8 mg, kcal 40 (0·17 MJ), vitamin A 3,000 μg, B_1 0·17 mg, B_2 0·13 mg, nicotinic acid 0·7 mg, vitamin C 25 mg—per 100 g. (FAO.)

Dark Adaptation. This is the change that takes place in the retina of the eye to assist vision in dim light. In dark adaptation a pigment, visual purple or rhodopsin, is formed from retinol (vitamin A aldehyde) and a protein. This is bleached in bright light. When body stores of retinol are inadequate **poor dark adaptation** — night blindness — results. This is the earliest indication of vitamin A deficiency. (Sebrell.)

Dasheen. W. Indian name for Taro.

Date-Plum. *See* Persimmon.

Dates. The fruit of the date palm, *Phoenix dactylifera;* there are hundreds of varieties classed as sweet, mild sweet and dry. The mild sweet are eaten fresh and the dry

or camel date is pressed whole or ground into flour and forms the staple diet of the Arabs.

The variety normally found on the world markets is the sweet type.

Composition of dried date: water 20%, protein 2%, carbohydrate 69%; kcal 284 (1·2 MJ), Fe 2 mg, vitamin A 30 μg, B_1 0·07 mg, B_2 0·04 mg, nioctinic acid 2·2 mg, vitamin C nil—per 100 g. (TND.)

D.B.D. Process. *See* Dry-blanchdry process.

D.E. Dextrose Equivalent Value, *which see.*

Defibrinated Blood. *See* Blood, defibrinated.

Degumming Agents. Used in refining of fats to remove mucilaginous matter consisting of gum, resin, proteins and phosphatides. Include hydrochloric and phosphoric acids, and phosphates. (Bailey.)

Dehydration. Scientific term for drying, but tends to be used for factory-dried materials as distinct from wind-dried.

Dehydroacetic Acid. Also Sodium Salt (DHA-S). Active against moulds but not a permitted additive.

Chemically can be regarded as the condensation product of acetic and acetoacetic acids, or 3-acetyl-6-methyl-1-pyran-2·4 dione.

Dehydroascorbic Acid. Oxidised form of vitamin C which can readily be reduced to the ordinary form, and is therefore biologically active. (Hawk.)

Dehydrocanning. A process in which 50% of the water is removed from a food before canning.

The advantages are that the texture is retained by the partial dehydration and there is a saving in bulk and weight.

Dehydrocholesterol. *See* Vitamin D.

Dehydrofreezing. A process for preservation of fruits and vegetables by evaporation of half to two-thirds of the water before freezing. The texture and flavour are claimed to be superior to either dehydration or freezing alone, and rehydration more rapid than with dehydrated products.

Dehydrogenases. Enzymes that carry out oxidations in the living cell by removing hydrogen from the substrate. They can only function by passing this hydrogen on to another substance, called the intermediate hydrogen acceptor. It is ultimately passed on to oxygen to form water.

There are specific dehydrogenases for each substrate, e.g. succinic dehydrogenase, lactic, malic, glucose, etc. *See also* Intermediate hydrogen carrier *and* Oxidases. (WHSS.)

Dehydrogenation. *See* Oxidation, Oxidases, *and* Intermediate hydrogen carrier.

Dehydroretinol. Formerly termed Vitamin A_2.

Demersal Fish. Usually called white fish; live on the sea bottom. Cod, haddock, whiting, hake, ling, saithe, halibut, sole, bream. Contain little fat, 1–4%. *See* Pelagic Fish.

Denaturation. (1) A reversible change in proteins that precedes coagulation (*which see*); the solubility is reduced and free –SH groups appear. Denaturation can be effected by changes in pH, heat, ultra-violet irradiation and violent agitation.

There is no change in nutritive value, but pharmacological activity is often lost.

(2) When the term is applied to alcohol it means the addition of denaturing agents, such as methyl violet and pyridine (as in methylated spirits) to render it unpleasant and so prevent its consumption.

Dendritic Salt. A form of ordinary table salt, sodium chloride, with the crystals branched or star-like (dendritic) instead of the normal cubes. The advantages claimed are the lower bulk density, rapid solution, and unusual capacity for absorbing moisture before becoming wet.

Deodorization. Generally applied to the removal of flavour (as in deodorized fish meal) but more specifically to the deodorization of fats during refining. Superheated steam is bubbled through the hot oil under vacuum, when most of the flavoured substances are distilled off. (Bailey.)

Depectinization. Removal of pectins from fruit pulp to produce a clear thin juice instead of a viscous, cloudy liquid; achieved by the use of enzyme preparations.

Derbyshire Neck. *See* Iodine *and* Goitre.

Desoxyribonucleic Acid. *See* Nucleic acids.

Detoxication. Destruction of a toxic compound, or, more usually, alteration of a chemical group to produce a non-toxic product.

71

In the body detoxication is effected by oxidation, reduction, hydrolysis, or by combination (conjugation) with glycine, glucuronic acid, glutamine, cysteine, or by methylation. E.g. the toxic substance benzoic acid is excreted in the urine as a complex with glycine, namely hippuric acid. (Hawk.)

Deuterium. Or heavy hydrogen; isotope of hydrogen with atomic weight 2. The isotope of atomic-weight 3 is tritium.

Devitalized Gluten. *See* Gluten.

Dewberry. A large variety of blackberry, but different in flavour.

Dexedrine. *See* Anorectic drugs.

Dextran. A polysaccharide composed of linked fructose units; unwelcome in the sugar factory but valuable clinically for blood transfusion (plasma extender). Produced by the action of *Betacoccus arabinosaceous* on sugar.

Dextrin, limit. *See* Limit dextrin.

Dextrins. Mixture of soluble compounds formed by partial breakdown of starch by heat, acid or enzymes; (complete breakdown yields maltose). Formed when bread is toasted.

Nutritionally equivalent to starch; industrially used as adhesives in the sizing of paper and textiles, and as gums. *See also* Amylases. (BDS.)

Dextrorotatory. *See* Optical activity.

Dextrose. Alternative name for glucose. Commercially the term glucose is often used to mean corn syrup (a mixture of glucose, sugars and dextrins) and pure glucose is called dextrose.

Dextrose Equivalent Value. A term used to indicate the degree of hydrolysis of starch into glucose syrup (*which see*). It is defined as the total reducing sugar content, expressed as dextrose, calculated as a percentage of the dry solids content (i.e. the higher the D.E. the more sugar and the less dextrins are present).

Liquid glucoses are commercially available ranging from 26 D.E. to 65 D.E. A complete acid hydrolysis converts all the starch into glucose but produces bitter degradation products.

Dhals. Indian term for split peas of various kinds, e.g. pigeon pea (*Cajanus indicus*), khesari (*Lathyrus sativus*), red dahl or Massur dahl the lentil (*Lens esculenta*). (TND.)

Diabetes, Alloxan. *See* Alloxan.

Diabetes Mellitus. Or Sugar Diabetes. A metabolic disorder affecting mainly carbohydrate metabolism; an inability to metabolise glucose which therefore appears in the urine. Usually due to a deficiency of insulin and is treated by insulin injections (also possibly due to increased destruction of insulin in the body, treated by oral drugs such as tolbutamide).

Impaired glucose metabolism leads to excessive fat breakdown with the accumulation of the penultimate products of fatty acid oxidation—namely acetoacetic acid, betahydroxybutyric acid and acetone (the so-called ketone bodies). These can cause diabetic coma. *See also* Sugar tolerance *and* Insulin. (BDS.)

Diabetes, Renal. The appearance of glucose in the urine without undue elevation of the blood sugar. It is due to a reduction of the renal threshold which allows the blood glucose to be excreted. *See also* Phlorrhizin.

Diabetes Test. *See* Glucose tolerance.

Di-acetate, Sodium and Calcium. Used to inhibit the growth of moulds in foods. Permitted in U.S.A. but not U.K. Chemical formula $CH_3COONa.CH_3COOH.\frac{1}{2}H_2O$ (equimolecular compound of acetic acid and sodium acetate).

Diacetyl. $CH_3CO.CO.CH_3$. The flavour-aroma agent in butter formed during the ripening stage by the organism *Streptococcus lactis cremoris*. Added as a synthetic compound to margarine as "butter flavour". (Tanner.)

Dialysis. Separation of small molecules from larger in solution by virtue of their different rates of diffusion through a membrane. Membranes are natural, such as pig bladder, or artificial, such as cellulose derivatives or collodion.

The solution is usually placed in a bag of the membrane and this immersed in water. The small molecules diffuse out into the water leaving the larger molecules inside the bag. This is a frequent method of separating proteins from solutions of salts. *See* Membranes, semi-permeable. (BDS.)

Diaphorase. A flavoprotein enzyme in the cell respiratory system; function is to accept hydrogen from NADH. (WHSS.)

Diastase. *See* Amylases.

Diastatic Activity. Of flour: a measure of its ability to produce sugar from its own starch under the influence of its own diastase. This sugar is needed for the growth of the yeast during the fermentation. Measured as "maltose figure". *See also* Amylograph. (KJ.)

Dicoumarin. Toxic substance found in spoiled sweet clover; causes haemorrhage (haemorrhagic sweet clover disease) by interfering with the synthesis of prothrombin in the liver, i.e. has an anti-vitamin K action. Used clinically to prevent post-operative thrombosis. (BDS.)

Diethyl Pyrocarbonate. Preservative that kills bacteria and yeasts (not moulds) and is rapidly hydrolysed to ethyl alchol and carbon dioxide; particularly suitable for beverages. Level of use is 50–300 ppm and hydrolysis is complete after several days.

Dietetic Foods. Foods prepared to meet the particular nutritional needs of persons whose normal processes of assimilation or metabolism are modified, or for whom a particular effect is to be obtained by a controlled intake of foods or certain nutrients. They may be formulated for persons suffering from physiological disorders or for healthy people with additional needs. (AEB.)

Dietitian, Dietician. According to the U.S. Dept. of Labour, Dictionary of Occupational Titles —one who applies the principles of nutrition to the feeding of individuals and groups; plans menus and special diets; supervises the preparation and serving of meals; instructs in the principles of nutrition as applied to the selection of foods. *See also* Nutritionist.

Diets. *See under individual entries:* Salt-free diets, Ketogenic diet, Salisbury cure, Hay diet, Karell diet, Kempner diet, Lenhartz diet, Meulingracht diet, Sippy diet.

Diets, Therapeutic. *See* Therapeutic Diets.

Differential Cell Count. *See* Leucocytes.

Digester. Alternative name for Autoclave or Pressure cooker.

Digestibility. The proportion of a foodstuff absorbed from the digestive tract into the bloodstream, normally 90–95%. It is measured as the difference between intake and faecal output, making allowance for that part of the faeces which is not derived from undigested food residues (such as shed lining of the intestinal tract, bacteria, residues of digestive juices).

Digestibility measured in this way is referred to as "true digestibility" as distinct from the approximate measure of "apparent digestibility" which is simply the difference between intake and output.

Digestion. The breakdown of a complex into its constituent parts. Most frequently refers to the digestion of food which means the breakdown by the digestive enzymes of proteins to amino acids, starch to glucose, fats to glycerol and fatty acids—these simple breakdown products are then absorbed into the bloodstream.

Digestion is also applied to the acid hydrolysis of a protein; the Kjeldahl digestion is the complete breakdown of a nitrogenous compound to ammonia by sulphuric acid. *See also* Intestinal juice and individual digestive enzymes. (BDS.)

Digestive Juices. *See* Pancreatic juice, Succus entericus, Gastric secretion, *and* Bile.

Dilatation of Fats. When fats change from solids to liquid at the same temperature there is an increase in volume. Measurement of this increase, dilatometry, may be used to estimate the amount of solid fat present in a mixture at any given temperature. The precise measure is the difference between the volumes of the solid and the liquid fat measured in microlitres per 25 g of fat.

Dill. Dried ripe fruit of *Anethum graveolens* (parsley family); leafy tops also used. Contains 15% fixed oil and 2–4% essential oil containing carvone, limonene and terpenes. Used in pickles and soups. (Jacobs, Merory.)

Diose. *See* Disaccharides.

Dipeptide. *See* Polypeptide.

Diphenyl. This, and orthophenyl phenol, are used for treatment of fruit after harvesting to prevent mould growth. Permitted in citrus fruits, diphenyl up to 100 ppm, OPP up to 70 ppm. Apples, pears and pineapples may contain 10 ppm, peaches 20 ppm, and melons 125 ppm of OPP. (Bell.)

Diphosphopyridine Nucleotide. *See* Nicotinamide adenine dinucleotide.

Diphosphothiamine. *See* Cocarboxylase.

Dipsa. Foods that cause thirst. Dipsetic—tending to produce thirst.

Dipsesis. Also Dipsosis. Extreme thirst, craving for abnormal kinds of drinks. Dipsomania—imperative morbid craving for alcoholic drink.

Dipsogen. Thirst-provoking agent.

Direct Extract. *See* Meat extract.

74

Disaccharide Intolerance. Impaired ability to digest maltose, sucrose or lactose, which may be inherited. Generalised lactose intolerance may be an adaptation to the absence of milk from the diet, and can be secondary to various inflammatory and degenerative diseases of the small intestine.

Treatment is by omitting the offending sugar from the diet. (AEB.)

Disaccharides. Sugars composed of two monosaccharide molecules combined, with the elimination of a molecule of water. E.g. glucose, $C_6H_{12}O_6$, plus fructose, $C_6H_{12}O_6$, produces sucrose, $C_{12}H_{22}O_{11}$. Conversely, when a disaccharide is hydrolysed, either by acid or enzymically, a molecule of water is added and two monosaccharides result.

Also known as **dioses** or **disaccharoses.** (BDS.)

Disaccharose. *See* Disaccharides.

Disc mill. One or more revolving circular plates between which substances, e.g. foodstuffs, are ground. The discs are separated by projecting teeth or pins; used to grind grain, fruit, sugar, chocolate, pastes, etc.

Distillers' Solubles. *See* Spent wash.

Diuresis. Loss of water from the body as urine. (BDS.)

Diuretics. Substances that increase the secretion of urine; include organic mercury compounds, xanthines (therefore also coffee and tea) and substances that alter the alkaline reserve of the blood, such as urea, potassium nitrate, potassium chloride. (Clark.)

DNA. Desoxyribonucleic acid. *See* Nucleic acids.

Dockage. Name given to foreign material in wheat which can be readily removed by a simple cleaning procedure.

Do-Maker Process. For continuous breadmaking. Ingredients are automatically fed into continuous dough mixer, the yeast suspension being added in a very active state. (FM.)

Dough Cakes. Term includes crumpets, muffins and pikelets, all made from flour, water and milk; batter is raised with yeast and baked on a hot plate. Crumpets have sodium bicarbonate added to the batter, muffins are thick and well aerated, less tough than crumpets, pikelets are made from crumpet batter that has been thinned down. (FM.)

Douglas Bag. Inflatable bag for collecting expired air. Energy usage can be determined from the oxygen and carbon dioxide analysis, i.e. by indirect calorimetry. *See also* Spirometer. (BDS.)

DPN. *See* Nicotinamide adenine dinucleotide.

Dripping. Unbleached and untreated fat from the fatty tissues or bones of sheep or oxen.

Drupes. Botanical name for fruit that is a single seed, surrounded by stony and fleshy pericarp, e.g. apricot, cherry, plum.

Dry-blanch-dry Process. A method of drying fruit so as to retain the bright colour and flavour; it is faster than drying in the sun and preserves flavour and colour better than hot air drying.

The material is dried to 50% water at about 82°C, blanched for a few minutes then dried at 68°C over a period of 6–24 hours to 15–20% water content.

75

Dryers. *See* Rotary louvre dryer, Spray dryer, Pneumatic dryer, Roller dryer, Fluid bed dryer.

"Dry Frying." Frying without the use of fat by using an anti-sticking agent of silicone or a vegetable extract.

Dry Ice. Solid carbon dioxide; has a temperature of —79°C; used to refrigerate foodstuffs in transit, for carbonation of liquids, and for cold traps in the laboratory.

Sublimes from the solid stage to a gas without liquefying; latent heat at subliming temperature 246 B.T.U. per lb; available refrigeration per lb nearly twice that of ice. (Loes.)

Drying, Azeotropic. *See* Azeotrope.

Drying Oil. A highly unsaturated oil that absorbs oxygen and, when in thin films, polymerizes to form a skin. Linseed and tung oil are examples of drying oils used in paints and in the manufacture of linoleum.

Nutritionally these oils are similar to edible fats, but when polymerized, are toxic. *See also* Iodine value.

Du Bois Formula. *See* Surface area.

Ductless Glands. *See* Hormones.

Dulcin. Synthetic material, paraphenetylurea (para-phenetolcarbamide), 250 times as sweet as sugar but not permitted in foods. Discovered 1883, also called sucrol and valzin.

Dulcite. Dulcitol.

Dulcitol. A six-carbon sugar-alcohol formed by reduction of galactose. Occurs in Madagascar manna (*Melampyrum nemorosum*), and also known as melampyrin, dulcite and galacticol.

Dulse. Purplish-red edible seaweed eaten raw or cooked.

Dun. In salted fish refers to the brown discoloration caused by mould growth.

Dunst. Very fine semolina (i.e. starch from the endosperm of the wheat grain) approaching the fineness of flour. Also called break middlings (not to be confused with middlings which is the branny offal). (KJ.)

Duodenum. First part of the small intestine, between the stomach and the jejunum. Pancreatic juice and bile are secreted into the intestine and the major part of digestion takes place there. (BDS.)

Durian. *Durio zibethinus;* tropical fruit with disgusting odour; weighs 6–8 lb., consumption restricted largely to S.E. Asia. No information about composition. (OF.)

Durum Wheat. A hard type of wheat of the species *Tricitum durum* (most bread wheats are *Tricitum vulgare*); largely used for the production of semolina intended for the preparation of macaroni. (KJ.)

Dutch Oven. Semi-circular metal shield which may be placed close to an open fire, and is fitted with shelves on which food is roasted. It may also be clamped to the fire bars.

Dynamic Equilibrium. Name given to the process whereby living tissues are continually being broken down and resynthesised so that their structure remains constant. Hence the need for food that supply new materials for tissue construction even in the mature, fully-grown adult. (BDS.)

Dyox. Trade name for chlorine dioxide used to treat flour. *See* Aging.

Dyspepsia. Any pain or discomfort associated with eating. Dyspepsia may be a symptom of gastritis, peptic ulcer, gall-bladder disease, etc., or, if there is no structural change in the intestinal tract it is called "functional dyspepsia". Treatment includes a bland diet. (DP.)

E

Earthnuts. *See* Peanuts.

Éau-de-Vie de Miel. Or honey brandy, made by distilling mead (which, in turn, is made by fermenting honey).

Eck Fistula. *See* Fistula.

Ectomorph. Description given to a tall, thin individual, possibly with underdeveloped muscles. (*See also* Mesomorph *and* Endomorph.)

Écuelle. Device for obtaining peel oil from citrus fruit. Consists of a shallow funnel lined with spikes on which the fruit is rolled by hand. As the oil glands are pierced the oil and cell sap collect in the bottom of the funnel. (Brav.)

Eddo. W. Indian name for Taro.

Edifas. Trade name (Imperial Chemical Industries); Edifas A —methyl ethyl cellulose; Edifas B —sodium carboxymethylcellulose.

Edosol. Trade name (Trufood Ltd.) for a low-sodium milk substitute.
Protein 30·3%, fat 26·4%, carbohydrate 37·9%; Ca 846 mg, Fe 0·6 mg, sodium 43 mg (dried milk, sodium 400 mg), kcal 510 (2·1 MJ)—per 100 g. (M&W.)

E.D.T.A. *See* Ethylenediamine tetraacetic acid.

EFA. Essential fatty acids, *which see*.

Egg. Hens' eggs are graded according to quality and size (European Economic Community). Quality: A—fresh, A extra—packed less than 7 days ago, B—less fresh than A, preserved or refrigerated, C—fit for food manufacture only.
Sizes: Grade 1, 70 g and over, then grades 2 to 6 at 5 g intervals, with grade 7 under 45 g.
Composition whole egg per 100 g: 12·1 g protein, 12·5 g fat, 160 kcal (0·69 MJ), 57 mg calcium, 2·5 mg iron, 330 μg vitamin A, 0·1 mg B_1, 0·36 mg B_2, 0·07 mg nicotinic acid, 4·5 μg D, 470 mg cholesterol.
Yolk: 16·4 g protein, 31 g fat, 350 kcal (1·47 MJ), 130 mg calcium, 6 mg iron, 1,000 μg vitamin A, 0·32 mg B_1, 0·36 mg B_2, 0·02 mg nicotinic acid, 12·5 μg D, 1·8 g cholesterol.
White: 9·3 g protein, 40 kcal (0·16 MJ), 0·1 mg iron, 0·36 mg B_2, 0·09 mg nicotinic acid.
Useful in food preparation to thicken sauces and custards, as an emulsifier, to hold air in meringues and sponges, and as a binder in croquettes. (FAO, FB.)

Egg Albumin. *See* Egg-white.

Egg, Dehydrated. Protein 47%, fat 43%; kcal 605 (2·5 MJ), Ca 186 mg, Fe 9·3 mg, vitamin A 100 μg, B_1 0·34 mg, B_2 1·08 mg, nicotinic acid 0·2 mg, vitamin C nil—per 100 g. (FAO.)

Egg Plant. *See* Aubergine.

Egg Proteins. *See under separate headings:* Ovalbumin, ovomucin, ovomucoid, ovoglobulin, conalbumin, and vitellin.

Egg Substitute. Name formerly used for golden raising powder. *See* Baking Powder.

Egg-white. 87·8% water, 10·8% protein, 0·6% ash. Composed of outer layer of thin white, layer of thick white, richer in ovomucin, and inner layer of thin white surrounding the yolk. Eggs vary in ratio of thick to thin white, depending on the individual hen. Higher percentage of thick white desirable for frying and poaching (helps the egg to coagulate into small firm mass instead of spreading); thin white produces larger volume of froth when beaten than does thick.

Proteins are ovomucin, ovalbumin, ovomucoid, ovoglobulin and conalbumin. (B. & R.)

Egg-white Injury. *See* Biotin.

E.H. Equilibrium Humidity, *which see.*

Einkorn. A type of wheat, the wild form of which, *Triticum boeoticum,* was probably one of the ancestors of all cultivated wheats. Still grown in some parts of S. Europe and Middle East, usually for animal feed.

The name Einkorn, "one seed", derives from the single seed found in each spikelet.

Eiweiss Milch. *See* Protein milk.

Elastin. Insoluble protein uniting muscle fibres in meat, not changed on heating; the cause of tough meat. *See also* Connective tissue *and* Albuminoids. (Hawk.)

Electronic Heating. *See* High frequency heating.

Electrophoresis. The movement of electrically charged particles when a current is passed through the solution.

The electric charge on proteins is sufficient to make them migrate under the influence of a current, the rate depending on the type of proteins. Electrophoresis is therefore a useful method for the analytical separation of proteins and can be applied to minute quantities in paper electrophoresis. Valuable in examination of blood proteins for diagnostic purposes.

Electropure Process. A method of pasteurizing milk by passing a low-frequency, alternating current. (Davis.)

Elements, Minor. *See* Trace elements.

Elute. To wash off or remove. Rather specifically applied to the removal of adsorbed chemicals from the substance that has adsorbed them, as in chromatography.

Embden Groats. *See* Groats.

Embden - Meyerhof - Parnas Scheme. Name for the first series of steps in the breakdown of glucose in the tissues, as far as pyruvic acid, i.e. the glycolytic part as distinct from the subsequent oxidation. *See* Glucose metabolism. (WHSS.)

Emblic. Berry of the S.E. Asian malacca tree, *Emblica officinalis;* similar in appearance to the gooseberry. Also known as Indian gooseberry. Rich source of vitamin C, 600 mg per 100 g. (TND.)

Emmer. A type of wheat known to be used more than 8,000 years ago; tetraploid (4 sets of 7 chromosomes). Wild emmer is *Triticum dicoccoides* and true Emmer is *T. dicoccum.* Nowadays usually grown for animal feed.

Emprote. Trade name (Eustace Miles Foods Co., Bucks.) for a dried milk and cereal preparation consumed as a beverage. 33% protein.

Emulsifying Agents. Substances like gums, egg yolk, albumin, casein, soaps, agar, lecithin, glycerol monostearate, alginates, Irish moss, that aid the uniform dispersion of oil in water, i.e. form emulsions like margarine, ice-cream, salad cream, etc. Stabilizers (*which see*) maintain these emulsions in a stable form. Also used in baking to aid the smooth incorporation of fat into the dough and to keep the crumb soft. (Jacobs.)

Emulsifying Salts. Sodium citrate, sodium phosphates and sodium tartrate, used in the manufacture of milk powder, evaporated milk, sterilized cream and processed cheese.

Emulsin. Mixture of glycosidase enzymes in bitter almond that decompose the glucoside amygdalin, to benzaldehyde, glucose and hydrocyanic acid.

Emulsion. An intimate mixture of two immiscible liquids, one being dispersed in the other in the form of fine droplets. E.g. oil and water. They will stay mixed only as long as they are stirred together unless an emulsifying agent (*which see*) is added to stabilize the emulsion.

Emulsoids. *See* Colloids, lyophilic.

Endergonic. Used of reactions (in living tissues) that require a supply of energy, such as the synthesis of complex molecules. (WHSS.)

Endive. A species of chicory, *Cichorium endivia;* the curly leaves are eaten as a salad. Called chicory in U.S.A.

Water 94%, protein 1·8%, fat mg, vitamin A 1,000 μg, C 12 mg —per 100 g.

Endocrines. *See* Hormones.

Endomorph. Description given to a stocky, fat individual. (*See also* Mesomorph *and* Ectomorph).

Endomysium. *See* Muscle.

Endopeptidases. Enzymes that split peptide bonds inside the protein molecule; i.e., according to the older nomenclature, they are proteinases, such as pepsin, trypsin and chymotrypsin. (WHSS.)

Endosperm. The inner and greater part of cereal grains. In wheat comprises about 83% of the grain, mainly starch, and is the source of semolina (*which see*).

Contains only about 10% of the thiamin, 35% of the riboflavin. 40% of the nicotinic acid, 50% of the pyridoxine and pantothenic acid of the whole grain. (KJ.)

Endotoxin. *See* Toxins.

Enema. *See* Nutrient enemata.

Energen Rolls. Trade name (Energen Foods Co. Ltd.) for a light bread roll of wheat flour plus added wheat gluten.

Protein 44%, fat 4·1%, carbohydrate 45·7%, Ca 47 mg, Fe 4 mg, kcal 390 (1·63 MJ)—per 100 g. (M&W.)

Energy. Defined as the ability to do work. Exists in several forms such as chemical energy in fuels and food; kinetic, potential, light and heat energy. Measured in joules; since various forms of energy are interconvertible often measured as heat in calories or British thermal units.

Total chemical energy in a food, as released in the bomb calorimeter, is **gross energy**. After allowance is made for the losses in the faeces the remainder is **digestible energy**. After allowance is made for loss in the urine (e.g. urea from dietary proteins) the remainder is **metabolisable energy**. Finally, after allowing for the loss by specific dynamic action the remainder is **net energy**.

Available energy in foods is calculated by use of the following factors: protein 17 kJ/g, fat 37 kJ/g, carbohydrate (calculated as monosaccharide) 16 kJ/g, alcohol 29 kJ/g.

Energy expenditure of average adult man: basal 1,700 kcal ($7 \cdot 1$ MJ) per day; light work, total 2,300 kcal ($9 \cdot 7$ MJ); medium work 3,000 kcal ($12 \cdot 6$ MJ); heavy work 3,500 kcal ($14 \cdot 7$ MJ). (DP.)

See also Atwater Factors, Rubner Factors *and* Phosphate Bond, Energy-rich.

Energy Conversion Factors. The amount of energy available in foodstuffs. When this was expressed in calories the factors were slightly different depending upon whether allowances were made for absorption (*see* Atwater Factors *and* Rubner Factors). With the change to the joule it was recognized that conversion factors for calculating the metabolizable energies of foods are relatively inaccurate and until

better values become available the following are used; protein 17 kJ/g, fat 37 kJ/g, carbohydrate (as monosaccharide) 16 kJ/g, ethyl alcohol 29 kJ/g. (AEB.)

Energy-rich Phosphate. *See* Phosphate bond, energy-rich.

Enfleurage. Method of extracting essential oils from blossoms, by placing them on glass trays covered with purified lard or other fat, which eventually becomes saturated with the oil. (Brav.)

Ennoblement. *See* Enrichment.

Enocianina. Desugared grape extract used to colour fruit flavours. Prepared by acid extraction of skins of red grapes; bluish when neutralized, turns red on acidifying. (Merory.)

Enolase. Enzyme that catalyses the conversion of 2-phosphoglyceric acid to phospho-enol-pyruvic acid, with the formation of an energy-rich phosphate bond. Important in the breakdown of glucose. (WHSS.)

Enrichment. Term applied to the addition of nutrients to foods. E.g. addition of vitamins A and D to margarine, extra vitamin C to fruit juices, iodide to table salt, B vitamins to flour and rice.

The terms ennoblement and fortification are also applied to these procedures. (AEB.)

Ensete. *See* Banana, False.

Enterogastrone. Hormone found in the small intestine which inhibits both motor and secretory activity of the stomach. Its secretion is stimulated by fat, hence fat in the diet inhibits gastric activity. (BDS.)

Enterokinase. An ingredient of the intestinal juice that activates the trypsinogen and chymotrypsinogen of the pancreatic juice to form trypsin and chymotrypsin, the active enzymes. (BDS.)

Entoleter. Machine used to disinfest cereals and other foods. The material is fed to the centre of a high-speed rotating disc carrying studs so that it is thrown against the studs and the impact kills any insects and destroys their eggs.

Enzymes. Catalysts produced by living cells. They are responsible for most of the reactions carried out in plants and animals. Composed of proteins and destroyed by heat and chemicals that coagulate proteins.

Some enzymes require the aid of coenzymes, most of which are members of the vitamin B complex.

See Specificity, Coenzymes, Substrate *and* Michaelis constant. (BDS, WHSS.)

Epicarp. *See* Flavedo.

Epinephrine. *See* Adrenaline.

Epoxy-. Prefix denoting an oxygen atom attached to two different atoms in a molecule.

Epsom Salts. Magnesium sulphate; acts as a purgative because the osmotic pressure of the solution causes it to retain water in the intestine and so increase the bulk of the faeces. (Clark.)

Equilibrium Humidity. The Relative Humidity of the atmosphere with which the substance under consideration is in equilibrium.

Equilibrium, Nitrogen. *See* Nitrogen balance.

Erepsin. Name given to a mixture of enzymes contained in the intestinal juice, including aminopeptidases and dipeptidases.

Ergocalciferol. *See* Vitamin D.

Ergosterol. Sterol isolated from yeast; when treated with ultraviolet light is converted to vitamin D_2 (ergocalciferol), this is the method of manufacture of the vitamin.

Ergot. Fungus that grows on grasses and cereal grains; the ergot of medical importance is *Claviceps purpurea* that grows on rye. The consumption of infected rye is harmful, causing the disease known as St. Anthony's Fire, and can be fatal.

The active principles in ergot are alkaloids, ergotinine, ergotoxine, ergotamine, ergometrine, etc. Hydrolysis of all of these produces lysergic acid, which is therefore believed to be the active component. Its effect is to increase tone and contraction of smooth muscle, particularly of the pregnant uterus. For this reason ergot is used in obstetrics, but pure ergonovine maleate and ergotonine tartrate are preferable.

Ergotism. Poisoning due to a mould infection of rye; *see* Ergot; occurs from time to time among peoples eating rye bread. Last outbreak in the United Kingdom was 1925 in Manchester when there were 200 cases. Symptoms appear when as little as 1% of ergotized rye is included in the flour.

Eriodictin. *See* Vitamin P.

Erucic Acid. Unsaturated fatty acid with one double bond at C9, $C_{21}H_{41}COOH$, comprising 30–50% of various varieties of rapeseed oil; small amounts in other vegetable and marine oils. Causes fatty infiltration of heart muscle of experimental animals and other changes. Generally accepted that

81

limited amounts of hardened rape seed oil may be tolerated in margarines.

Erythorbic Acid. *See* Ascorbic Acid.

Erythroamylose. Old name for amylopectin.

Erythrocytes. Red blood cells. *See under* Blood, red cells.

Erythropoiesis. Development of the red blood cells; takes place in the bone marrow. (BDS.)

Erythrosine BS. Red colour permitted in foods in most countries. Disodium or potassium salt of 2:4:5:7- tetraiodofluorescein. (In U.S.A. called Red No. 3.)

Used in preserved cherries, sausage and meat and fish pastes; unstable to light and heat.

Erythrotin. Obsolete name for vitamin B_{12}.

Escalopes. Thin pieces of meat or fish.

Essential Amino Acid Pattern, Provisional. The quantities of the essential amino acids considered desirable in the diet. (AEB.)

Essential Amino Acids. *See* Amino acid.

Essential Fatty Acids. Collective name for the two unsaturated fatty acids, linoleic (18 carbon chain, two double bonds) found in vegetable oils, and arachidonic (20 carbon chain, four double bonds) found in animal tissues. They are dietary essentials for experimental animals: formerly called vitamin F, they are also known as the polyunsaturates.

Deficiency in animals causes restriction of growth, abnormalities of skin and hair, damage to reproductive system, and abnor- mal composition of serum and tissue fatty acids. The need for EFA for man is not established (there are claims that babies suffer skin disorders in their absence). It has been claimed that a high dietary level of these unsaturated fatty acids lowers blood cholesterol levels and may therefore be beneficial in atherosclerosis.

EFA are poorly distributed in animal fats and occur mainly in vegetable oils especially safflower, sunflower and corn oils, hence the use of these oils in diets sometimes recommended for the treatment of atherosclerosis. (Sebrell, AEB.)

Essential Oils. Volatile, odorous oils found in plants. They bear no relation to the edible oils since they are not glycerol esters. They are inflammable, soluble in alcohol and ether but not water; used for flavouring foods. Examples are oil of spearmint, oil of bitter almonds, oil of citronella, spirits of turpentine. *See also* Terpenes.

Ester. Chemical name of compound of acid and alcohol, e.g. ethyl alcohol and acetic acid yield ethyl acetate—an ester.

Fats are esters of the trihydric alcohol, glycerol, and long-chain acids like stearic or oleic. *See also* Flavours, synthetic, *and* Waxes. (Cohen.)

Esterases. Name given to a group of enzymes that attack simple esters rather than fats; may be of low specificity as esterase itself, which attacks all simple esters, or of more specific nature such as choline esterase. (WHSS.)

Ester Value. Same as saponification value.

Ethylene. A gas of the formula CH_2CH_2, of interest in its use to assist the ripening of fruits, e.g. 0.4% accelerates the ripening of pears; 0.05% will convert green lemons to yellow in one week at 30–40°C. (Cohen.)

Ethylenediamine Tetra-acetic Acid. Forms stable complexes with metals, hence called sequestering agent or chelating agent. (Trade name Versene.)

Suggested for use in foods to sequester traces of metallic impurities that cause spoilage, and to inhibit certain bacteria. Level used 500 ppm. Not permitted in U.K.

Inhibits the oxidation of vitamin C by trapping the copper that may be present (in acid solution); prevents off-flavours in canned fruits; prevents blackening of asparagus, cauliflowers and potatoes; aids prevention of struvite formation in canned seafoods.

Ethyl Formate. $H.COOC_2H_5$.
Fumigant—used against raisin moth, dried fruit beetle, fig moth, etc.

Flavour—ingredient of lemon and strawberry flavour and artificial rum and arrack.

Chemical intermediate—in synthesis of vitamin B_1, sulphadiazine, etc.

Euglobulin. The name given to that fraction of serum globulin which is precipitated by dialysis of blood serum against distilled water. The name implies that this fraction is a typical globulin by reason of its insolubility in water.

Eukeratins. *See* Keratin.

Euler's Yeast Coenzyme. Nicotinamide adenine dinucleotide.

Eutectic Ice. The solid formed when a mixture of 76.7% water and 23.3% salt (by weight) is frozen. It melts at $-21°C$; 3 lb eutectic ice has the refrigeration effect equivalent to 1 lb solid carbon dioxide; particularly useful in icing fish on board trawlers.

Eutrophia. Normal nutrition.

Evaporation, Flash. A short, rapid application of heat so that a small volume (about 1%) is quickly distilled off carrying with it the greater part of the volatiles. The flash distillate is collected separately from the later distillate and added back to the concentrate to restore the flavour; applied to products such as fruit juices.

Evian Water. Non-gaseous, slightly mineralized; diuretic. (Hutch.)

Exergonic. Energy-supplying reactions, such as oxidation of foodstuffs. (WHSS.)

Exopeptidases. Enzymes that split peptide bonds near the terminal units, i.e. at the ends of the protein chain. According to the older nomenclature they were peptidases, such as aminopeptidase, carboxypeptidase and dipeptidases of the digestive juices. (WHSS.)

Exotoxin. *See* Toxins.

Expansion Ring. In relation to cans refers to the concentric rings stamped into the ends of the can to allow bulging during heat processing without straining the seams unduly. (Baum.)

Expeller Cake. Oilseed after removal of most of the oil by pressing: a valuable source of protein. (Cotton, coconut, groundnut, sunflower, sesame, etc.)

Extensograph. An instrument for measuring the stretching quality of a dough as an index of its baking quality; the dough is stretched in cylindrical form. (KJ.)

Extensometer. An instrument used to measure the stretching strength of a dough as an index of its baking quality. A ball of fermenting dough is fixed on two pins which are moved apart to stretch the dough. *See also* Alveograph. (KJ.)

Extraction Rate. Refers to the yield of flour obtained from wheat in the milling process. 100% extraction (or straight-run flour) is whole-meal flour containing all of the grain; lower extraction rates are the whiter flours from which more of the bran and the germ are excluded, down to a figure of 72% extraction which is the normal white flour of commerce.

"Patent" flours are of lower extraction rate, 30 to 50%, and so comprise mostly the endosperm of the grain.

Analysis: 72% extraction—protein 8–12·5%, fibre 0·1–0·2%; vitamin B_1 0·1 mg, B_2 0·06 mg, nicotinic acid 0·8 mg; Fe 1·5 mg —per 100 g.

80% extraction—protein 9–12·5%, fibre 0·2–0·3%; vitamin B_1 0·25 mg, B_2 0·07 mg, nicotinic acid 1·6 mg; Fe 1·7 mg—per 100 g.

100% extraction (wholemeal) —protein 10–14%, fibre 1·5–2·0%; vitamin B_1 0·4 mg, B_2 0·13 mg, nicotinic acid 5·5 mg; Fe 3·0 mg—per 100 g.

70–72% extraction flour is now fortified to be equivalent to 80% flour and must contain not less than 0·24 mg vitamin B_1, 1·6 mg nicotinic acid, and 1·65 mg iron per 100 g flour. Also fortified with 14 oz *creta praeparata* (chalk) per 280 lb flour. (KJ.)

Extract of Malt. *See* Malt.

Extract of Meat. *See* Meat extract.

Extract of Yeast. *See* Yeast extract.

Extrinsic Factor. *See* Intrinsic factor.

F

Factor I. Obsolete name for vitamin B_6.

Factor U. Cabagin, anti-ulcer factor reported in cabbage leaves, believed to be methyl sulphonium salt of methionine. *See also* Folic Acid.

Factor W. Obsolete name for biotin.

Factor X. Obsolete name for vitamin B_{12}.

Factor Y. Obsolete name for vitamin B_6.

Factor 3. First described in 1941 as an unknown agent present in wheat germ, wheat bran and whey, which protected rats against dietary necrosis of the liver. Also protected against multiple sclerosis in mice, exudative diathesis in chicks and muscular dystrophy in mink. So-called since it was the third agent, the others being vitamin E and cystine, that was shown to be protective.

Now known to be an organic derivative of selenium, and the

protective action of cystine is due to the presence of selenium contamination. Selenium compounds differ in their potency; selenate, selenite, selenium analogues of cystine, cystathione and methionine are effective at 2–3 micrograms per 100 g diet, Factor 3 is effective at 0·7 micrograms; one atom of selenium in this form is equivalent to 700–1000 molecules of vitamin E. Importance to man unknown.

F.A.D. *See* Flavine adenine dinucleotide.

Faeces. Composed of undigested food residues, remains of digestive secretions not reabsorbed, bacteria from the intestinal tract, cells and mucus from the intestinal lining, substances excreted into the intestinal tract. Average 100 g per day. Principal pigment stercobilin. (Hawk.)

Faggot. 1. Small bundle of parsley, thyme, marjoram and bay leaf tied together with cotton and added to the dish being cooked. Also known as Bouquet garni.
2. Dish of liver, chopped, seasoned and baked.

F.A.O. Food and Agriculture Organisation of the United Nations.

Farex. Trade name (Glaxo Laboratories) of an infant cereal food. Protein 12·9%, fat 2·3%, carbohydrate 73%, Ca 885 mg, Fe 24 mg, kcal 348 (1·46 MJ), vitamin B_1 1·4 mg, B_2 1·6 mg—per 100 g. (M&W.)

Farfals. *See* Alimentary pastes.

Farina. General term for starch. More specifically in Gt. Britain refers to potato starch; in U.S.A. is defined as the starch obtained from wheat other than Durum wheat; starch from the latter is semolina.

Farina Dolce. Italian flour made from dried chestnuts.

Farinograph. An instrument for measuring the physical properties of a dough. It measures the time taken for the dough to attain standard consistency in a high-speed mixer, the time it can maintain this consistency and the extent to which the dough falls on further mixing. (KJ.)

Farlene. Trade name (Farley's Infant Food, Plymouth) for a high protein baby food in the form of a dried powder. Composed of wheat flour, high protein wheat flour, soya, peas, milk, wheat gluten and egg, fortified with vitamins and minerals.
Protein 25%, fat 5·5%, carbohydrate 61·5%; kcal 390 (1·6 MJ), Ca 0·8 g, Fe 12 mg, vitamin A 840 μg, B_1 0· 8mg, B_2 0·6 mg, nicotinic acid 15 mg, vitamin C 70 mg, D 18μg—per 100 g.

Fat, Blood. About 590 mg per 100 ml plasma; 150 mg neutral fat, 160 mg cholesterol, 200 mg phospholipid. (BDS.)

Fat-extenders. Substances that permit a reduction of fat content without altering the texture; used in baked products, e.g. glyceryl monostearate.

Fat, Neutral. The triglyceride fats; used in distinction from other lipids, as, for example, in blood, where the subdivision is neutral fat, cholesterol and phospholipid. (BDS.)

Fats. (1) Chemically fats are substances which are insoluble in water but soluble in organic solvents such as ether, chloroform and benzene, and are actual or potential esters of fatty acids. The term includes triglycerides, phospholipids, waxes and sterols; also termed lipids.

(2) In the more general use the term fats refers to the neutral fats which are mixtures of esters of fatty acids with glycerol, i.e. triglycerides. (BDS.)

Fats, High Ratio. Shortenings with a greater proportion of mono- and diglycerides, i.e. superglycerinated (*see also* Superglycinerated fats). These shortenings disperse more readily into doughs, and allow the use of a higher ratio of sugar to flour than with ordinary shortening. *See also* Flour, high ratio. (Bailey.)

Fats, Hydrogenated. *See* Hydrogenated oils.

Fat-soluble Vitamins. Vitamins A, D, E and K; occur in food in solution in the fats. Are stored in the body to a greater extent than the water-soluble.

The distinction into fat-soluble and water-soluble is of historical interest and is convenient for chapter headings in text-books, but otherwise has no significance.

Fatty Acids. Organic acids consisting of carbon chains with a carboxyl group at the end. Simplest is formic acid, $H \cdot COOH$, then acetic acid, CH_3COOH, propionic, butyric, etc.

Longer-chain fatty acids include those found in soap, such as stearic, palmitic and oleic. (BDS.)

They may be saturated fatty acids, in which every carbon atom carries its full quota of hydrogen atoms, or unsaturated, in which there is a shortage of hydrogen atoms compensated for by a double instead of a single bond

linking two adjacent carbon atoms. Such double bonds are susceptible to the addition of oxygen and hence unsaturated fatty acids (and unsaturated fats made from them) are less stable than fully saturated ones. Fats with a large number of double bonds, i.e. highly unsaturated, readily oxidise to resin-like consistency and are the so-called "drying oils" such as linseed and tung oil, used in paints.

Two of the unsaturated fatty acids, namely linoleic and arachidonic, are dietary essentials. *See* Essential fatty acids, *also* Drying oil, Hydrogenated oils *and* Iodine value.

Fatty Acids, Essential. *See* Essential fatty acids.

Fatty Acids, Free. (1) Liberated from triglycerides when subjected to hydrolytic rancidity, therefore determination of FFA is an index of quality of fats.

(2) *See also* Non-esterified Fatty Acids.

Fecula. Name given to foods which are almost solely starch; prepared from roots and stems by grating, e.g. tapioca, sago and arrowroot. *See under separate entries.*

Favism. Acute haemolytic anaemia induced in sensitive subjects by eating broad beans (*Vicia faba*) or by contact with the pollen. Very rare indeed in Western Europe. Due to an inherited metabolic defect, namely a deficiency of the enzyme glucose-6-phosphate dehydrogenase in the red blood cells, causing a reduction in the glutathione level.

Fehling's Solution. *See* Fehling's test.

Fehling's Test. For reducing substances, mostly used to distinguish

86

reducing from non-reducing sugars. Depends upon the reduction of blue cupric hydroxide to yellow cuprous oxide on heating the alkaline solution.

Fehling's solution A is copper sulphate, and solution B is alkaline tartrate; mixed immediately before use to prevent deterioration. *See also* Benedict's test. (Hawk.)

Fennel. *Foeniculum vulgare* (parsley family): seeds contain 10% fixed oil and 6% essential oil, containing anethole, fenchone and terpenes. Leaves used in fish dishes and sauces. (Jacobs, Merory.)

Fenugreek. *Trigonella feonumgraecum.* Leguminous plant eaten as vegetable, seeds used for flavouring. Consumed by women in Orient to help gain weight.

Composition of seeds per 100 g: 29 g protein, 5 g fat, 50 g carbohydrate, 355 kcal (1·46 MJ), 180 mg calcium, 22 mg iron, 0·4 mg B_1, 0·3 mg B_2, 1·5 mg nicotinic acid. (OF, Platt.)

Ferguzade. Trade name (Ferguzade Ltd.) for a glucose beverage.

Ferment. As a noun, the old name for enzyme. As a verb, **to carry** out the process of fermentation.

Fermentation. The transformation or metabolism of compounds without the use of oxygen.

The breakdown of sugar by yeast to carbon dioxide and alcohol is a fermentation, as also is the production by micro-organisms of substances like lactic acid, citric acid, riboflavine. From the point of view of the organism it is an anaerobic method of liberating energy.

In mammalian muscle the first stage in glucose metabolism is anaerobic breakdown to pyruvic acid, followed by oxidation. *See also* Glucose metabolism. (WHSS.)

Fermented Milks. *See* Milks, fermented.

Fermentograph. An instrument for measuring the gas-producing power of a dough. The fermenting dough is contained in a balloon immersed in water and as gas is produced the balloon expands and rises in the water, the rise being measured continuously. (KJ.)

Ferric Ammonium Citrate. Form in which iron is sometimes added to foods. Occurs as brown-red scales (16·5–18·5% iron) and as green scales (14·5–16% iron).

Ferritin. A ferric-hydroxide-phosphate-protein complex (containing 23% iron) present in the cells of the intestinal mucosa, liver, spleen and bone marrow, as a storage form of iron. *See also* Haemosiderin. (BDS.)

Ferrum Redactum. *See* Iron, Reduced.

FFA. Free Fatty Acids. *See* Fatty Acids, Free.

Fibre. General term given to indigestible parts of food. According to the Fertiliser and Feeding Stuffs Act, 1932, fibre is defined as the residue left after successive extractions with petroleum ether, boiling 1·25% sulphuric acid, and 1·25% caustic soda, minus the ash.

Fibrin. (1) *See* Fibrinogen.

(2) Discarded name for one of the muscle proteins, once called "albumin" and "fibrin".

Fibrinogen. One of the proteins of the blood plasma that is responsible for the clotting of blood. Under the influence of thrombin it is converted to fibrin, which is deposited as strands that trap the red cells and form the clot. *See also* Blood, defibrinated, *and* Coagulation, blood. (BDS.)

Fibrous Proteins. *See* Albuminoids.

Ficin. Proteolytic enzyme from the fig.

Fig. *Ficus carica;* eaten fresh, dried (when they contain 50% sugars) and preserved; have mild laxative properties, e.g. syrup of figs is a medicinal preparation.

Composition per 100 g: 1·3 g protein, 11 g carbohydrate, 49 kcal (0·2 MJ), 1 mg iron, 24 μg vitamin A, 0·05 mg B_1, 0·05 mg B_2, 0·4 mg nicotinic acid, 2 mg C.

Dried figs: 4 g protein, 63 g carbohydrate, 269 kcal (1·1 MJ), 200 mg calcium, 4 mg iron, 30 μg vitamin A, 0·1 mg B_1, 0·08 mg B_2, 1·7 mg nicotinic acid, zero vitamin C. (OF, Platt.)

FIGLU Test. Measure of folic acid status of a subject by giving a test dose of histidine. When there is a deficiency of the vitamin formimino glutamate (FIGLU) is excreted in the urine. (AEB.)

Filix Mas. Male fern; contains organic acids, including filicic acid, which have a selective action on, and therefore used in treatment for, tapeworm. (Clark.)

Filled Milk. *See* Milk, filled.

Film Yeasts. *See* Yeast.

Filth Test. Name given to a test originated in U.S.A. for determining the contamination of a food with rodent hairs and insect fragments as an index of the hygienic handling of the food. (KJ.)

Filtrate Factor. *See* Pantothenic acid.

Fines Herbes. A mixture of chopped parsley, chervil, chives and tarragon.

Fining Agents. Substances used to clarify liquids by precipitating and carrying down suspended matter, e.g. egg albumin, casein, bentonite, isinglass, gelatin, etc.

Finnan Haddock. Smoke-cured haddock. (Findon in Scotland.) (Tressler.)

F.I.R.A. Food Industries Research Association.

Fireless Cooker. *See* Haybox.

Fire Point. A term used with reference to frying oils; the temperature at which the fat will sustain combustion. It ranges between 340 and 360°C for different fats. *See also* Smoke point *and* Flash point. (Bailey.)

Firkin. A quarter of a barrel of beer, i.e. 9 imperial gallons; also 56 lb of butter.

Firming Agents. Fresh fruits contain insoluble pectins as a firm gel around the fibrous tissues and keep the fruit firm. Breakdown of cell structure allows conversion of pectin to pectic acid, with loss of firmness. Addition of calcium salts (chloride or carbonate) forms calcium pectate gel which protects the fruit against softening; these are known as firming agents.

Alum is sometimes used to firm pickles. *See also* Pectin. (Jacobs.)

Fish. The composition of all nonfatty fish, such as cod, hake, haddock, flatfish, is similar. *See* Cod; *see also* Fish, fatty.

Fish, Fatty. All fatty fish, such as herring, salmon, trout, mackerel, tuna, have similar composition.

Fillet: 20% protein, 10% fat; 180 kcal, 40 mg Ca, 1·2 mg Fe; 30 μg vitamin A, 0·08 mg

B_1, 0·21 mg B_2, 2·7 mg nicotinic acid—per 100g.

Round: 10% protein, 5% fat; 90 kcal, 19 mg Ca, 0·6 mg Fe; 15 μg vitamin A, 0·04 mg B_1, 0·1 mg B_2, 1·4 mg nicotinic acid —per 100 g. (FAO.)

Fish Ham. Japanese product made from a red fish such as tuna or marlin, pickled with salt and nitrite, mixed with whale meat and pork fat and stuffed into a large sausage-type casing.

Fish Meal. Surplus fish, waste from filleting (fish-house waste) and fish unfit for human consumption are dried in vacuum, by steam, or hot air, and powdered.

The resultant fish meal is a valuable source of protein as animal feedingstuff, or, after deodorisation, as human food, since it contains about 70% protein of biological value up to 75.

That made from white fish is termed white fish meal as distinct from the oily type. The latter is sometimes of very poor quality and is then used as fertilizer.

Fish Paste. Legally must contain not less than 70% fish. (Bell.)

Fish Protein Concentrate. Deodorised, decolourised, defatted fish meal also known as fish flour. Cheap source of protein for enrichment of foods. (FM.)

Approximately 75% protein, BV 75–80.

Fish Sausage. Japanese product made from chopped fish fillet, spiced, flavoured and with preservatives, plus fat and starch, and the whole packed into sausage casing.

Fistula. A short-circuiting connection. E.g. an Eck fistula is a surgical joining of the portal vein to the inferior vena cava, so that the liver is short-circuited. Used as an experimental technique for examining the function of the liver. (BDS.)

Flamber. To light spirit poured over a dish, e.g. brandy on the Christmas pudding.

Flash Evaporation. *See* Evaporation, flash.

Flash-pasteurization. Process in which the material is held at a higher temperature than in normal pasteurization, but for a shorter period. There is less development of the cooked flavour in the shorter period.

For milk, ordinary pasteurization involves heating to 60°C for 30 seconds; in the flash process 74°C for only a few seconds. *See also* Pasteurization.

Flash Point. With reference to frying oils, the temperature at which the decomposition products can be ignited, but will not support combustion. When they will support combustion, this is the fire point. Cottonseed oil: smoke point 232°C, flash point 330°C, fire point 363°C. These points are lowered by the presence of free fatty acids.

Flash point varies with different fats and ranges between 290 and 330°C. (Bailey.)

Flash 18. A method of canning foods (Swift & Co., U.S.A.) under pressure 18 pounds per square inch above atmospheric pressure. The food is sterilised at 121°C and then canned at that temperature, not requiring further heat.

The advantages claimed are improved taste and texture compared with conventional canning, and the possibility of using large containers without overheating the food.

Flat Sours. Bacteria that render canned food sour, without gas production, i.e. the ends of the can are not swelled out but remain flat. They are thermophilic, facultative anaerobes, that attack carbohydrates with the production of acids, lactic, formic, acetic, but without gas formation.

Economically they are the most important of the thermophilic spoilage agents; some species can grow slowly at 25°C and thus spoil products after long storage periods. Type species is *Bacillus stearothermophilus*. (Baum.)

Flavanols. *See* Flavonoids.

Flavanones. *See* Flavonoids.

Flavedo. The coloured outer peel layer of citrus fruits, also called the epicarp or zest. It contains the oil sacs and numerous yellow plastids (green in the unripe fruit, containing chlorophyll; yellow in the ripe fruit, containing carotene and xanthophyll). (Brav.)

Flavin. Also called quercitron. Colour obtained from the quercitron bark (species of oak, *Quercus tinctoria*); legally permitted in food in most countries. Insoluble in water but soluble in alkalies to give yellow colour, changed to brown in air. (Jacobs.)

Flavin. Adenine Dinucleotide. Or FAD. A coenzyme in cellular oxidation consisting of the vitamin riboflavin, attached to two phosphate molecules, and ribose and adenine. *See* Flavoproteins. (WHSS.)

Flavins. Derivatives of iso-alloxazine, as in riboflavin (the 6·7 dimethyl derivative).

Flavone. *See* Flavonoids.

Flavonoids. Compounds widely distributed in nature as pigments in flowers, fruit, vegetables and tree barks.

Structurally the **flavone** nucleus consists of a benzenoid ring fused to gamma-pyrone carrying a second benzenoid ring and bearing a number of hydroxyl groups. **Flavonoids** are flavone glycosides with rhamnose or rhamnoglucose attached at position 3 or 7.

Flavonoids divided into **Flavonols**: hydroxyl group replaces H in flavone nucleus; **Flavanones**—one double bond reduced in the 2 = 3 position; **Flavanals**—hydroxyl group in place of the 0 and reduction of double bond at 4 and reduction of 2 = 3 double bond; **Isoflavones**—benzenoid ring attached to C3 instead of C2.

The term **"bioflavonoid"** is sometimes used instead of vitamin P, *which see*.

Flavonols. *See* Flavonoids.

Flavoproteins. A group of oxidizing enzymes composed of conjugated proteins containing riboflavin (vitamin B_2) as the prosthetic group. There are two classes, those containing flavin mononucleotide, and those containing adenineflavin dinucleotide. The protein itself differs in each specific enzyme.

Examples, amino acid oxidase (which oxidizes amino acids to ketonic acids), cytochrome reductase (part of the oxidation chain in the cell), diaphorase and Warburg's yellow enzyme (also part of the oxidation chain). (WHSS.)

Flavour Potentiator. Substance that enhances the flavours of other substances without itself imparting any characteristic flavour of its own, e.g. mono sodium glutamate, ribotide, as well as small quantities of sugar, salt and vinegar.

Flavour Profile. Method of judging flavour of foods by examination of a list of the separate factors into which the flavour can be analysed—the so-called character notes. (Griswold.)

Flavours, Synthetic. Mostly mixtures of esters, e.g. banana oil—ethyl butyrate and amyl acetate; apple oil—ethyl butyrate, ethyl valerianate, ethyl salicylate, amyl butyrate, glycerol, chloroform and alcohol; pineapple oil—ethyl and amyl butyrates, acetaldehyde, chloroform, glycerol, alcohol. (Jacobs, Merory.)

Flipper. *See* Swells.

Florence Oil. Name given to high grade of olive oil.

Floridean Starch. A glucosan resembling glycogen, obtained from red algae (*Florideae*).

Flour. Generally refers to the ground wheat berry although also used for other cereals and applied to powdered dried materials such as fish flour (deodorized dried fish) potato flour, etc.

The ground wheat berry yields wholemeal flour (100% extraction), whiter flours are obtained by separation of the bran and the germ from the starchy endosperm, (*see* Extraction rate).

The white flour as used in the ordinary white loaf is 70–72%

extraction fortified to contain not less than $0 \cdot 24$ mg vitamin B_1, $1 \cdot 6$ mg nicotinic acid, and $1 \cdot 65$ mg iron per 100 g plus 14 oz of *creta praeparata* (chalk) per 280 lb sack of flour. *See also* Aging, Extraction rate *and* Wheatmeal, National. (KJ.)

Flour, Aging. *See* Aging.

Flour, Bleaching. *See* Aging.

Flour Enrichment. The addition of certain vitamins and minerals to flour: flour must contain not less than:

U.K., mg per 100 g: Vitamin B_1 $0 \cdot 24$, B_2 not added, nicotinic acid $1 \cdot 6$, calcium 14 oz per 280 lb sack as creta.

U.S.A., mg per 100 g: Vitamin B_1 $0 \cdot 44$–$0 \cdot 56$, B_2 $0 \cdot 26$–$0 \cdot 33$, nicotinic acid $3 \cdot 6$–$4 \cdot 4$, iron $2 \cdot 9$–$3 \cdot 7$, calcium not specified. (AEB.)

Flour, Extraction Rate. *See* Extraction rate.

Flour, High Ratio. Flour of very fine and more uniform particle size, treated with chlorine to reduce the gluten strength. Used for making cakes since it is possible to add up to 140 parts of sugar to 100 parts of this flour, whereas only half this quantity of sugar can be incorporated into cakes with ordinary flour. (KJ.) *See* Flour strength.

Flour Improvers. *See* Aging.

Flour, National. *See* Wheatmeal, national.

Flour, Patent. *See* Extraction rate.

Flour, Self-raising. Flour to which have been added chemicals that produce carbon dioxide in the presence of water and heat; the dough is thus aerated without prolonged fermentation. Usually "weaker" flours are used. (*See* Flour Strength.)

91

4

Chemical agents used: sodium carbonate (3 lb 4 oz per 280 lb sack); calcium acid phosphate or sodium pyrophosphate (4¼ lb); or a mixture of these two. Legally self-raising flour must contain not less than 0.4% available carbon dioxide. *See* Baking Powder. (KJ.)

Flour Strength. A property of the flour proteins enabling the dough to retain gas during fermentation to give a "bold" loaf. "Strong" flour is higher in protein content, has greater elasticity and resistance to extension, and greater ability to absorb water.

A "weak" flour gives a loaf that lacks volume. (KJ.) *See also* Farinograph *and* Extensometer.

Flour, Whole Meal. *See* Wholewheat meal.

Fluid Balance. *See* Water balance.

Fluid Bed Dryer. A bed of solid particles is supported on a cushion of hot air jets (fluidized) and the material may be conveyed in this way, while being dried. The method achieves intimate mixing without mechanical damage: it is applicable to particles of a size sufficiently small to become impervious when packed closely and sufficiently large to float on an air cushion (as distinct from fine powders), e.g. cereals, tabletting granules, salt, coffee and dried vegetables.

Flummery. Another name for frumenty.

Fluorescence. The ability to absorb light at one wavelength and radiate part of it at another wavelength. Is used analytically for quantitative measurement by fluorimetry; the intensity of fluorescence being proportional to the amount of material present. For example, vitamin B_2 and thio-chrome, prepared from vitamin B_1, fluoresce. (Hawk.)

Fluoridation. Process of adding traces of fluoride to drinking water to arrest or prevent dental decay. *See* Fluorine.

Fluorimetry. *See* Fluorescence.

Fluorine. An element of the same family as chlorine, bromine and iodine (the halogens). Although it ordinarily occurs in small amounts in plants and animals it is not thought to be essential to either and no deficiency symptoms have ever been produced.

Drinking water ranges in fluoride content between 0.05 and 14 parts per million, and water containing concentrations around 1 ppm helps to protect teeth from decay, although the mechanism of this effect is unknown. Quantities of this order are added to drinking water in enlightened areas to confer this protection. In larger amounts it causes chalky white patches to appear on the surface of the teeth, known as mottled enamel. Excessive doses are toxic and give rise to fluorosis. (GMW.)

F.M.N. Flavine mononucleotide.

Foam-mat Drying. A method of drying food. The liquid concentrate is whipped to a foam with the aid of a foaming agent, spread on a tray and dried in a stream of warm air. It reconstitutes very rapidly with water because of the fine structure of the foam. It has the further advantage that the foam-dried materials hold less water at a given relative humidity than do spray-dried foods and are less liable to cake.

Folacin. *See* Folic Acid.

Folic Acid. Vitamin essential in the synthesis of purines and pyrimidines and certain amino acids. Deficiency causes many symptoms, specifically megaloblastic anaemia. Occurs in foods as a variety of derivatives of pteroylglutamic acid; the active form appears to be formyltetrapteroylglutamic acid (previously called **folinic acid** and **citrovorum factor** or **CF**).

The various forms isolated have given rise to a number of names including **Wills factor, Lactobacillus casei factor, Streptococcus lactis R factor** or **rhizopterin, leucovorin, vitamin M, vitamin B$_c$, factors U, R** and **S.**

The nomenclature adopted by the International Union of Pure and Applied Chemistry does not agree with that of the International Union of Nutritional Sciences (given in brackets).

Generic description **folic acid (folacin).**

Specific compounds, pteroylglutamic acid (folic acid); pteroyldiglutamic acid (folic acid glutamate (2)); pteroyltriglutamic acid (folic acid diglutamate (3)); tetrapteroylglutamic acid (tetrahydrofolic acid).

Found in fresh, dark green vegetables, kidney and liver. The assay is uncertain and amounts are expressed as folate equivalent, being the amount of folic acid activity measured by L. casei assay without pre-treatment to liberate combined forms. Recommended intake according to U.S. National Research Council 0·4 mg per day. (AEB, Sebrell.)

Folinic Acid. *See* Folic acid.

Fondant. Minute sugar crystals in a saturated sugar syrup; used as the creamy filling in chocolates and biscuits and for decorating cakes. Prepared by boiling sugar solution with addition of confectioners' glucose or an inverting agent and cooling rapidly while stirring.

Food. Substances taken in by mouth which maintain life and growth, i.e. supply energy, and build and replace tissue.

Food Additives and Contaminants Committee. Advisory body to Ministry of Agriculture, Fisheries and Food.

Food Industries Research Association. Formerly British Food Manufacturing Industries Research Association—carries out food research for the industry.

Food Phosphate Factor. A term applied to the resistance of bacteria to thermal destruction; defined as the ratio of resistance to heat when present in a food, to the resistance when in phosphate buffer (at pH 6·98). The protective action of the ingredients of food renders the bacteria more resistant than in buffer.

Factor 360 is the thermal death time at 100°C of the most resistant strain of *Clostridium botulinum* that has been isolated. (Baum, Tanner.)

Food Poisoning. May be due to (1) contamination with harmful bacteria; (2) toxic chemicals; (3) allergic reaction to certain proteins; (4) chemical contamination.

The commonest bacterial contamination is due to salmonellae, staphylococci and *Clostridium welchii.* Staphylococcal poisoning causes rapid symptoms within 2–4 hours of abdominal cramp, nausea, vomiting and diarrhoea; recovery is rapid.

Salmonellae produce an endotoxin which is not destroyed by cooking and causes acute gastroenteritis after 12–24 hours. It is not often fatal but nausea, vomiting and diarrhoea may persist several weeks.

Very rarely food poisoning is due to *Clostridium botulinum*, i.e. botulism, *which see.* (Baum, Tanner.)

Food Scientist. One who studies the basic chemical and physical, biochemical and biophysical properties of foods and their constituents.

Food Standards Committee. Advisory body to Ministry of Agriculture, Fisheries and Food.

Food Technologist. One who applies food science to the processing of foods to preserve them, improve flavour, texture, appearance and other desirable properties, and manufactures foods from basic materials.

Food Yeast. *See* Yeast.

Foots. *See* Soapstock.

Force. Trade name (Fincken and Co. Ltd.) for a breakfast cereal made from wheat flakes. Not fortified with added vitamins, natural content 0·07 mg vitamin B_1 and 0·07 mg vitamin B_2—per 100 g.

Forcemeat. Savoury seasoned stuffing for fish, meat and poultry made of sage, parsley, onion and thyme.

Formula 21. "Slimming" preparation (Greenwood Laboratories Ltd.) composed of methyl cellulose and glucose, with flavour and colour, plus vitamin B_1 1·1 mg, B_2 2·7 mg, nicotinic acid 10·9 mg, reduced iron 10·9 mg, Ca 675 mg —per oz.

Fortifex. Protein-rich baby food (30% protein) developed in Brazil; made from maize, defatted soya flour with added vitamins A, B_1, B_2, calcium carbonate and methionine.

Fortification. *See* Enrichment.

Fovantini. *See* Alimentary pastes.

FPC. Fish Protein Concentrate.

Fractional Test Meal. Method of examining secretion of gastric juices of patients. The stomach contents are sampled at intervals via a stomach tube after a test meal of gruel. It is usual to test for total and free acidity, and in addition peptic activity may be measured. (BDS.)

Frangipane. Originally a jasmine perfume, which gave its name to an almond cream flavoured with the perfume. The term is used for cake-filling made from eggs, milk and flour with flavouring; and also for the pastry filled with an almond-flavoured mixture. (GH.)

Frankfurters. *See* Sausage.

Frappé. Egg-white and sugar syrup whipped until so aerated that the density reaches 5 lb per gallon.

Freeze Concentration. Concentration of a liquid by freezing out pure ice leaving a more concentrated solution; of interest in the concentration of fruit juices, vinegar and beer.

Freeze Drying. A method of drying in which the material is frozen and subjected to high vacuum. The ice sublimes off as water vapour without melting. Materials dried in this way are damaged little if at all.

Freeze-dried food is very porous since it occupies the same volume as the original and so rehydrates rapidly. There is less loss of flavour and texture than with most other methods of drying. Controlled heat may be applied to the process without melting the frozen material—this is **accelerated freeze drying.**

Freezerburn. A change in the texture of frozen meat, fish and poultry during storage due to sublimation of the ice.

French Dressing. Temporary emulsion of oil and acid in distinction to mayonnaise which is a stable emulsion. Heavy French Dressing is a similar product stabilized with pectin or vegetable gum.

Frenching. Breaking up the fibres of meat by cutting, usually diagonally or in a criss-cross pattern.

French Mustard. *See* Mustard.

Fricassée. *See* Cooking.

Frigi-canning. A process of preserving food by controlled heating, sufficient to destroy the vegetative form of micro-organisms (and possibly to damage spores sufficiently to prevent germination) followed by sealing aseptically and storing at a low temperature but not at freezing point.

Froment. Trade name (John H. Heron Ltd.) for a wheat germ preparation. Protein 28·5%, fat 7·7%, carbohydrate 44·4%, kcal 360 (1·5 MJ), vitamin B_1 0·45 mg, B_2 0·2 mg, E 8 mg, Fe 2·7 mg—per 100 g.

Fructofuranose. Fructose formulated as the five-membered furan ring. (BDS.)

Fructopyranose. Fructose formulated as the six-membered pyranose ring. (BDS.)

Fructosan. A complex built up of units of fructose. E.g. Inulin.

Fructose. A six-carbon sugar—$C_6H_{12}O_6$—differing from glucose in containing a ketonic group (on carbon 2) instead of an aldehydic group (which glucose has on carbon one).

Found as the free sugar in some fruits and in honey and combined with glucose as sucrose. Prepared by the hydrolysis of inulin from the Jerusalem artichoke. Alternative names fruit sugar and laevulose; 173% as sweet as sucrose.

Fructose rotates polarized light to the left hence the name laevulose, in distinction from glucose which rotates polarized light to the right. *See also* Invert sugar. (Hawk.)

Fruit. Fleshy seed-bearing part of plants (including tomato, usually called a vegetable). Contain negligible protein and fat; carbohydrate varies from 3% in melon to 25% in banana. Carbohydrate occurs as glucose, fructose, sucrose, starch, pectin and cellulose. Cellulose adds bulk to the diet; pectin gives jelling power to fruit.

During ripening of fruit starch changes to sugars. Fruits are a good source of potassium and vitamin C, and some are a useful source of carotene and iron. (FB.)

Fruit, Canned. The fruit is usually canned in a sugar solution (*see* Syrup) and hence the energy content is greater than that of the fresh fruit.

For example fresh peaches (without stones) 9·1% carbohydrate, 37 kcal (0·15 MJ), per 100 g; canned, 17·2% carbohydrate, 66 kcal (0·27 MJ) per 100 g.

Vitamin loss is about 50%, e.g. peaches lose half of the carotene, B_1, B_2, nicotinic acid and vitamin C in canning. (M&W.)

Fruit Cordials. *See* Soft drinks.

Fruit, Dried. (Dried figs, dates, prunes and raisins, all have similar analyses).

Protein 2·5%, fat 0·6%; 255 kcal (1·06 MJ), Ca 73 mg, Fe 2·7 mg, vitamin A 21 μg, B_1 0·11 mg, B_2 0·1 mg, nicotinic acid 1·5 mg, vitamin C nil—per 100 g. (FAO.)

Fruit Drinks. *See* Soft drinks.

Fruit-squash. *See* Soft drinks.

Frumenty. Whole wheat stewed in water for 24 hours until the grains have burst and set in a thick jelly, then boiled with milk. (GH.)

Frying. Involves rapid evaporation of water. In the case of meat nearly all the extractives are left in the meat and the losses are smaller than in roasting. (*See also* Connective tissue.) About 10–20% loss of vitamin B_1, 10–15% loss of B_2 and nicotinic acid.

Fish loses 20% B_1. (Johnson.)

Fudge. Caramel in which crystallization of the sugar (graining) is deliberately induced by the addition of fondant (saturated syrup containing sugar crystals).

Fumeol. Refined smoke with the bitter principles removed; used for preparing "liquid" smokes for dipping foods such as fish to give them a smoked flavour. *See also* Smoking.

Fungi. Sub-division of *Thallophyta*, plants without differentiation into root, stem and leaf; cannot photosynthesise, all are parasites or saprophytes. Varieties of penicillium, aspergillus etc. are the cause of deterioration in foods in the presence of oxygen and relative humidity of at least 70%. On the other hand varieties of penicillium such as *P. cambertii* and *P. rocquefortii* are desirable in certain cheeses.

Among the edible fungi are mushrooms, *Agaricus campestris*.

Experimentally, varieties such as Graphium, Fusarium and Rhizopus are grown on waste carbohydrates as a potential food; their fibrillar structure offers textural advantages in foods manufactured from them. (Baum, FM.)

Fusel Oil. Alcoholic fermentation produces about 95% alcohol and 5% fusel oil—a mixture of organic acids, higher alcohols (propyl, butyl and amyl), aldehydes and esters.

Present in low concentration in wines and beer, and higher concentration in pot-still spirit. On maturation of the liquor the fusel oil changes and imparts the special flavour to the spirit. (Clark.)

Fussol. Monofluoroacetamide—a systemic insecticide for treating fruit.

Fustic. Colouring matter obtained from the tree *Chlorophora tinctoria* or *Maclura tinctoria*. Two colour agents present, morin, sparingly soluble in water but soluble in alcohol, and maclurin, more soluble. Both are yellow but altered by alkali and metals. (Jacobs.)

G

Gaffelbitar. "Semi-preserved" herring product in which microbial growth is checked by the addition of salt at a concentration of 10–12%, and sometimes by the addition of benzoic acid as preservative.

Anchovy is a similar product.

Galacticol. Dulcitol, *which see*.

Galactomin. Trade name (Trufood Ltd.) for preparation free from lactose and galactose used for patients suffering from lactose intolerance. (AEB.)

Galactosaemia. Inherited inability to metabolize the sugar galactose beyond the formation of its phosphate. Unless galactose is excluded from the diet the subject suffers mental retardation, growth failure, vomiting and jaundice. Special baby foods are therefore prepared entirely free from lactose. (AEB.)

Galactose. A six-carbon sugar differing from glucose only in the position of the hydroxyl group on carbon four.

It occurs mainly linked with glucose to form lactose (milk sugar), and is also present in the galactolipids of nerve tissue. Has 32% of the sweetness of sucrose *See also* Cerebrosides. (Hawk.)

Galantine. A dish of white meat or poultry, boned, rolled, cooked with herbs, glazed with aspic jelly and served cold. (GH.)

Galenicals. Crude drugs, infusions, decoctions, and tinctures prepared from medicinal plants.

Gallates. Salts and esters of gallic acid, found in many plants. Used in making dyes and inks and medicinally as an astringent.

Propyl, octyl and dodecyl gallates are legally permitted antioxidants; 100 ppm permitted in fats and vitamin oils, 80 ppm in butter-fat for manufacturing, 1,000 ppm in essential oils for flavouring. (Bell.)

Gall-bladder. Organ situated in the liver that stores the bile manufactured by the liver. (BDS.)

Gallon. Imperial gallon is 4.546 litres:(= 10 lb of water at 17°C.).

U.S. gallon is 3·7853 litres: Imperial gallon = 1·2 U.S. gallons.

Gallstones. Stones formed in the gall bladder or in the bile duct. In the latter they obstruct the flow of bile and the result is jaundice. The stones consist of cholesterol and calcium salts of bilirubin, carbonate or phosphate; also called biliary calculi. Treatment includes a low-fat diet. (BDS.)

Game. Non-domesticated (i.e. wild) animals and birds.

Gammon. Hind legs of bacon pig, cured while still part of carcass.

Garbanzo. Chickpea (*Cicer arietinum*).

Garlic. Bulb of *Allium sativum* of the lily family. Grows wild in Sicily, Italy and S. France. Has a pungent odour and strong taste and is used in various types of sausage and cold meat.

The bulb has expectorant and antiseptic properties and contains an antibiotic, allicin.

Garlic salt is dried powdered garlic mixed with salt with the addition of starch to prevent caking.

Gas Storage. Method of storing fruit and vegetables in fresh condition, applied mostly to apples and pears. Storage in gas at $4 \cdot 5°C$ doubles the "life" of the fruit compared to $4 \cdot 5°C$ without gas.

Gas mixture varies with type of fruit. Bramley seedlings produce their own gas by respiration; Cox's Orange Pippin requires $2 \cdot 5\%$ oxygen, 5% carbon dioxide and 92% nitrogen. Some varieties require good ventilation and cannot be gas-stored.

Eggs can be stored 9 months in 60% carbon dioxide. Control of growth of micro-organisms also achieved by gas, e.g. obligate aerobes, like moulds, inhibited by storage in nitrogen or vacuum; addition of carbon dioxide limits growth of bacteria in cold store and delays germination of mould spores.

Chilled beef in 10% carbon dioxide can be stored 60–70 days. Ozone useful in storage of eggs and soft fruits at level of few parts per million. (Baum.)

Gastric Secretion. Gastric juice consists of the enzymes pepsin, rennin and lipase, together with mucin and hydrochloric acid. The acid is secreted by the parietal cells at a strength of $0 \cdot 16 N = 0 \cdot 5 - 0 \cdot 6\%$ acid.

The pepsin is secreted by the chief cells, and the mucin by the mucous cells. Pepsin requires an acid medium to function and breaks down proteins to proteoses.

Sole function of rennin is to coagulate milk. The small amount of lipase present splits only a very small proportion of the fat. *See also* Fractional test meal. (BDS.)

Gastrin. Hormone secreted by the pyloric antrum of the stomach under the influence of certain foods (especially meat) and by distension of the stomach. The gastrin enters the blood stream and stimulates the secretion of gastric juice. (BDS.)

Gastro-Intestinal Tract. Term covering the whole of the digestive tract, from the mouth to the anus. Average length $4 \cdot 5$ metres (15 feet). (BDS.)

Gefillte Fish. Also spelled gefilte and gefültte. Literally German for stuffed fish. The dish is of Russian or Polish origin, where it is commonly referred to as Jewish fish. The whole fish is served and the filletted portion chopped and stuffed back between the skin and the backbone. More frequently today, the fish is simply chopped into a pulp and made into balls.

In the United Kingdom has been legally referred to as "fish cutlets in fish sauce" instead of a fish cake.

Gel. A sol or colloidal suspension that has set to a jelly. (Hawk.)

Gelatin. A water-soluble protein prepared from collagen by boiling with water, or from bones (*see* Ossein gelatin). There are several grades used for different purposes, e.g. 40 mesh for confectionery; crumble gelatin for meat canning; sheet gelatin for table jellies; 10 mesh for pharmaceutical capsules.

As a protein it is of poor nutritive value since it lacks tryptophan. (Jacobs).

Gelatin Sugar. Glycine.

Gelometer. *See* Bloom gelometer.

Generic Descriptor. *See* Vitamin.

Genetic Disease. Inherited disease due to a metabolic defect such as the absence of a particular enzyme; termed an **inborn error of metabolism.** Some can be treated by dietary means such as phenylketonuria, galactosaemia, maple syrup urine disease, cystic fibrosis, disaccharide intolerance and coeliac disease. *See under separate entries, see also* Alcaptonuria *and* Tyrosinosis.

Genetic Disease. In connection with food, the inherited inability to metabolise certain dietary factors, often with harmful results. *See* Phenylketonuria, Galactosaemia, Alcaptonuria, Tyrosinosis.

Gentiobiose. Two molecules of glucose joined 1·6′—beta.

Gerber Test. Test for fat in milk. When sulphuric acid and milk are mixed, heat develops, the organic matter dissolves, but not the fat. This separates, aided by the addition of amyl alcohol. The reaction is carried out in a Gerber bottle with a thin, graduated neck, in which the fat collects, and is measured. Used for routine analyses of milk. (Davis.)

Germ. In reference to cereals that part of the grain which gives rise to the new plant; comprises 2·5–3·5% of the berry (except maize —8%). Consists of the embryo proper (plumule and radicle) and the scutellum, a membrane separating the germ from the endosperm.

Composition 6–11% fat, 17–27% protein, 4–5% ash, 2–4% fibre. Rich in vitamins of the B group and E. The scutellum contains the greater part of the thiamin of the grain (about 50%) but only small amounts of the riboflavin and nicotinic acid.

In low-extraction flours much of the germ is removed with consequent reduction in the nutritive value. Certain speciality loaves, e.g. Hovis, include extra wheat germ. (KJ.)

Ghee. Clarified butter fat after the evaporation of the water; made from the milk of cow, buffalo, goat or sheep.

Widely used in India; the Egyptian equivalent is samna or semnah. Does not turn rancid as quickly as butter. (Davis & Mac.)

Gherkin. *Cucumis anguria.* Young green cucumber of small variety, used for pickling.

Gibberellins. Derivatives of gibberellic acid, originally found in the fungus *Gibberella fujikuroi* growing on rice. Causes mutant dwarf forms of plants to revert to normal size; accelerates germination and used in brewing to accelerate the germination of barley.

Gin. An alcoholic spirit distilled from grain fermentation and flavoured with juniper berries. The name is derived from the French, Genièvre, meaning juniper. There are two main kinds of English gin, dry and sweetened.

Ginger. Rhizome of *Zingiber officinale;* used as a flavouring; pungency due to non-volatile compounds including gingerol, zingerone and shogool. Preserved ginger made from young fleshy rhizomes boiled with sugar and packed in syrup.

Composition per 100 g: 2·5 g

99

protein, 0·8 g fat, 11 g carbohydrate, 2·1 g fibre, 63 kcal (0·26 MJ), 2·5 mg iron, 0·8 mg nicotinic acid, 4 mg vitamin C. (Merory, Platt.)

Glasgow Magistrate. Term for Red Herring, *which see.*

Gliadin. One of the proteins of wheat, differentiated by its solubility in 70% alcohol; a prolamin.

Globins. Basic proteins that differ from histones since they are rich in histidine, deficient in isoleucine and contain average amounts of arginine and tryptophan.

Globins are simple proteins themselves (i.e. free from non-protein substances) but are often found as the protein portion of conjugated proteins, e.g. globin from haemoglobin. (Hawk.)

Globulins. Class of proteins that are heat-coagulated and soluble in dilute solutions of salts; they differ from albumins in being insoluble in water. They occur in blood, i.e. serum globulins, in milk, i.e. lactoglobulins, and edestin from hemp seed and amandin from almond are also globulins. (Hawk.)

Glossitis. *See* Ariboflavinosis.

Glucagon. A hormone secreted by the pancreas which causes an increase in blood sugar probably by increasing the breakdown of liver glycogen. (DP.)

Glucaric Acid. Alternative name for saccharic acid, the dicarboxylic acid derived from glucose.

Glucide. Name occasionally used for saccharine.

Glucitol. Or **Glycitol.** Obsolete names for sorbitol.

Glucoascorbic Acid. Homologue of ascorbic acid containing an extra CHOH group. Acts as an antagonist to the vitamin; its administration can cause scurvy in animals that do not normally require the vitamin in the diet. (Hawk.)

Glucocorticoids. Obsolescent term for the steroid hormones of the adrenal cortex which affect carbohydrate metabolism. *See* Adrenal glands. (BDS.)

Glucofuranose. Glucose formulated as the five-membered furan ring. (BDS.)

Gluconeogenesis. Formation of glucose and glycogen from non-carbohydrate sources via glucose. (BDS.)

Gluconic Acid. The acid derived from glucose by oxidizing the hydroxyl group on carbon atom number one. The acid produced when carbon six is oxidized is glucuronic acid; the oxidation of both carbons one and six yields saccharic acid. (BDS.)

Glucono-delta-lactone. Lactone of gluconic acid; slowly liberates acid at a controlled rate; used in chemically leavened bread, i.e. to liberate carbon dioxide from bicarbonate instead of using yeast. (*See* Bread, aerated.) Also used in bland-flavoured sherbets and to reduce fat-absorption in products such as doughnuts.

Glucopyranose. Glucose formulated as the six-membered pyran ring. (BDS.)

Glucosamine. Amino derivative of glucose. Constituent of many complex polysaccharides. (BDS).

Glucosan. A complex of glucose molecules, e.g. starch, cellulose and glycogen. Inulin is a complex of fructose molecules and is a fructosan. The general name for the polysaccharide complexes made up from simple hexose units is hexosans.

Glucose. Also known as dextrose, grape sugar and blood sugar.

A simple six carbon sugar (hexose) $C_6H_{12}O_6$, occurring naturally in plant tissues and formed by the hydrolysis of starch. It is the major product of the digestion of carbohydrates in the intestine and is the form in which the carbohydrate is absorbed into the bloodstream. During digestion sucrose is hydrolysed to glucose and fructose, lactose to glucose and galactose, and starches and maltose to glucose.

Normal levels in blood lie between 80 and 100 mg per 100 ml, any surplus being converted to glycogen and stored as such in the liver and muscles. Glycogen is broken down to glucose when required for energy.

Energy is liberated by the oxidation of glucose to carbon dioxide and water at the rate of 3·9 kcal per g or 686 kcal per gram-mol.

Used in the manufacture of confectionery since its mixture with fructose prevents sucrose from crystallizing (*See* Boiled sweets) and it is less sweet than sucrose being 74% as sweet. *See also* Glucose syrup *and* Glucose metabolism. (BDS.)

Glucose, Liquid. *See* Glucose syrup.

Glucose Metabolism. Process through which glucose is broken down in living tissues to provide energy. The overall reaction follows the equation:—

$$C_6H_{12}O_6 + 6O_2 = 6\ CO_2 + 6\ H_2O + 3·9\ \text{kcal per gram}$$

of glucose, but in detail the process involves about 20 stages.

The first series of stages does not require oxygen and is referred to as **glycolysis** or glucose fermentation. The glucose is converted through a number of sugar phosphates to 3-carbon sugars (trioses) and then to pyruvic acid.

The latter is oxidized in a series of reactions known as the **Krebs** or **tricarboxylic acid cycle** ultimately to carbon dioxide and water. The energy is liberated from the glucose at certain of these stages.

Surplus blood glucose is stored in the muscles as glycogen, and when energy is required the latter is converted first to glucose and then follows the metabolic pathway outlined above. (WHSS.)

Glucose Oxidase. *See* Notatin.

Glucose Syrup. A clear, viscous, colourless syrup produced by the partial hydrolysis of starch, usually maize or potato. The product is of variable composition depending upon the degree of hydrolysis and includes glucose, maltose, dextrins and trisaccharides.

Widely used as a sweetening agent in confectionery, and particularly useful in sugar confectionery since it prevents crystallization of the sugar on cooling. Also known as **corn syrup** (especially in U.S.A.), **starch syrup, confectioner's glucose** and **liquid glucose.** *See also* Dextrose Equivalent Value. (Jacobs.)

Glucose Tolerance. The ability of the body to deal with a large dose of glucose; used as a test for *diabetes mellitus.*

The fasting subject ingests 50 g of glucose and the blood sugar is measured at intervals. In the normal individual the fasting sugar level is approx. 80–100 mg per 100 ml, rises to about 150 mg, and returns to the starting level within 1–1½ hours. In diabetics the sugar rises to higher levels and takes longer to return. The plotted results form a glucose-tolerance curve. (BDS.)

Glucose-Tm. A term used in measuring the efficiency of the kidneys; it is the maximum rate of reabsorption of glucose by the kidney tubules. Tm is the maximum reabsorptive capacity. (BDS.)

Glucosides. Complexes of substances with glucose. General name for such complexes with other sugars is glycosides. (BDS.)

Glucostatic Mechanism. Theory that appetite depends on the difference between arterial and venous levels of glucose; when the difference falls to 8 mg %, the hypothalamus is stimulated and hunger results.

Glucuronic Acid. The acid derived from glucose by the oxidation of the group on carbon atom number six. Many toxic substances are excreted from the body combined with glucuronic acid as glucuronides. It is also present in various complex polysaccharides. (BDS.)

Glutamate, Sodium. Sodium salt of the amino acid, glutamic acid. First introduced as a flavouring agent under the Japanese name of **Aginomoto.** Enhances the flavour of some foods, especially meat and vegetables, apparently by stimulating the taste buds. Frequently added to soup mixes and meat products. Commercially manufactured from sugar beet pulp and wheat gluten.

Glutamic acid has two acidic groups and it is the mono sodium salt, known as **MSG,** that has this flavour property.

Glutamic Acid. A non-essential amino acid; amino glutaric acid. Involved in transamination reactions in the body; its amide is glutamine. The sodium salt, monosodium glutamate or MSG, originally known as Aginomoto, is used to enhance the flavour of savoury dishes and is frequently added to canned meat and soups. (BDS, AEB.)

Glutamine. Amide of the amino acid, glutamic acid; formed by the addition of ammonia to glutamic acid.

Occurs in plants, where it appears to function as a storage depot for ammonia, and as part of the urea cycle in animals. (WHSS.)

Glutathione. A tripeptide of glycine, glutamic acid and cysteine; occurs in animal tissues and believed to function as an oxidation-reduction system. (BDS.)

Glutelins. Proteins insoluble in water and neutral salt solutions but soluble in dilute acids and alkalies, e.g. wheat glutenin. (Hawk.)

Gluten. Name given to protein fraction of wheat; the part of the flour that has the extensible properties essential for bread making. Too much gluten gives too strong a dough and it is "weakened" by the addition of an enzyme, or malt flour rich in the enzyme, to break down a limited amount of the gluten.

Prepared from flour by washing out the starch. Gluten in the undamaged state with its extensible properties is called **vital gluten.** Overheating destroys these properties and the result is **devitalized gluten.** (KJ.)

Gluten-free Foods. Formulated without any wheat or rye protein (although the starch may be used) for subjects suffering from coeliac disease, *which see.* (AEB.)

Glutose. A hexose sugar carrying a keto group on carbon 3; not metabolized and non-fermentable.

Glycamines. Derivatives of sugar alcohols in which the CH_2OH group is replaced by CH_2NH_2, e.g. ethanolamine, and ribamine (part of vitamin B_2).

Glycerides. Esters of glycerol with fatty acids. As glycerol possesses three hydroxyl groups it can combine with three molecules of fatty acid to form a **triglyceride** or simple fat.

If all three molecules of fatty acid are the same, a simple triglyceride is formed, e.g. tristearin, triolein; mixed glycerides may be formed such as distearo-olein and stearo-oleo-palmitin. *See also* Glycerol, Superglycinerated fats, *and* Fats.

Glycerides, Partial. *See* Acetoglycerides *and* Superglycinerated fats.

Glycerine. *See* Glycerol.

Glycerol. A trihydric alcohol, chemically 1, 2, 3 propane triol, $CH_2OH.CHOH.CH_2OH$, popularly called **glycerine.**

Simple or neutral fats are esters of glycerol with three molecules of fatty acid, i.e. triglycerides.

Glycerol is a clear, colourless, odourless, viscous liquid, sweet to taste; it is made from fats by alkaline hydrolysis (saponification). Used as a solvent for flavours, as humectant to keep foods moist, and in cake batters to improve texture and slow down staling.

See also Superglycinerated Fats *and* Glycerides. (Bailey.)

Glycerose. Simple, three-carbon sugar, derived from the corresponding alcohol, glycerol. Formula $CHO.CHOH.CH_2OH$. (BDS.)

Glyceryl Lacto-stearate. Also known as lacto-stearin. Formed by glycerolysis of hydrogenated soya bean oil followed by esterification with lactic acid, which results in a mixture of mono and di-glycerides and their lactic mono esters. Used as an emulsifier in shortenings.

Glyceryl Monostearate. *See* Superglycinerated fats.

Glycine. A non-essential amino acid, chemically amino acetic acid, CH_2NH_2COOH. Clinically used as a buffer for gastric acidity. (BDS.)

Has 70% of the sweetness of sucrose and is sometimes used mixed with saccharine as a sweetening agent.

Glycinin. Globulin protein in soya bean.

Glycitol. Obsolete name for sorbitol.

Glycocholic Acid. *See* Bile.

Glycocoll. Obsolete name for the amino acid glycine.

Glycogen. Storage form of carbohydrate in the animal body, in the liver and muscles. Composed of glucose units; is synthesized from the blood sugar and broken down to blood sugar as required. Sometimes referred to as animal starch.

In an adult the glycogen stored in the muscles is about 250 g and in the liver about 100 g.

Since glycogen is rapidly broken down to glucose immediately an animal is killed, meat and animal liver do not contain glycogen, the

103

only dietary sources are oysters, cockles, muscles, scallops, clams, whelks and winkles that are eaten virtually alive and contain about 5% glycogen. (BDS.)

Glycogenesis. Synthesis of glycogen from glucose, as, for example, occurs in the muscle where glucose is stored as glycogen; facilitated by insulin. (BDS.)

Glycogenolysis. Breakdown of glycogen to glucose when this is required for the production of energy. (WHSS.)

Glycoleucine. Obsolete name for norleucine.

Glycolysis. There are two parts to the total breakdown of glucose, the first is anaerobic and called glucose fermentation or glycolysis. This ends at the formation of pyruvic acid. The second part is an oxidation and the series of reactions is the Krebs' tricarboxylic acid cycle, or the citric acid cycle. This completes the breakdown to carbon dioxide and water. *See also* Glucose metabolism. (BDS.)

Glycoproteins. Conjugated proteins, e.g. mucins, proteins containing a uronic acid, found in vitreous humour; mucoids, contain a polysaccharide such as polymerized glucosamine-mannose, e.g. serum mucoid, ovomucoid; sulphomucins, contain sulphuric acid, uronic acid and either chondrosamine or glucosamine, e.g. found in cartilage, cornea, gastric mucosa. (Hawk.)

Glycosides. Compounds consisting of a sugar attached to another molecule. When glucose is the sugar they are called glucosides. A wide variety occur in plants and some are useful medicinally, such as digitalis and rutin. (BDS.)

Glycosuria. Appearance of glucose in the urine, as in diabetes and after the administration of drugs that lower the renal threshold. *See also* Phlorrhizin. (Hawk.)

Glycyrrhiza. Liquorice, *Glycyrrhiza glabra.* Extract of root long used to flavour medicines because of sweet taste due to calcium and potassium salts of glycyrrhizic acid.

Glycyrrhizin. Triterpenoid glycoside (a saponin of the corresponding glycyrrhetinic acid with an attached disaccharide) from liquorice root. 50–100 times as sweet as sucrose but with undesirable after-taste.

GMS. Abbreviation for glyceryl monostearate. *See* Superglycerinated fats.

Goitre. Enlargement of the thyroid gland, seen as a swelling in the neck, due to deficiency of iodine in the diet and to the presence of "goitrogens" in certain foods such as *Brassicas* and peanuts.

Supplementation with an iodide often prevents the condition, hence the use of iodized salt. (BDS, AEB.) *See also* Thyroid Gland *and* Cretinism.

Gold Thioglucose. Chemical used to cause obesity in experimental animals by stimulation of the appetite through damage to the hypothalamus.

Gooseberry. Berry of shrub, *Ribes grossularia.* Protein 1·0%, fat 0·4%, kcal 42 (0·18 MJ), Ca 22 mg, Fe 0·5 mg, vitamin A 90 μg, B_1 0·04 mg, B_2 0·02 mg, nicotinic acid 1 mg, vitamin C 33 mg—per 100 g. (FAO.)

Gooseberry, Cape. Fruit of *Physalis peruviana,* also called Golden Berries. *See* Berry, Golden.

Gooseberry, Indian. *See* Emblic.

Gossypol. Toxic substance found in cottonseed, which must be removed before the seed-cake can be used as foodstuff. It is a bright-yellow pigment of undetermined composition found in pigment gland in the seed. If present in chick diet it causes the eggs to discolour on storage. (Bailey.)

Gourds. Vegetables of the family *Cucurbitaceae*, including cucumber, marrow, pumpkin, squash, gourd and melon.

Calabash or bottle gourd (*Lagenaria vulgaris*), ash gourd (*Benicasa hispida*), snake gourd (*Trichosanthes anguina*), cucumber (*Cucumis sativus*), vegetable marrow (*Cucurbita pepo*), pumpkin, (*Cucurbita moschata*), squash (*Cucurbita maxima*), coocha or chayote (*Sechium edule*), cantaloupe melon (*Cucumis melo*), water melon (*Citrullus vulgaris*).

All contain more than 90% water and about 1% protein and have little food value apart from vitamin C at 10 mg per 100 g. In addition yellow pumpkin contains 900 μg vitamin A per 100 g. Melons are sometimes grown for their seeds which contain 20–40% oil and 20% protein. (TND.)

Graham Bread. Whole-wheat bread in which the bran is very finely ground. Graham cakes are made from whole meal flour and milk. The name is that of a miller of whole-meal flour who advocated its use in the United States (Treatise on Bread and Bread Making, 1837).

Gram-negative and Gram-positive. Bacteria fall into two groups depending on whether or not they retain crystal-violet dye after staining and decolorizing with alcohol. Named after Danish botanist Gram. (Baum.)

Grams, Indian. Name given to small dried peas, e.g. green gram (*Phaseolus aureus*), black gram (*Phaseolus mungo*), red gram (*Cajanus indicus*). (TND.)

Granadilla. *See* Passion fruit.

Grapefruit. Fruit of *Citrus maxima*. Protein 0·4%, fat 0·1%, kcal 25 (0·1 MJ), Fe 0·3 mg, vitamin A 3 μg, B$_1$ 0·03 mg, B$_2$ 0·01 mg, nicotinic acid 0·2 mg, vitamin C 28 mg—per 100 g. (FAO.)

The pith contains a bitter glucoside naringin, *which see*.

Grapefruit, Bitter Principle. *See* Naringin.

Grapenuts. Trade name (Alfred Bird and Sons Ltd.) for a breakfast cereal made from wheat.

Protein 11·7%, fat 3·0%, carbohydrate 75·2%; Ca 48 mg, Fe 5·6 mg, kcal 358 (1·5 MJ)—per 100 g. (M&W.)

Grapes. Fruit of the vine (*Vitis* species). Protein 0·7%, fat 0·4%; kcal 62 (0·26 MJ), Fe 0·6 mg, vitamin A 20 μg, B$_1$ 0·06 mg, B$_2$ 0·04 mg, nicotinic acid 0·2 mg, vitamin C 4 mg—per 100 g. (FAO.)

Grape Sugar. Alternative name for glucose.

GRAS. "Generally regarded as safe". Designation given to food additives when further evidence is required before the substance can be classified more precisely (U.S.A. usage).

Grass Tetany. Magnesium deficiency in cattle. *See* Magnesium.

Gratin, Au. This term added to the name of the dish means that it has been sprinkled with breadcrumbs

105

or cheese and browned under a hot grill. Cheese is not essential. (GH.)

Green Butter. *See* Vegetable butters.

Green S. Food colour also known as Wool green S and Brilliant acid green BS; sodium salt of di-(p-dimethyl-aminophenyl)-2-hydroxy-3 : 6-disulphonaphthylmethanol anhydride.

Grilling or Broiling. Rapid roasting on a gridiron. With meat the expressed juices mostly evaporate before they have time to drip away, and so leave most of the extractives on the surface.

Grilling causes minimum losses of vitamins.

Losses: meat—B_1 30%, B_2 15%, nicotinic acid 20%; fish—50% B_1. (Johnson.)

Grissini. Italian "finger rolls" or stick bread 6–18 inches long.

Grist. Cereal for grinding.

Grits, Corn. *See* Hominy.

Groats. Oats from which the husk has been entirely removed; when crushed, Embden groats result. (Hutch.)

Groundnuts. *See* Peanuts.

Guanine. *See* Purines *and* Nucleic acids.

Guarana. Dried paste prepared from the seeds of the climbing shrub, *Paullinia cupana* (S. America); rich in caffeine; used in S. America as a beverage similar to cocoa.

Guar Gum. Obtained from the seeds of the leguminous plant, *Cyamopsis tetragonaloba*, grown in India, Pakistan and S.W. of United States. A polysaccharide of galactose and mannose, used as a stabilizer in ice-cream mixes, salad dressings, processed cheese, etc., and as a "cloud" stabilizer in fruit drinks.

Guava. Fruit of *Psidium guajava*, tropical shrub (Central and South America), eaten raw or preserved as guava jelly.

Water 80%, protein 1%, fat 0·4%, carbohydrate 13%, kcal 58 (0·25 MJ), Fe 1 mg, vitamin A 60 μg, B_1 0·05 mg, B_2 0·04 mg, nicotinic acid 1·0 mg, C 200 mg—per 100 g. (Platt.)

Gum Acacia. *See* Gum arabic.

Gum Arabic. Exudate from the stems of several species of Acacia, also known as **gum acacia** (best product comes from *Acacia senegal*). Used as thickening agent, as stabiliser often in combination with other gums, in gum drops and soft jelly gums and to prevent crystallization in sugar confectionery. (Jacobs.)

Gum, British. Dextrin—partly hydrolysed starch.

Gum, Chewing. Based on chicle, the partially evaporated milky juice of latex of the Sapodilla tree, plus sugar, balsam of Tolu and flavour. (Jacobs.)

Gums. Substances that can disperse in water to form a viscous, mucilaginous mass. Used in food processing to stabilize emulsions (such as salad dressings, processed cheese) as a thickener and in sugar confectionery.

Extracted from seeds (guar gum, locust, quince, psyllium), sap or exudates (gum arabic, karaya (or sterculia), tragacanth, ghatti, bassora or hog gum, shiraz, mesquite, anguo) and seaweeds (agar, kelp, alginate, Irish moss) or they may be made from starch or cellulose (dextrins and methyl-, carboxymethyl-, etc. cellulose) or they may be synethetic, such as vinyl polymers.

Most of these (apart from dextrins) are not digested and have no food value.

Gum Tragacanth. Obtained from the trees of *Astralagus* species; used as stabiliser.

Gut Sweetbread. *See* Pancreas.

G.Y.E. Guinness Yeast Extract, *see* Yeast Extract.

Gynaminic Acid. *See* Sialic acid.

Gynolactose. *See* Allolactose.

H

Haem. The iron-containing pigment which, in combination with protein, forms the haemoglobin of the red blood cell. (The iron is in the ferrous state.) (BDS.)

Haemagglutinins. Toxic substances naturally present in many legumes which cause the red blood cells to agglutinate. Also called phytoagglutinins or lectins.

Found in jack beans, hyacinth beans, soy beans, sweet pea, etc. and destroyed on heating.

Haematin. Formed by the oxidation of haem, the non-protein part of haemoglobin; the iron is oxidized from the ferrous to the ferric state. (BDS.)

Haemin. The hydrochloride of haematin, derived from haemoglobin. The crystals are readily recognizable under the microscope and used as a test for blood. (BDS.)

Haemoglobin. The red colouring matter of the red blood cell composed of the protein, globin, combined with an iron-containing pigment, haem.

Haemoglobin combines reversibly with oxygen which it carries from the lungs to the tissues, and with carbon dioxide, which it carries from the tissues to the lungs where it is excreted.

In iron-deficiency anaemia there is a deficiency of haemoglobin and impaired oxygenation. (BDS.)

Haemoglobinometer. Instrument to measure the amount of haemoglobin in blood by direct colorimetry or after conversion to another coloured compound. (Hawk.)

Haemopoietic Factor. *See* Intrinsic factor.

Haemosiderin. Brown granular pigment composed of iron-protein complex, present in various tissues. It is a storage form of iron that can be mobilized for haemoglobin synthesis but is only present when there are ample stores of ferritin. It accumulates in the spleen, liver and bone marrow in diseases where there is excessive destruction of blood. Siderosis also occurs on poor diets rich in iron. (BDS.)

Haff Disease. A paralysis due to the excessive consumption of various freshwater fish (probably inadequately cooked) which contain the anti-vitamin antithiamin. Occurs in Sweden and is the human equivalent of Chastek's paralysis which effects foxes. (DP.)

107

Hagberg Test. Measure of alpha-amylase activity of flour derived from the change in viscosity of flour paste. (FM.)

Haggis. Traditional Scottish dish. Made from liver, heart and lungs of sheep, cooked with suet, oatmeal and seasoning, then filled into a bag made from sheep's stomach and boiled for several hours.

Said to have been originated by the Romans when campaigning in Scotland; when breaking camp in an emergency the food was wrapped in the sheep stomach. (GH.)

Hake. *See* Codfish.

Half-life. In the field of radioactive isotopes this term means the period of time in which half of the original material has decomposed.

In biochemistry it refers to the time taken for half of the body tissue in question to be replaced. The tissues are continuously being degraded and rebuilt even in the mature adult, and the half-life is used as a quantitative measure of this "dynamic equilibrium". The half-life of human liver and serum proteins is 10 days, and of the total body protein 80 days.

Halibut-liver Oil. One of the richest natural sources of vitamins A and D; contains 5 g vitamin A and 8 mg vitamin D per 100 g.

Halophilic Bacteria. Able to grow in high concentrations of salt (25%). Colon group of bacteria inhibited at 8–9% salt, *Clostridia* at 7–10%, food-poisoning staphylococci at 15–20%, *Penicillium* 20%; film-forming yeasts can grow in 24% brine. (Baum.)

Halva. Also spelled halwa, halawa and chalva. A sweetmeat composed of an aerated mixture of glucose, sugar and crushed sesame seeds; because of the seeds, the sweet contains 25% fat.

Ham. The whole hind leg of the pig removed from the carcase and cured individually, sometimes the process is secret.

Hams cured or smoked in different ways have different flavours—York, Bradenham, Suffolk and Westphalian hams.

After cooking: Protein 16%, fat 40%, carbohydrate nil; kcal 435 (1·8 MJ), Fe 2·5 mg, B_1 0·5 mg, B_2 0·2 mg, nicotinic acid 3·5 mg—per 100 g. (M&W)

Hammarsten's Casein. Casein prepared by the method of Hammarsten. Fat-free milk diluted with water and precipitated with acetic acid. Washed three times with water by decantation; dissolved in ammonium hydroxide and reprecipitated, this repeated twice. The final precipitate washed with alcohol and ether and finally extracted with ether in a Soxhlet. (Davis.)

Hammer Mill. Mill in which material is powdered by impact from a set of hammers; a continuous process.

Hardening of Oils. *See* Hydrogenated oils.

Hardness of Water. *See* Water hardness.

Hashish. *See* Indian hemp.

Haslet. Pigs' offal, minced with herbs and spices and baked.

Haybox Cooking. The food is cooked for only a short time, then placed in a well-lagged container, the haybox, where it remains hot for many hours and so cooking continues without further usage of fuel. Also known as the **fireless cooker.** (Hutch.)

Hay Diet. A system of eating based on the fallacy that carbohydrates and proteins should not be eaten at the same meal. Since protein, in the absence of adequate carbohydrate, is oxidized to provide energy and therefore not available for tissue building, this diet is not only faddish but foolish. (Hutch.)

Haze. Term in general use in brewing to indicate cloudiness of the beer. Chill haze appears at 0°C and disappears at 20°C; permanent haze remains at 20°C but there is no fundamental difference. Due to gums derived from the barley, leucoanthocyanins from the malt and hops, and glucose, pentoses and amino acids.

Headcheese. Chopped, cooked edible parts of meat or meat products, also known as Mock brawn.

Health Foods. Substances whose consumption is advocated by various reform movements including vegetable foods, whole grain cereals, food processed without chemical additives, foods grown on organic compost, "magic" foods (honey, molasses, yogurt, etc.) and pills and potions.

Heart Sugar. Inositol.

Heat Exchanger. Equipment for heating or cooling liquids rapidly by providing a large surface area and turbulence for the rapid and efficient transfer of heat. Used for continuous pasteurization and also for the subsequent cooling.

Heat of Combustion. Energy released by complete combustion, as, for example, in the bomb calorimeter. Values can be used to predict energy available physiologically only if an allowance is made for material not oxidized in the body. E.g. the end products of protein oxidization in the body are carbon dioxide, water and urea; the latter contains non-available energy.

Hedonic Scale. Term used in tasting panels where the judge indicates the extent of his like or dislike for the food. (Griswold.)

Heifer. Young cow that has never had a calf.

Hemataminic Acid. *See* Sialic acid.

Hemeralopia. Inability to accomodate the vision to intense light: often (incorrectly) used as a symptom of night blindness (nyctalopia)—which is a symptom of vitamin A deficiency.

Hemicelluloses. Complex carbohydrates composed of polyuronic acids combined with xylose, glucose, mannose and arabinose. Found together with cellulose and lignin in plant cell walls; most gums and mucilages belong to this group of compounds.

Heparin. Substance isolated from liver, lung, muscle, heart and blood that prevents blood coagulation by acting as an antiprothrombin and an antithrombin. *In vivo* disappears rapidly from the bloodstream, but *in vitro* 10 mg prevents the coagulation of 100 ml of blood. (BDS.)

Hepatectomy. Surgical removal of the whole liver. The animal survives only a short time; during this time the manufacture of urea ceases, indicating that the liver is the seat of urea synthesis. (BDS.)

Hepatoflavin. Name given to substance isolated from liver, shown later to be riboflavin.

Herbs. Not clearly distinguished from spices except that it usually refers to the whole of the soft-stemmed aromatic plant while spices are only part of the plant.

Hermesetas. Trade name (Crookes-Anestan Ltd.) for saccharine tablets.

Herring Family. Herring is *Clupea harengus*; young herrings are sild. Sprat is *Clupea sprattus*; young are brislings. Pilchard is *Clupea pilchardus*; young are sardines. Kippers, bloaters and red-herrings are salted and smoked herrings; bucklings are hot-smoked herrings. Gaffelbitar are preserved herring.

For analysis, *see* Fish, fatty.

Hesperidin. At one time called vitamin P since it affects the fragility of the capillary walls. Found in the pith of the unripe orange and other citrus fruits; chemically a complex of glucose and rhamnose with the flavanone, hesperitin. (Brav.)

Hess Test. A test for capillary fragility in scurvy. A slight pressure is applied to the arm for five minutes and a shower of petechiae appear on the skin below the area of application. (DP.)

Heterosides. *See* Holosides.

Heterotrophes. *See* Autotrophes.

Hexamic Acid. A synthetic sweetening agent; trade name (Abbott Laboratories) for cyclohexyl sulphamic acid (the free acid of cyclamate): 27 × as sweet as sugar, used in effervescent drinks.

Hexoestrol. Synthetic oestrogenic hormone, does not occur naturally. *See* Oestrogens.

Hexosans. The general name for complex polysaccharides built up from simple units of hexose sugars, *see* Glucosan *and* Fructosan.

Hexose. A six-carbon sugar such as glucose and fructose.

Hexose Monophosphate Shunt. An alternative pathway in the metabolism of glucose to the Embden-Meyerhof-Parnas pathway.

The glucose-6-phosphate formed in the main route can be converted to phosphogluconic acid, then to pentose phosphate and to sedoheptulose-7-phosphate. The latter then joins the main pathway.

Since pentoses are formed it is also referred to as the pentose cycle and the direct oxidative pathway. (WHSS.)

Hexuronic Acid. The acid derived from a hexose sugar by the oxidation of the group on carbon atom number six. The hexuronic acid derived from glucose is glucuronic acid. (BDS.)

HF Heating. *See* High frequency heating.

High Frequency Heating. Heat results from the passage of a high frequency current, i.e. radio frequency at 5 million cycles per second. If a foodstuff (nonconductor) is placed between the electrodes heat is generated inside the material due to the very high electrostatic stresses and molecular movement.

The process, in effect, heats from the inside outwards in contrast to normal oven heating and is applied, for example, to biscuits after baking to reduce the final moisture content. Also called radio frequency heating and electronic heating.

High-ratio Fats. *See* Fats, high ratio.

High-ratio Flour. *See* Flour, high ratio.

High-ratio Shortenings. *See* Fats, high ratio.

Hiochic Acid. Growth factor isolated 1956 in Japanese rice wine (saké) and later shown to be identical with mevalonic acid, *which see.*

H ion. *See* pH.

Hirudin. Blood anticoagulant found in the buccal glands of the leech. Functions by interfering with thrombin. (BDS.)

Hi-soy. Trade name (British Arkady) for full-fat soya flour.

Histamine. Compound formed from the amino acid histidine by decarboxylation and also found in ergot.

Has powerful pharmacological effects on the body; constricts the smooth muscle of the bronchioles as in asthma (hence the use of antihistamines in this condition), lowers blood pressure by dilating the vessels, and powerfully stimulates secretion of acid in the stomach (used as a test for achlorhydria). (Hawk.)

Histidine. An amino acid essential to the growing rat but not to adult man. It is assumed that it is essential to the growing child. Chemically amino iminazole propionic acid.

Decarboxylation produces histamine. (DP.)

Histohaematin. Or myohaematin, earlier name for cytochrome, *which see.*

Histones. Proteins soluble in water but insoluble in dil. ammonia; yield precipitates with solutions of other proteins; on hydrolysis yield large quantities of arginine and lysine. E.g. scombrone from mackerel sperm, thymus histone. (Hawk.)

HMS. *See* Hexose monophosphate Shunt.

HMT. Hexamethylene tetramine. Preservative permitted in some countries.

Hogget. One-year-old sheep.

Hogshead. For beer or cider contains 54 gallons, for wine contains $52\frac{1}{4}$ gallons.

Holocellulose. Mixture of cellulose and hemicellulose in wood, the fibrous residue that remains after the extractives, the lignin, and the ash-forming elements, have been removed.

Holosides. Name given to complexes of sugars (or osides) that yield only sugars on hydrolysis. As distinct from heterosides that yield other substances as well as sugars on hydrolysis, e.g. tannins, anthocyanins, nucleosides.

Hominy. Prepared maize kernels. Lye hominy—pericarp and germ removed by soaking in caustic soda. Pearled hominy—degermed hulled maize.

Corn grits are ground hominy. (Loes.)

Homocysteine. The demethylated form of the amino acid methionine, $SH.CH_2.CH_2.CHNH_2.COOH$. Does not occur in foods and is not of nutritional importance, but of great biochemical interest as an intermediate in cell reactions. The non-essential amino acid, cystine, is made from the essential methionine via homocysteine. (Hawk.)

Homogenization. Emulsions usually consist of a suspension of globules of varying size. Homogenization reduces these globules to a smaller and approximately equal size.

In homogenized milk the smaller globules adsorb more of the milk protein, which is a stabilizer, and the cream does not rise to the top. (Jacobs.)

Homogenizer, Ultrasonic. *See* Ultrasonic homogenizer.

Homoiotherms. Animals that maintain constant body temperature irrespective of the surrounding temperature; also known as warm-blooded animals.

Honey. Syrupy liquid manufactured by bees from the nectar of flowers (essentially sucrose). The flavour and colour depend on the flowers from which the nectar was obtained and the composition also varies with the source.

Average composition: water 18% (12–26%), invert sugars, i.e. glucose and fructose, 74% (69–75%), sucrose 1·9% (0–4%), ash 0·18% (0·1–0·8%) organic acid 0·1–0·4%.

If the ratio of fructose to glucose is high there is a tendency for the honey to crystallize.

Honeydew Honey. During periods of prolonged drought bees may supplement their nectar supplies with honeydew, the sweet fluid excreted on leaves by leaf-sucking insects. The resultant honey is dark with an unpleasant taste.

Hop. A perennial climbing plant, *Humulus lupulus*. The female flowers contain bitter resins and essential oils used in brewing beer. *See* Humulones. (Matz.)

Hordein. A protein in barley; one of the prolamines. (Hawk.)

Horlick's. Trade name (Horlick's Ltd.) for a preparation of malted milk, for consumption as a beverage when added to milk.

Protein 14·4%, fat 8·0%, carbohydrate 70·8%; Ca 272 mg, Fe 1 mg, kcal 400 (1·7 MJ)— per 100 g. (M&W.)

Hormones. Chemical agents produced in the body, also known as **endocrines.** Thyroxine and tri-iodothyronine from the thyroid, adrenaline from the adrenals, insulin from the pancreas and a variety of hormones from the pituitary gland. They are secreted directly into the bloodstream from these ductless glands and act as chemical messengers which stimulate other tissues. *See also* Hormones, sex *and* Oestrogens. (BDS.)

Hormones, Sex. Male hormones, or androgens, include testosterone and androsterone; female hormones, or oestrogens, include oestradiol, oestrone and progesterone. Chemically all are steroid in structure.

The synthetic female hormones, stilboestrol and hexoestrol, are similar in biological activity but quite different chemically. Apart from clinical use the oestrogens have been widely used in chemical caponization of cockerels and to enhance the growth rate of cattle. *See also* Oestrogens. (BDS.)

Horsemeat. Protein 15%, fat 3%; kcal 94 (0·4 MJ); Ca 8 mg, Fe 1•8 mg; vitamin A nil, B_1 0·05 mg, B_2 0·08 mg, nicotinic acid 3·2 mg, vitamin C nil—per 100 g. (FAO.)

Horse Radish. Root of *Armoracia lapathifolia.* Pungency due to volatile oil (including allyl isothiocyanate and butyl sulphocyanide) liberated by the enzyme myrosinase from the glucoside sinigrin. Used as a condiment. (Jacobs.)

Hortvet Freezing Test. Test for the adulteration of milk with water by measuring the depression of freezing point; normal range −0·53 to −0·55°C.

Hot Breads. Americanese for waffles and pancakes.

Hot Sauce. A tomato sauce with hot flavour due to cayenne.

Hot Springs Conference. International Conference held in 1943 at which the Food and Agriculture Organization of the United Nations originated.

Hovis. Trade name (Rank-Hovis-McDougall Ltd.) of a wheat germ-enriched loaf.
    Protein 9%, fat 2·3%, carbohydrate 47·6%: Ca 107 mg, Fe 2·7 mg, kcal 237 (1 MJ), vitamin B_1 0·29 mg, nicotinic acid 2·0 mg—per 100 g.
    Phytic acid phosphorus 38% of total P (which is 200 mg per 100 g of the bread) compared with white bread, in which phytic acid P is 15% of total P (which is 80 mg per 100 g bread. (M&W.)

H.T.S.T. High Temperature Short Time Pasteurization—*see* Pasteurize.

Huckleberry. *See* Bilberry.

Humectant. Substance that absorbs moisture and used to maintain the water content of materials like tobacco, glue, inks, baking products, soaps, textiles. E.g. glucose syrup, invert sugar, honey, dried whey, glycerol, sorbitol. They allow the addition of sugar without adding more water and so prevent the growth of moulds.

Humulone. One of the two resins found in hops, the other being lupulone. Humulone is a mixture of humulone, cohumulone and adhumulone. The resins are responsible for the bitter flavour of the hops used in brewing. (Matz.)

Hursting Mill. Horizontal stone grinders once used for grain milling.

Husk or Hull. In reference to cereal grain this is the outer woody cellulose covering. In wheat it is loosely attached and removed during threshing; in rice it is firmly attached.
    High in fibre content and of limited use as animal feed.

Hyaluronic Acid. (*See also* Hyaluronidase.) The mucopolysaccharide, which, in animal tissues, binds water in the interstitial spaces, and holds the cells together and acts as a shock-absorber in the joints; also present in the vitreous humour of the eye.
    Its viscosity is reduced by the enzyme hyaluronidase by which it is depolymerized. (BDS.)

Hyaluronidase. Group of carbohydrase enzymes that depolymerize mucopolysaccharides such as hyaluronic acid. Found in beesting, bacteria, testes, leeches.
    Also known as spreading factor because the enzyme breaks down the hyaluronic acid under the skin

and permits the spread of substances there. For this reason it is used clinically to aid the absorption of drugs administered subcutaneously or intramuscularly, and to permit the subcutaneous injections of relatively large volumes of solution as, for example, in glucose feeding by this route. (BDS.)

Hydrocooling. Vegetables are washed in cold water then, while still wet, subjected to vacuum. The evaporation of the water chills the vegetables for transport. The term is also applied to vegetables washed in ice water without the vacuum treatment.

Hydrogen Acceptor. *See* Intermediate hydrogen carrier.

Hydrogenated Oils. Liquid oils can be hardened by hydrogenation. Treatment with hydrogen in the presence of a nickel catalyst causes "saturation" of the double bonds of the fatty acid chain and a rise in melting point. Cottonseed, maize, sunflower, and whale oils are commonly hardened and used in margarine and cooking fats. (Bailey.)

Hydrogen Carrier. *See* Intermediate hydrogen carrier.

Hydrogen, Heavy. Or deuterium; the isotope of hydrogen with atomic weight 2 instead of 1. Tritium has atomic weight 3.

Hydrogen-ion Concentration. Measure of the acidity or alkalinity of a solution by the concentration of hydrogen ions present. *See* pH.

Hydrogen Peroxide. Anti-microbial agent; can be used at $0 \cdot 1\%$ to preserve milk (Buddeized milk), but destroys vitamin C, methionine and tryptophan. Not permitted in U.K.

Formula H_2O_2, readily loses active oxygen, the effective sterilizing agent, and so forms water.

Hydrogen Swells. *See* Swells.

Hydrolyse. To split a substance and add the OH and the H of the water to the two halves. E.g. cane sugar, $C_{12}H_{22}O_{11}$, is hydrolysed to glucose $C_6H_{12}O_6$ and fructose $C_6H_{12}O_6$; proteins are hydrolysed to amino acids. Acid or alkali is usually needed as catalyst.

Hydrostatic Sterilizer. A continuous sterilizer used for the large-scale (8,000 per minute) production of canned foods. The principle is that the pressure is developed beneath an adequate depth of water.

Hydroxybenzoic Acid Esters. Methyl, ethyl, propyl and butyl esters and sodium salts used as preservatives in some countries at 500–1,200 ppm.

In U.K. methyl- and propyl-*p*-hydroxybenzoates or sodium salts may be used only as alternative to benzoic acid where, and at the level at which, that is permitted. (Bell.)

Hydroxycholecalciferol. *See* Vitamin D.

Hydroxyproline. A non-essential amino acid. Chemically hydroxypyrrolidine carboxylic acid. (BDS.)

Hydroxyproline Index. Biochemical test for protein malnutrition; ratio of urine hydroxyproline to creatinine.

Hygroscopic. Readily absorbing water, as when table salt becomes damp. Materials like calcium chloride and silica gel absorb water so readily that they are used as drying agents.

Hypercalcaemia. Increased levels of calcium in the blood; affects infants and can be fatal. The cause is not established but is believed to be due to hypersensitivity to vitamin D leading to excessive absorption of calcium into the bloodstream. Symptoms include loss of appetite, vomiting, wasting, constipation, flabby muscles; there can be abnormal calcification of the kidneys. (AEB.)

Hyperchlorhydria. Excess of hydrochloric acid in the stomach, due, not to higher concentration in the gastric juice, but to a greater volume of secretion. (Hawk.)

Hyperthyroidism. Overactive thyroid gland causing increased basal metabolic rate, i.e. increased caloric usage. (BDS.)

Hypertonic. A solution more concentrated than isotonic, *which see.*

Hypervitaminosis. Overdosage with vitamins. In most cases there is no ill-effect, but hypervitaminosis A and also D have ill-effects; overdosage with nicotinic acid causes flushing of the face and neck.

Hypokalaemia. A fall in the level of blood potassium. (Latin name *kalium.*)

Hypophysectomy. Surgical removal of the pituitary gland (the hypophysis).

Hypoproteinaemia. Total plasma protein level less than $5 \cdot 5$ g per 100 ml (normally $6 \cdot 7 – 7 \cdot 7$). (BDS.)

Hyposite. Low-calorie food.

Hypothermia. Literally low temperature; used in connection with reduction of the body temperature (down to 28°C) to permit surgery of the heart or brain.

Hypothyroidism. Underactivity of the thyroid gland. *See* Cretinism *and* Thyroid gland.

Hypotonic. A solution more dilute than isotonic, *which see.*

Hypoxanthine. *See* Purines *and* Nucleic acids.

I

Ice-cream. A frozen confection of fat, milk and sugar. In the U.K. legally must contain not less than 5% fat and 7% milk solids-not-fat.

"Non-drip" ice-cream contains $0 \cdot 06 – 0 \cdot 75\%$ added mixed triglycerides (mono and di) which holds together the looser globules of water and gives a "drier" non-drip product.

Typical analysis: water 62%, protein 4%, fat 11%, sugar 20%; kcal 196 ($0 \cdot 82$ MJ), Ca 137 mg. *See also* Overrun. (Bell, M&W.)

Ichthyosarcotoxin. Poisoning from eating fish.

I.E.P. Iso-electric point.

Ileum. Last portion of the small intestine, after the jejunum and before the small intestine joins the large intestine or colon. (BDS).

Illipé Butter. *See* Vegetable butters.

Immunization. *See* Toxins,

IMP. Integrating motor pneumo-tachograph. Apparatus for measuring energy expenditure indirectly from oxygen consumption. It meters the expired air and removes a proportion for analysis. (BDS.)

Improvers, Flour. *See* Aging.

Inanition. Exhaustion and wasting due to complete lack of or non-assimilation of food; a state of starvation.

Inborn Errors of Metabolism. *See* Genetic Disease.

Incaparina. A protein-rich dietary supplement developed by the Institute of Nutrition of Central America and Panama (INCAP). One version consists of 38% cottonseed flour, 29% ground corn, 39% sorghum, 3% Torula yeast, 1% calcium carbonate and 1350 μg vitamin A per 100 g. Incaparina 9A includes 58% maize and 38% cottonseed flour; in formula 14 the cottonseed is replaced by soya. All versions contain 27·5% protein. (AEB.)

Indian Corn. Maize, *which see.*

Indian Hemp. Or hashish, *Cannabis indica*; active principle unknown, stimulates and deranges the mental processes. (Clark.)

Indian Rice Grass. Perennial, growing wild in U.S.A., *Oryzopsis hymenoides;* tolerant to drought.
Seeds resemble millet, small, round, dark in colour, covered with white hairs. Used by N. American Indians for flour; now used almost exclusively for forage. (Matz 2.)

Indican. Indoxyl potassium sulphate. *See* Indoxyl.

Indicator. Usually refers to a pH indicator. Various dyes such as litmus, methyl orange, phenol-phthalein, change colour at a specific degree of acidity or alkalinity and this colour change is used as an indicator of pH. (Hawk.)

Indigo Carmine. Blue food colour, disodium salt of indigotin-5:5′-disulphonic acid. Indigotin is the colouring principle of natural indigo obtained from the Indigo fern. Permitted food colour in most countries but its use is limited by its low stability and solubility.

Indoxyl. A substance found in the urine which is a metabolic derivative of the amino acid tryptophan. It is excreted as indoxyl potassium sulphate, known as indican, and is thus one of the means whereby sulphur is excreted from the body. (BDS.)

Induction Period. Frequently used in connection with fats. It is the lag period during which the fat shows stability to oxidation because of its content of antioxidants, natural or added, which are preferentially oxidized. After this induction period there is a sudden and large consumption of oxygen and the fat becomes rancid. *See* Antioxidants. (Bailey.)

Inhibition, Competitive. With reference to enzymes means inhibition by a substance chemically similar to the substrate, which competes with the true substrate for the active surface of the enzyme. Thus malonic acid competitively inhibits succinic dehydrogenase, of which the true substrate is the chemically similar succinic acid.

116

The inhibition is reversed with a sufficiently high concentration of the true substrate.

Sulphanilamides act as bacteriostats because they compete for a vitamin essential to the bacteria, namely, para-amino benzoic acid. (WHSS.)

Inorganic. Denoting of mineral as distinct from animal and vegetable origin. Apart from carbonates and cyanides inorganic chemicals are those that contain no carbon.

Inosite. Obsolete name for inositol.

Inositol. Essential nutrient for micro-organisms and many animals and so classed as a vitamin, although there is no evidence of its essentiality for man. Deficiency causes alopecia in mice and "spectacle eye" (denudation around the eye) in rats.

Chemically hexahydrocyclohexane $(CHOH)_6$; there are nine stereoisomers of this compound but only one, meso- or myoinositol, is of major interest. It occurs widely in plant and animal tissues as an essential part of the structure and in combination in phosphatides. Its hexaphosphoric acid ester is phytic acid, *which see*.

Obsolete names inosite and meat sugar. The insecticide gammexane is hexachlorocyclohexane, and appears to function by competing with inositol. (Sebrell.)

Instant. Used with reference to dried foods that reconstitute rapidly when added to water, e.g. instant milk, tea, coffee, soups.

Instant tea and coffee are simply the dried forms of the liquid preparations. Instant milk is the dried form that has been further treated, "instantized", so that it reconstitutes more rapidly than ordinary dried milk. The treatment consists of moistening the dried product and redrying.

Instant coffee was first prepared in 1906 by Mr. G. Washington, an Englishman living in Guatemala, and marketed in 1909.

Insulin. Hormone that controls carbohydrate metabolism; secreted by the pancreas gland. Diabetes mellitus (*which see*) is due to under-production or over-destruction of insulin. The hormone is a protein and is digested if given by mouth so must be administered by injection.

Cannot be synthesized and is prepared from animal pancreas. There are four types used clinically; standard (quick-acting), protamin-zinc-insulin (12–14 hours), globin insulin (8–10 hours), and modified protamin insulin (28–30 hours). *See also* Glucose tolerance. (BDS.)

Interesterification. Fats are mixtures of triglycerides with various fatty acids esterified to the glycerol. By dry heat at 45–95°C there is an exchange of the fatty acids between the glycerol molecules—interesterification—with a consequent change in physical properties of the fat. E.g. lard is not a good creaming fat until it has been so treated. (Bailey.)

Intermediate Hydrogen Carrier. The oxidation of many substances in the living cell involves their loss of hydrogen. The hydrogen is passed on to an intermediate hydrogen acceptor, under the influence of an enzyme, and thence along a chain of acceptors to the ultimate hydrogen acceptor, which is oxygen (thus forming water).

For example, lactic acid is dehydrogenated (oxidized) to pyruvic acid, under the influence of a specific enzyme, and the hydrogen is passed on to Coenzyme I (an intermediate hydrogen carrier) thence to cytochrome (another intermediate hydrogen carrier) and finally to oxygen. (WHSS.)

International Units. Used as a measure of the comparative potency of natural substances, such as vitamins, before they are obtained in sufficiently pure form to measure by weight.

An international unit (i.u.) is arbitrarily defined in terms of a reproducible standard, e.g. 1 i.u. of vitamin A was originally 1 microgram of the purest then known preparation of carotene, later 0·6 microgram of beta-carotene.

Intestinal Juice. Also called succus entericus. Digestive juice produced by the intestinal glands lining the small intestine. Contains the enzymes "erepsin" (aminopeptidase and dipeptidase), amylase, maltase, lactase, sucrase, lipase, esterase, nucleases, nucleotidase, and the activator enterokinase (activates trypsinogen and chymotrypsinogen of the pancreatic juice to trypsin and chymotrypsin). (BDS.)

Intestine. Loosely used to describe the whole of the gastro-intestinal tract; more specifically that part after the stomach—comprising small intestine (duodenum, jejunum, and ileum) and large intestine. (BDS.)

Intestine, Small. That part lying between the stomach and the large intestine, comprising duodenum, jejunum and ileum. The site of the greater part of digestion of food and absorption of the products. Only water is absorbed in the large intestine. (BDS.)

Intrinsic Factor. Vitamin B_{12} from the diet (formerly known as the extrinsic factor) appears to require an unidentified substance from the gastric mucosa (known as intrinsic factor) either to aid its absorption or to form a complex called the haemopoietic factor. This complex or the B_{12}, is stored in the liver and is essential for the synthesis of the nucleoproteins of the red blood cells.

In pernicious anaemia there appears to be a deficiency of the intrinsic factor and the vitamin B_{12} is not absorbed. Treatment is by administering B_{12} intravenously, or orally in conjunction with dried hog mucosa (which contains intrinsic factor) or by injecting the complete haemopoietic factor as liver extract. (BDS, DP.)

Inulin. A polysaccharide composed of fructose units; produced in the dahlia tuber and Jerusalem artichoke as a storage carbohydrate. It is used as a test of renal function. *See* Kidney clearance test. (BDS.)

Inversion. Applied to sucrose, means its hydrolysis to glucose and fructose. *See* Optical activity.

Invertase. Enzyme that splits sucrose into the invert sugars, glucose and fructose. Also known as sucrase or saccharase.

Saccharases are widely distributed in plant tissues and the digestive juice of animals and are of two types, glucosaccharases (in animals and the mould, Aspergillus) and fructosaccharases (in yeast). They respectively attack the glucose and the fructose end of complex sugars. As sucrose is glucose-fructoside, it is attacked by any of the saccharases. (BDS.)

Invert Sugar. Mixture of glucose and fructose produced by hydrolysis of sucrose. (*See* Optical activity.) 130% sweetness of sucrose. Important in the manufacture of sugar confectionery (*see* Boiled sweets) since the presence of 10–15% of invert sugar prevents the crystallization of cane sugar. (Hawk.)

In Vitro. Literally "in glass"; used to indicate an observation made experimentally in the test-tube, as distinct from the natural living conditions, *in vivo.*

In Vivo. In the living state, as distinct from *in vitro*—in the test-tube.

Iodine. A trace element required at the level of 150 micrograms per day. It is part of the hormone thyroxine produced by the thyroid gland, and a prolonged shortage of iodide in the diet leads to goitre.

It is plentifully supplied by sea foods and by vegetables grown in soil containing iodide. In certain areas where the soil water is deficient in iodide, goitre occurs in defined geographical regions. For example, in England it occurs in Derbyshire, where it is known as **Derbyshire neck,** and in Oxfordshire; there are goitrous areas in most countries, e.g. Switzerland, U.S.A., New Zealand.

Iodine is not essential to plant growth but is present in plants in amounts varying with the level in the soil. *See also* Iodized salt, Goitre *and* Thyroid gland. (DP, AEB.)

Iodine Number. *See* Iodine value.

Iodine, Protein-bound. *See* Thyroglobulin.

Iodine Solution, Hübl's. A solution of iodine and mercuric chloride used to determine the iodine number of unsaturated compounds. (Hawk.)

Iodine Value. Or iodine number; measure of the degree of unsaturation of a fat by the extent of the uptake of iodine (grams iodine per 100 g of fat) by the unsaturated double bonds in the fatty acid chain.

Examples of iodine values: butter 22–38, lard 54–70, coconut oil 8–10, cottonseed 104–114, linseed 170–202. Drying oils (*which see*) are highly unsaturated and have high iodine numbers, as linseed oil. (Hawk.)

Iodized Salt. Contains added potassium (or sodium) iodide, 433 to 725 micrograms per ounce (as well as a small amount of magnesium carbonate to improve the free-running qualities); i.e. 15–30 parts of iodide per million of salt.

Ion-exchange Resins. Various resins, such as Permutit, Zeocarb, Amberlite, Dowex, will adsorb ions under one set of conditions and release them under other conditions. The best-known example is in water-softening, where the calcium ions are removed from the hard water by the resin, and liberated from the resin by the addition of salt (regeneration).

The ion-exchange resins are used for purification of chemicals, metal recovery and analysis. *See also* Amberlite.

Ionization. When a salt such as sodium chloride is put into solution, the NaCl splits into positively charged Na ions (cations) and negatively charged Cl ions (anions). Salts ionize readily, many organic compounds do not ionize.

119

The degree of ionization of an acid determines its strength (*see* pH).

Ionizing radiation is that which ionizes the air or water through which it passes, e.g. X-rays and gamma-rays. (Hawk.)

Irish Moss. *See* Carageenan.

Iron. A mineral essential to the body; the average adult has 4–5 grams of iron of which 60–70% is present as haem in the circulating haemoglobin, and the remainder present in various enzymes (e.g. catalase, cytochrome oxidase), in muscle myoglobin or stored. About 15% of the iron is stored in the liver as ferritin, in other tissues as haemosiderin, and as the blood transport complex called transferrin (average blood level 50–180 micrograms of iron per 100 ml plasma).

Iron balance: losses in faeces 0·3–0·5 mg per day, in sweat as skin cells 0·5, traces in hair and urine, total loss 0·5–1·5 mg per day; diet contains 10–15 mg of which 0·5–1·5 mg is absorbed.

Recommended intake 12 mg for adults, 15 mg during pregnancy and lactation and for adolescents, 7·5–10·5 mg for children rising to 13·5 mg in 11–14 year old group. Absorption aided by vitamin C and reduced by phosphate and phytic acid.

Content of foods: liver, 6–14 mg per 100 g, cereal, up to 9 mg, nuts 1–5 mg, eggs 2–3 mg, meat 2–4. Added to flour so that it contains not less than 1·65 mg per 100 g. Fortified cereals provide 35% of the iron of British diets.

Prolonged deficiency gives rise to nutritional anaemia. (Gil., DP.)

Iron Ammonium Citrate. *See* Ferric ammonium citrate.

Iron Caseinate. Preparation of iron and casein; also known as iron nucleo-albuminate.

Iron Chink. Machine used to behead and eviscerate salmon before canning (in the early days the work was done by Chinese labour). (Loes.)

Iron, Reduced. Metallic iron in finely divided form produced by reduction of iron oxide. The form in which iron is sometimes added to foods, such as bread. Latin name *ferrum redactum*.

Iron, Storage. *See* Ferritin *and* Haemosiderin.

Iron, Transport. *See* Siderophilin.

Iron Vitellinate. Preparation of egg yolk and iron.

Irradiation. In respect of food, apart from ultra-violet irradiation (*which see*), refers to ionizing radiation which kills off various micro-organisms—so-called cold sterilization. Complete sterilization requires high dosage that causes changes in flavour, colour and texture. Smaller doses useful to inactivate Salmonellae in egg, parasites in meat, for disinfestation of grain. Also useful to prolong storage life by suppression of sprouting in potatoes and root vegetables.

Isinglass. Protein membrane from the swim bladder of certain species of sturgeon; practically pure collagen. When specially prepared is used to clarify beer, as it slowly precipitates and carries with it any suspended particles. (Tressler.)

Islets of Langerhans. Areas of the pancreas from which the insulin is secreted.

Isoascorbic Acid. *See* Ascorbic Acid. Also known as erythorbic acid, a geometric isomer of ascorbic acid with only slight vitamin C activity.

Isoelectric Point. Proteins and amino acids carry both negative and positive charges on the molecule, and are therefore called amphoteric. At a certain degree of acidity, depending on the particular protein or amino acid, the substance becomes electrically neutral, i.e. the isoelectric point.
Proteins are usually least soluble and therefore precipitated from solution at the **I.E.P.** (BDS.)

Isoenzymes. A mixture of several different enzymes with similar biological activity. E.g. tissue lactic acid dehydrogenase contains at least five components.

Isoflavones. *See* Flavonoids.

Isoleucine. An essential amino acid, rarely limiting in foods. Chemically aminomethyl valeric acid. (BDS, DP.)

Isomaltose. Two molecules of glucose joined 1·6′—alpha, as distinct from maltose in which the bond in 1·4′—alpha.

Isomers. Molecules containing the same atoms but differently arranged. They can be quite different compounds or closely related, as citric and isocitric acids, leucine and isoleucine.

Iso-osmotic. *See* Isotonic.

Isoprene. The unit that forms part of the structure of the terpenes and the carotenoids,
$$CH_2 = C—CH = CH_2.$$
$$|$$
$$CH_3 \qquad \text{(Cohen.)}$$

Isoriboflavin. An analogue of riboflavin containing the two methyl groups in the 5,6 instead of the 6,7 positions. It competes with the vitamin and so inhibits growth. (Hawk.)

Isotonic. Two solutions are iso-osmotic (isosmotic) when they have the same total osmotic pressure. They are isotonic, relative to a particular semi-permeable membrane, when their effective osmotic pressures are the same, i.e. the osmotic pressure of their non-permeating ions.
If two isotonic solutions are separated by a semi-permeable membrane, there is no net movement of water across the membrane. E.g. human blood plasma is isosmotic with 0·945% sodium chloride, and isotonic with 0·935% sodium chloride, since part of the osmotic pressure of the blood is due to its proteins, which are non-permeating. (BDS.)

Isotopes. Elements with the same chemical properties, differing only in their atomic weights. Thus carbon can exist as four isotopes, carbons 11, 12, 13 and 14. C12 and C13 are stable isotopes and detected by the mass spectrometer; C11 and C14 are radioactive, i.e. they continually break down with the emission of radioactive particles or radiation. These isotopes are detected through the radiation emitted.
Isotopes incorporated into physiological substances, such as amino acids, enable those substances to be traced in their reactions in the body. *See* Labelled substances *and* Radioactivity. (BDS.)

I.U. International Unit. *which see.*

121

J

Jaggery. Coarse dark sugar made from the sap of the coconut palm; or raw sugar cane juice, used in India as sweetening agent—also known as gur.

Used also to prevent oxidative rancidity of fats since it contains a natural antioxidant.

Jake Paralysis. Effect of poisoning by tri-ortho-cresyl phosphate in a product called "Jamaica ginger". It was the widespread occurrence of this poisoning that helped to stimulate new food laws in the United States. (DP.)

Jak Fruit. Tropical fruit that grows from the trunk and large boughs of *Artocarpus integrifolia, heterophyllus* and *integra*. Both pulp and seeds are eaten.

Pulp: carbohydrate 10%, protein 2·5%, vitamin A 130 μg, B_1 0·1 mg, nicotinic acid 0·4 mg, vitamin C 10 mg—per 100 g. Seeds: carbohydrate 30%, protein 3·5%. (TND.)

Jam. Fruit preserve set to a gel by reaction between acid, pectin and added sugar. The solution of pectin in the fruit is caused to conglomerate by the sugar and forms a network of fibres enclosing liquid, i.e. a jelly. This only occurs under acid conditions, pH 2·5–3·5, optimum sugar concentration 67·5%. Normally 0·5–1% pectin used in jam manufacture.

Legally jam must contain not less than 68% soluble solids (or 65% if hermetically sealed). Minimum fruit content: blackberry, strawberry and greengage, 38%; blackcurrant 25%; damson, redcurrant, strawberry - and -

gooseberry 35%; gooseberry, raspberry, loganberry, 30%; marmalade 20%. *See also* Pectin. (Bell, Jacobs.)

Jamaica Pepper. *See* Allspice.

Jejunum. Second portion of the small intestine, between the duodenum and the ileum.

Jelly. A colloidal suspension that has set; may be made from gelatin, pectin, agar, usually flavoured with fruit juice or synthetic flavour.

Jerked Beef. Dried meat of S. America, similar to biltong. *See also* Charqui.

Jesuit's Bark. Cinchona bark, source of quinine. (Clark.)

Job's Tears. Adlay, *which see*.

Jonathan. Calcined, ground oat chaff used as adulterant for maize and other cereals (mid-nineteenth century).

Joule. Unit of energy; used to express energy content of foods and energy expenditure of man and animals. Gradually adopted as replacement for the calorie from about 1970 in accordance with International System of Units.

4·184 J = 1 calorie. 1,000 J = 1 kJ = 0·239 kcal; 1,000 kJ = 1 MJ.

Jower. Indian name for millet, *which see*.

Judas Goat. Sheep cannot readily be driven to slaughter but will follow a goat. A Judas goat is used to lead the sheep to the killing pens.

Julienne. Vegetables cut into thin, match-like strips. Also a clear, vegetable soup.

Junket. Precipitated protein of milk (casein only) carrying the fat with it and leaving behind the clear whey. The precipitation is carried out with the enzyme rennin.

K

Kaffir Beer. A beer brewed from Kaffir corn grain (sorghum), kaffircorn malt, and various maize products.

Kaffir Corn. Variety of millet, *which see*.

Kaoliang. Sorghum.

Karaya Gum. Obtained from East Indian trees of the genus *Sterculia*. Used as stabilizer, e.g. in frozen water ices, also used in combination with other stabilizers, sometimes used as a laxative.
Also called sterculia gum.

Karell Diet. For patients with severe cardiac failure. It is a low-calorie fluid diet consisting of 800 ml milk given in four feeds; it provides 550 kcal (2·3 MJ), 28 g protein, and 0·45 g (20 mEq) of sodium and is given for only two or three days. (DP.)

Karo Syrup. Trade name (Corn Products Refining Co., U.S.A.) for a dextrimaltose preparation made from maize starch, used as a carbohydrate modifier in milk preparations for infant feeding. Consists of a mixture of dextrin, maltose, glucose and sucrose.

Kasha. *See* Buckwheat.

Katadyn Process. *See* Oligodynamic.

Katemfe. *Thaumatococcus Daniellii.* Intensely sweet African fruit, called katemfe in Sierra Leone and miraculous fruit of the Sudan (not the same as Miracle Berry). Active principle, protein named **thaumatin**, 1,600 times as sweet as sucrose on weight basis, 100,000 times as sweet on molar basis.

Kathepsins. *See* Cathepsins.

Kcal. Kilo calorie, *see also* Calorie.

Kebab. General name (Muslim) for meat usually two or three kinds, grilled on charcoal; the pieces of meat are interspersed with vegetables.

Kebobs. Indian dish; slices of mutton or fowl dipped in eggs and cooked on skewer.

Kedgeree. Indian dish of rice, split pulse, onions, eggs, etc.; European dish of fish, rice, eggs, etc. (Hindustani, *khichri*.)

Kefir. *See* Milks, fermented.

Kellogg's Special K. Trade name (Kellogg's Ltd.) for enriched breakfast cereal based on maize.
Composition per 100 g.: 18 g protein, 0·8 g fat, 73 g soluble carbohydrate, 0·4 g fibre, 360 kcal (1·5 MJ), 7 mg iron, 1·4 mg B_1, 1·8 mg B_2, 19 mg nicotinic acid.

Kempner Diet. Or rice diet. A diet low in salt comprising rice, fruit, fruit juices, sugar and vitamins, containing about 2,000 kcal (8·4 MJ), 15–30 g protein and 100–150 mg sodium per day for patients suffering from congestive heart failure, cirrhosis of the liver, hypertensive disease, toxaemias of pregnancy and certain kidney disorders.

See also Salt-free diets.

Kephalins. Or cephalins; phosphatides similar to lecithins but composed of glycerol, fatty acids, phosphoric acid and ethanolamine (instead of choline). Found in brain and nerve tissue, part of cell structure. (BDS.)

Keratin. Insoluble protein of hair, horns, hoofs, feathers and nails. See Albuminoids.

Not hydrolysed by digestive enzymes, therefore useless as food. Used as fertilizer since it is slowly broken down by soil bacteria. Steamed feather meal is used to some extent as supplement for ruminants.

These proteins not digested by proteases have been designated eukeratins, as distinct from pseudokeratins of skin and eye lens which are digested by proteases and contain less cystine. (Hawk.)

Kesp. Trade name (Courtauld's Ltd.) for textured vegetable protein made from spun fibres from field bean (*Vicia faba*). Marketed frozen in wet form.

Ketchup. See Tomato ketchup.

Ketogenic Diet. A diet poor in carbohydrate (20–30 g) and rich in fat; causes accumulation of the ketone bodies in the tissues; used to be used in the treatment of epilepsy. (BDS.)

Ketonaemia. Accumulation in the blood of ketone bodies, *which see*.

Ketone Bodies. Name given to the penultimate products of fatty acid metabolism — acetoacetic acid, betahydroxybutyric acid and acetone. They can be oxidized at only a limited rate, and when their production rate is excessive, as in diabetes and starvation, they accumulate in the blood (ketonaemia), and are excreted in the urine (ketonuria). (BDS.)

Ketonic Rancidity. Certain moulds of *Penicillium* and *Aspergillus* species attack fats containing short carbon chains and produce ketones with a characteristic odour and taste—so-called ketonic rancidity. Fats such as butter, coconut and palm kernel are most susceptible.

Ketonil. Trade name (Merck, Sharp & Dohme, U.S.A.) for protein-rich food low in phenylalanine for feeding patients with phenylketonuria. (AEB.)

Ketonuria. See Ketone bodies.

Ketosis. Clinical condition in which ketone bodies (*which see*) accumulate in the blood and appear in the urine.

Khushkhash. Israeli term for the bitter orange. See Orange, bitter.

Kidney Clearance Test. Test of kidney function by measuring the ability to excrete inulin, urea, or a dye, in the urine. The quantity excreted per minute divided by the amount present in 1 ml of plasma is the urinary clearance. (Clark.)

Kieves. Irish term for mash tuns, *which see*.

Kilocalorie. See Calorie.

Kinetic Energy. See Energy.

Kipper. Herring that has been lightly salted and smoked (*see also*

124

Red herring); invented by John Woodger, a fish curer of Seahouses, Northumberland, 1843.

Analysis, without bones and skin, baked, protein 23·2%, fat 11·4%, carbohydrate nil, kcal 200 (0·8 MJ), Ca 65 mg, Fe 1·4 mg—per 100 g. (M&W).

Kitol. An inactive form of vitamin A found in whale liver (kitos, Greek for whale) which is converted into retinol by heating at 200°C.

Kjeldahl Determination. Widely used method of determining total nitrogen in a substance by digesting with sulphuric acid and a catalyst in a Kjeldahl (long-necked) flask. The nitrogen is converted to ammonia which is then measured.

In foodstuffs most of the nitrogen is protein, and the term crude protein is the total "Kjeldahl nitrogen" multiplied by the factor 6·25. (Hawk.)

Klim. Trade name (Borden Co., U.S.A.) for dried milk.

Klipfish. Salted and dried cod mainly produced in Norway. The fish is boned, stored in salt for a month, washed and dried slowly. It is known as bacalao in S. America.

Kofranyi-Michaelis Spirometer. *See* Spirometer.

Koji. A fungal proteolytic enzyme preparation from the mould *Aspergillus oryzae* traditionally grown on steamed rice. Used to prepare products such as miso by the proteolysis of soya and soya sauces. Introduced from China to Japan 1700 years ago. Introduced to the U.S.A. 1890 by Dr. Takamine and used as a digestive aid called Takadiastase.

Now prepared on a commercial scale for treating flour proteins.

Kosher. The selection and preparation of foods in accordance with traditional Jewish ritual and dietary laws.

The only kosher flesh foods are from animals that chew the cud and have cloven hoofs, such as cattle, sheep, goats and deer, and the hindquarters must not be eaten. The only fish permitted are those with fins and scales; birds of prey and scavengers are not kosher. Moreover, the animals must be slaughtered according to ritual before the meat can be considered kosher. From Hebrew 'Kosher' meaning 'right'. (Deuteronomy, chap. 14.)

Krebs' Cycle. *See* Citric acid cycle.

Krebs' Solution. Solution of inorganic salts with ionic composition similar to that of mammalian blood serum; with the addition of glucose, tissue slices continue to respire in such a solution. (Contains, Na, Ca, Mg, K, Cl, PO_4, SO_4, HCO_3, CO_2.) (Hawk.)

Kreis Test. For oxidative rancidity of fats. Fat treated with a solution of phloroglucinol in ether and hydrochloric acid—a pink colour develops in rancid fat, due to the presence of epihydrin aldehyde.

Kryptoxanthin. Alternative spelling of cryptoxanthin, *which see.*

Kuban. *See* Milks, fermented.

Kumiss. *See* Milks, fermented.

Kümmel. A liqueur prepared from caraway seeds, fennel and orris root.

Alcoholic strength varies from 60–75% of proof spirit.

125

Kumquat. A citrus fruit of the genus *Fortunella*; widely distributed in S. China; resemble citrus fruits, but very small, acid pulp, and sweet, edible skin. (Brav.)

Kurrat. Plant closely related to leek.

Kwashiorkor. A form of malnutrition in infants due to shortage of protein associated with adequate or near adequate carbohydrate intake. Occurs in infants weaned on to a low-protein diet and the name is from the Ga language of Ghana used to describe the sickness of the first child when a second child is born (and the first one has to be weaned on to an inadequate diet). It is common in most tropical countries in the age-group 1–3 years.

Symptoms include poor growth, oedema, wastage of the muscles, mental apathy, fatty infiltration of the liver. (TDN.)

L

l-. Obsolete prefix indicating laevorotatory, now replaced by (-) *see* Optical activity.

L-. *See* D-

Labelled Substances. To follow the progress of a substance, foodstuff or drug, through the body, it is sometimes marked or labelled so that it can readily be distinguished. Such labels may be chemical radicals that are abnormal and can therefore be distinguished, e.g. the introduction of phenyl groups into fatty acids, or, more recently, the use of radioactive substances. *See* Radioactivity *and* Isotopes.

Laccase. Enzyme in bacteria, potato, and mushrooms that converts polyphenols to quinones.

Lacquer. In reference to tinned foods—a layer of gum and gum resin coated on to the tin-plate and hardened with heat. The layer of lacquer protects the tin lining from attack by acid fruit juices.

Lactalbumin. One of the proteins of milk; casein 3%, lactalbumin 0·5%, lactoglobulin 0·25%. Not precipitated from acid solution as casein is, hence during cheesemaking the whey contains the lactalbumin and lactoglobulin. They are precipitated by heat, and a whey cheese can be made in this way.

Lactaminic Acid. *See* Sialic acid.

Lactase. Enzyme that splits milk sugar, lactose, into glucose and galactose; present in the pancreatic juice. (BDS.)

Lactic Acid. The acid produced by the fermentation of milk sugar and responsible for the flavour of sour milk and precipitation of the casein curd in cottage cheese.

Also produced by fermentation in silage, pickles, sauerkraut, cocoa, tobacco—its value here is in suppressing the growth of unwanted organisms.

In mammalian muscle metabolism the first stages of breakdown of glucose end at pyruvic acid. In severe exercise this is reduced to lactic acid which can accumulate in the muscles. Similarly formed in meat muscle from glycogen immediately after death.

Used as an acidulant (as well as citric and tartaric acids) in sugar confectionery, soft drinks, pickles and sauces. *See also* Pickling *and* Sarcolactic acid. (WHSS, Jacobs.)

Lactein Bread. Another name for milk loaf, i.e. loaf to which skim milk powder has been added.

Lactide. Compound formed by reaction between two molecules of an alpha-hydroxy acid, with the loss of two molecules of water and the formation of a ring compound containing two oxygen atoms in the ring. (Cohen.)

Lactobacillus casei **Factor.** *See* Folic Acid.

Lactobiose. Lactose.

Lactochrome. Pigment in milk.

Lactoflavin. Obsolete name for vitamin B_2; so named because it was isolated from milk.

Lactoglobulin. *See* Lactalbumin.

Lactollin. Protein found recently (1962) in small traces in bovine milk; of unusual composition, lacking methionine and with little alanine.

Lactometer. Floating device used to measure the specific gravity of milk ($1 \cdot 027$–$1 \cdot 035$).

Lactone. Compound formed by loss of water from a molecule of a hydroxy acid to form a ring compound or inner ester, e.g. gluconic acid forms gluconolactone. (Cohen.)

Lac-tone. Protein-rich baby food (26% protein) made in India from peanut flour, skim milk powder, wheat flour and barley flour with added vitamins and calcium.

Lacto-ovo-vegetarian. One whose diet is composed of vegetables, fruit, milk and eggs but no flesh foods.

Lactose. Milk sugar, $4 \cdot 8\%$ of milk. A disaccharide that is hydrolysed by acid or the enzyme lactase, to glucose and galactose. Fermented by micro-organisms to lactic acid hence the souring of milk by lactobacilli.

Used pharmaceutically as tablet filler and as medium for growth of micro-organisms.

Ordinary lactose is alpha lactose (16% of the sweetness of sucrose); if crystallized above 93°C is changed to the beta form, which is more soluble and sweeter than the alpha form.

Lactose Intolerance. *See* Disaccharide Intolerance.

Lacto-serum. Grandiloquent word for whey.

Lactostearin. *See* Glyceryl lactostearate.

Lactulose. Disaccharide ketose, galactosidofructose, found in human milk; stimulates growth of *Lactobacillus bifidus* in intestine of babies fed on breast milk and so termed bifidus factor.

Ladies Fingers. *See* Okra; also a short kind of banana.

Laevorotatory. *See* Optical activity.

Laevulose. Alternative name for fructose.

Lager. *See* Beer.

Lamb. Meat from sheep younger than 12–14 months. Genuine spring lamb, 3–6 months; spring lamb up to 1 year.

Protein $12 \cdot 8\%$, fat $7 \cdot 1\%$; kcal 119 ($0 \cdot 5$ MJ), Ca 7 mg, Fe $1 \cdot 5$ mg, vitamin A nil, B_1 $0 \cdot 12$ mg, B_2 $0 \cdot 15$ mg, nicotinic acid $3 \cdot 8$ mg, vitamin C nil—per 100 g. (FAO.)

Hoggets are 1-year-old sheep; tegs are 2 years old; shearlings 15–18 months.

Langouste. *See* Lobster.

Lanoline. The fat from wool. Consists of a mixture of cholesterol oleate, cholesterol palmitate and cholesterol stearate and therefore not useful as food; used in various cosmetics.

Lard. Best quality from fat surrounding stomach and kidneys of pig, but also from sheep and cattle.
Neutral Lard No. 1—kidney and bowel fat rendered below 50°C; Neutral Lard No. 2—back fat rendered below 50°C; Leaf Lard—residues from top two qualities rendered in autoclave; Prime Steam Lard—fat from any part of the carcass rendered in the autoclave. (Bailey.)

Lard Compounds. Blends of animal fats, such as oleostearin or premier jus, with vegetable oils to produce products similar to lard in consistency and texture.
Vegetable shortenings made from mixtures of partially hardened vegetable fats with the consistency of lard are referred to as lard substitutes.

Lardine. *See* Margarine.

Larding. Method of adding fat to lean meat so that it does not dry during long slow cooking. Narrow strips of bacon fat, 1–1½ inches long and ¾ inch wide, are threaded into the surface of the meat with a special larding needle. The strips are called lardoons.
Barding is the process of tying a thin sheet of bacon fat over the meat.

Lard, Leaf. Made from the residue of kidney and back fat

after the preparation of neutral lard (at 50°C) by treating with water above 100°C in an autoclave. *See* Lard, neutral. (Hilditch.)

Lard, Neutral. Highest quality pig fat, prepared by agitating the minced fat with water at a temperature below 50°C. Kidney fat provides No. 1 quality; back fat provides No. 2 quality. (Hilditch.)

Lathyrism. Disease caused by excessive intake (50% of the diet) of the chick pea, *Lathyrus sativus*; characterized by degeneration of the spinal cord and thrombosis of the spinal artery; common in India. The cause is unknown, no toxic substance has been found in the chick pea, unlike the toxin found in the sweet pea that causes odoratism in the rat (*see* Odoratism).

Lauric Acid. One of the long chain fatty acids, $CH_3(CH_2)_{10}COOH$. Occurs as the triglyceride in seeds of the spice bush and to lesser extent in butter, coconut oil and palm oil.

Laver. Edible seaweed. Laverbread is made from the seaweed *porphyra* by boiling in salted water and mincing to a gelatinous mass. It is made into a cake with oatmeal or fried. Locally known in S. Wales as Bara lawr.

Lax or **Lox.** Scandinavian term for salmon; term used for smoked salmon in U.S.A.

Laxative. Substance that accelerates the passage of food through the intestine. If it alters peristaltic activity it is termed a purgative, other types stimulate or depress the muscular activity of the gut.
Cellulose acts as a purgative by

128

retaining water and increasing the volume of intestinal contents, Epsom salts function similarly through osmotic pressure. Castor oil is hydrolysed by lipase to liberate ricinoleic acid which irritates the intestinal mucosa. Drugs such as aloes, senna, cascara, rhubarb and phenol phthalein irritate the intestine. (Clark.)

Lead. Of no dietary interest except that it is toxic and its effects are cumulative. May be present in food from traces naturally present in the soil, from shell fish that have absorbed it from sea-water, as lead arsenate used as insecticide and from lead glazes on vessels. Traces are excreted in the urine. (GMW.)

Leaf Lard. *See* Lard, leaf.

Lean Body Mass. Measure of body composition excluding adipose tissue, i.e. cells, extracellular fluid and skeleton. (DP.)

Leaven. Sour dough, soured by wild yeast. Old method of fermenting bread before commercially prepared yeast was available. Still used in rye bread. *See also* Sauerteig. (KJ.)

Leben. *See* Fermented milk.

Lecithins. Fatty substances of the type called phosphatides; consist of glycerol, fatty acids, phosphoric acid and choline. Important in the body for fat transport.

Used in food technology as emulsifiers, e.g. in chocolate, help emulsification, save cocoa butter and prevent bloom, also used as anti-spattering agents in frying fats. Obtained commercially from soy-bean, peanut and corn.

From a dietary point of view lecithins form a very small fraction of the total fat intake, and may be considered simply as fats. (BDS, Jacobs.)

Leek. *Allium ampeloprasum* var. *porrum.*

Composition per 100 g: 1·9 g protein, 6 g carbohydrate, 30 kcal (0·13 MJ), 1 mg iron, 6 µg vitamin A (bulb only, leaves 300 µg), 0·1 mg B_1, 0·6 mg nicotinic acid, 18 mg C. (OF, M&W.)

Legumin. Globulin protein in pea, bean and lentil.

Lehmann Process. A method of treating straw to render it digestible by cattle. The straw is chopped and soaked in 1·5% sodium hydroxide when it is delignified. The process raises the starch equivalent 3–4 times. (Abrams.)

Lemon. Fruit of *Citrus limonis*; protein 0·5%, fat 0·3%, kcal 15 (0·06 MJ), Ca 25 mg, Fe 0·4 mg, vitamin A nil, B_1 0·02 mg, B_2 nil, nicotinic acid 0·1 mg, vitamin C 31 mg—per 100 g. (FAO.)

Lemon juice, a classical source of vitamin C, was first used to treat scurvy by Sir James Lancaster (1554–1618) who, between 1591 and 1603 ordered three teaspoons of lemon juice per day to sailors under his command trading with the East Indies. There appears to be no information as to his knowledge of the curative properties.

Lemon Curd. Cooked mixture of sugar, butter, eggs and lemons. Legally 4% fat, 0·33% citric acid, 1% dried egg or equivalent, 0·125% oil of lemon or 0·25% oil of orange, not less than 65% soluble solids. (Bell.)

Lemon Oil. The peel oil—0·15–0·3% of the weight of the fruit;

90% limonene, together with phellandrene, terpinene. camphene, bisabolene, cadinene, citral, etc. (Brav.)

Lenhartz diet. For peptic ulcer patients (originated 1915); mainly fluid diet including raw eggs, milk, boiled rice and vegetable purées fed at frequent intervals. (DP.)

Lentils. Seeds of many varieties of *Lens esculenta;* fall into the same group as peas and beans. There is a green variety and an orange-red variety that is commonly imported into Europe from Egypt and India. Frequently used as a soup thickener in the powdered form.

Composition: Protein 24%, fat 1·8%; kcal 346 (1·45 MJ), Ca 56 mg, Fe 6·1 mg, vitamin A 30 μg, B_1 0·5 mg, B_2 0·2 mg, nicotinic acid 1·8 mg, vitamin C 3 mg— per 100 g. (FAO.)

Lettuce. Leaves of the plant *Lactuca sativa.* Not a very valuable food: the vitamin C is only one-seventh of that of cabbage.

Protein 0·9%, fat 0·1%; kcal 10 (0·04 MJ), Ca 17 mg, Fe 0·3 mg; vitamin A 40 μg, B_1 0·03 mg, B_2 0·06 mg, nicotinic acid 0·1 mg, vitamin C 5 mg—per 100 g. (FAO.)

Leucine. An essential amino acid; rarely limiting in foods. Chemically amino isocaproic acid. (BDS.)

Leucocytes. White blood cells, normally 5,000–9,000 per cubic mm; includes polymorphonuclear neutrophils, lymphocytes, monocytes, polymorphonuclear eosinophils, and polymorphonuclear basophils. A "white cell count" determines the total; a "differ-

ential cell count" estimates the numbers of each type.

Fever, haemorrhage, violent exercise, cause an increase—leucocytosis; starvation and debilitating conditions cause a decrease—leucopoenia. (BDS.)

Leucocytosis. Increase in the white cells in the blood. *See* Leucocytes.

Leucopoenia. Decrease in the white cells in the blood. *See* Leucocytes.

Leucosin. One of the water-soluble proteins of wheat flour.

Leucovorin. Growth factor for *Leuconostoc citrovorum,* related to folic acid, *which see.*

Levitin. One of the proteins of egg yolk, about one-fifth of the total, the remainder being vitellin. Rich in sulphur and accounts for half of the sulphur in the yolk. (B. & R.)

Lieberkuhn, Crypts of. Glands lining the small intestine which secrete intestinal juice. (BDS.)

Liebermann-Burchard Reaction. Test for unsaturated sterols; green colour when treated with chloroform, acetic anhydride and conc. sulphuric acid. (Hawk.)

Lights. Butchers' term for the lungs of an animal.

Lignin. Associated with the carbohydrates of the cell wall of plants but not, itself, a carbohydrate, but a high molecular weight aromatic compound.

Lignocellulose. Alternative name for lignin.

Lignoceric Acid. Long-chain fatty acid containing total of 24 carbon atoms (tetracosanoic acid); present in the cerebrosides and sphingomyelins.

Lime. Fruit of *Citrus aurantifolia.* Source of vitamin C and the origin of the name "limeys" for the British sailors. A much poorer source of vitamin C than the lemon.

Protein 0·3%, fat 0·1%; kcal 16 (0·07 MJ), Ca 14 mg, Fe 0·2 mg, B_1 0·01 mg, B_2 nil, nicotinic acid nil, vitamin C 9 mg—per 100 g. (FAO.)

Limit Dextrin. When a branched polysaccharide such as glycogen is hydrolysed enzymically (e.g. by phosphorylase) glucose is split off step by step until the branch point is reached. The hydrolysis then stops leaving what is termed a limit dextrin. Further hydrolysis requires a different enzyme. (WHSS.)

Limiting Amino Acid. *See* Amino acid, limiting.

Limmisax. Trade name (Leas Cliff Products) for saccharine.

Limmits. Trade name (Leas Cliff Laboratories Ltd.) for a "slimming" preparation composed of wholemeal biscuits with a vitamin–methyl cellulose mixture as filling, containing vitamin A, B_1, B_2, nicotinamide, C and D with iron, calcium, iodine and phosphorus. Intended to replace a meal or meals with a reduced calorie diet. Six biscuits contain 1,050 kcal (4·2 MJ).

Limonin. Bitter principle in the albedo of the Valencia orange. Similarly isolimonin is the bitter principle of the navel orange. Both are present in a non-bitter,

water-soluble state, and are liberated into the juice during extraction. On standing they slowly hydrolyse and the juice becomes bitter. Not present in the ripe fruit. (Brav.)

Linoleic Acid. Straight-chain fatty acid with 18 carbon atoms and two double bonds (a diene): $C_{17} H_{31}$ COOH, double bonds at 9–10 and 12–13 carbons (octadecadienoic acid). *See* Essential fatty acids. (Cohen.)

Linolenic Acid. Straight-chain fatty acid of 18 carbon atoms with three double bonds; $C_{17}H_{29}$ COOH with double bonds at 9–10, 12–13 and 15–16 carbons (octadecatrienoic acid). It is a major component of linseed oil and its high degree of unsaturation is responsible for the drying properties of the oil.

At one time included with the essential fatty acids. (DP.)

Lintner Value. Measure of diastatic activity using soluble starch as a substrate and measuring the effect by Fehling's solution. Applied to flour, malt extract, etc. (KJ.)

Liothyronine. Alternative name for L-tri-iodo thyronine, the most potent of the hormones of the thyroid gland. Used as an aid to weight reduction by stimulating the metabolism of the body.

Lipase. Enzyme that hydrolyses fat to glycerol and fatty acid. Has a low specificity and will attack any triglyceride or long-chain ester. Present in the intestinal juice and in many seeds and grains. Sometimes responsible for development of rancidity in stored foods.

Lipases from different sources, e.g. digestive juices or seeds, appear to be similar but attack the

131

substrates at different rates. (BDS.)

Lipides. *See* Lipids.

Lipids. General term embracing fats and oils and waxes, as well as the complex compounds, the phosphatides and cerebrosides. i.e. all naturally-occurring compounds of fatty acids. Also referred to as lipides and lipins; the term lipoid is obsolete. (BDS.)

Lipins. *See* Lipids.

Lipocaic. Unidentified factor in the pancreas that prevents the deposition of fat in the liver.

Lipochromes. Plant pigments soluble in fats and organic solvents, e.g. chlorophyll, carotenoids.

Lipoic Acid. Essential growth factor for various micro-organisms; discovered in yeast and liver extracts and called by various workers, acetate replacement factor, pyruvate oxidation factor, thioctic acid and protogen. Chemically dithio-octanoic acid.

In combination with vitamin B_1, phosphate and coenzyme A, lipoic acid forms lipothiamide, essential for the oxidative decarboxylation in carbohydrate metabolism. (Sebrell.)

Lipolysis. The splitting of fats (to glycerol and fatty acid).

Lipolytic. Fat-splitting. Lipases are lipolytic enzymes.

Lipolytic Rancidity. Some micro-organisms produce lipases, and these fat-splitting enzymes are also present in tissues. In stored foods they hydrolyse the fats to free fatty acids—so-called lipolytic rancidity. As the enzyme is destroyed by heat this type of rancidity occurs only in uncooked foods.

Lipomul. Trade name (U.S.A.) for a mixture of 10% glucose and 40% vegetable oil.

Lipothiamide. *See* Lipoic acid.

Lipotropic Substances. *See* Liver, fatty infiltration of.

Lipovitellenin. A lipoprotein complex of egg comprising about one-sixth of the solids of the yolk.

Liqueurs. For alcohol content, *see* Alcoholic beverages. Prepared from distilled alcohol by the addition of fruit flavours and sugar.

Liquid Paraffin. *See* Medicinal paraffin.

Liquified Herring. Herring reduced to liquid state by enzyme action at slightly acid pH; used as protein concentrate for animal feed.

Liquorice. Liquorice root and extract are obtained from the plant, *Glycyrrhiza glabra;* stick liquorice is the crude evaporated extract of the root.

The plant has been grown in the Pontefract district of Yorkshire since sixteenth century, hence the name of Pontefract cakes for the sugar confection of liquorice.

Litchi. *Litchi chinensis*, also lychee; native of China; the size of a small plum with a translucent white jelly-like interior surrounding the seed.

Composition per 100 g: 0·9 g protein, 0·5 g fat, 16 g carbohydrate, 70 kcal (0·28 MJ), 0·5 mg iron, 0·04 mg B_1, 0·04 mg B_2, 0·3 mg nicotinic acid, 50 mg C. (OF, Platt.)

Liver. An extremely valuable source of nutrients. Fish liver oils are the major source of vitamins A and D.

Composition of animal liver (after cooking); protein 30%, fat 16%, carbohydrate 4%; kcal 280 (1·2 MJ), Fe 20 mg, vitamin A 13 mg, B_1 0·3 mg, B_2 3·5 mg, nicotinic acid 15 mg, vitamin C 20 mg, D 0·5 μg—per 100 g. (M&W.)

Liver Factor 2. Obsolete name for pantothenic acid.

Liver, Fatty Infiltration of. Under the influence of liver poisons, and in the absence from the diet of substances containing methyl groups, there is a flow of fats to the liver—the so-called fatty liver. This is prevented by lipotropic substances, which include choline, methionine, and a pancreatic extract called lipocaic.

The affliction is aggravated on a high-fat diet and is found clinically on chronic low-protein diets. (BDS.)

Liver Filtrate Factor. Obsolete name for pantothenic acid.

Livetin. A water-soluble protein fraction of egg yolk.

Lobster. Shellfish of various tribes of the suborder *Macrura*. True Lobster (with claws), species of *Homarus*.

Norway lobster, Scampi or Dublin Bay Prawn—*Nephrops norvegicus*.

Squat Lobster—family *Galatheidae*.

Crayfish, freshwater—families *Astacidae*, *Parastacidae* and *Austroastacidae*.

Crawfish, spiny lobster, rock lobster or sea crayfish

(without claws)—species of family *Palinuridae*.

Langouste—*P. vulgaris*.
Composition per 100 g: 21 g protein, 3·4 g fat, 119 kcal (0·5 MJ), 62 mg calcium, 0·8 mg iron, 0·05 mg B_2, 1·5 mg nicotinic acid. (M&W.)

Locasol. Trade name (Trufood Ltd.) for a low-calcium milk substitute.

Protein 22·8%, fat 19·9%, carbohydrate 51·9%; Ca 46 mg (dried milk Ca 960 mg), Fe 1·5 mg, kcal 474 (2·0 MJ)—per 100 g. (M&W.)

Locksoy. Fine drawn rice macaroni, Chinese.

Locust Bean. 1. Carob seed, *which see*. 2. African locustbean, *Parkia* spp; composition per 100 g: 26 g protein, 10 g fat, 47 g carbohydrate, 380 kcal (1·6 MJ), 300 mg calcium, 4 mg iron, 0·06 mg B_1, 0·2 mg B_2, 3 mg nicotinic acid. (Platt.)

Lofenalac. Trade name (Mead Johnson Ltd.) for food low in phenylalanine for treatment of phenylketonuria. (AEB.)

Loganberry. Cross between the European raspberry and the Californian blackberry (named after L. H. Logan). Vitamin C content 40 mg per 100 g.

Logarithmic Phase. In reference to bacteria means the most rapid period of growth when the numbers increase in geometric progression. Under ideal conditions bacteria can double in numbers every 20 minutes. (Baum.)

Lohmann Reaction. Transfer of phosphate, with its energy, from adenosine triphosphate to creatine, to form adenosine diphosphate and creatine phosphate.

The first source of energy on muscle stimulation is adenosine triphosphate, leaving the diphosphate. This is resynthesized to the triphosphate by creatine phosphate which thus serves as the reserve of energy. It is resynthesized during the recovery period by the Lohmann reaction. (WHSS.)

Lonalac. Trade name (Mead Johnson Co.) for a milk preparation free from sodium. (AEB.)

Loonzein. Rice from which the husk has been removed; also known as brown rice, hulled rice and cargo rice. (TND.)

Loquat. *Eriobotrya japonica*, also known as Japanese medlar; small pear-shaped fruit; member of apple family. (OF.)

Lotus. *Nelumbium nuciferum.* Sacred lotus of India and China; water plant whose rhizomes and seeds are used for food. Other water plants of the same family whose seeds and rhizomes are eaten are the water-lilies, *Nymphaea*.

Composition of rhizome per 100 g: $1 \cdot 7$ g protein, 11 g carbohydrate, 49 kcal ($0 \cdot 21$ MJ), $1 \cdot 5$ mg iron, $0 \cdot 05$ mg B_1, 20 mg C. (OF, Platt.)

Lovibond Comparator. Instrument for visual comparison of the depth of colour of a solution with a standard coloured glass slide.

A set of colour standards is usually made for each specific colour reaction, e.g. phosphate, pH determinations, etc. The comparator thus differs from the Tintometer (*which see*) as the latter is for general application and includes a range of colours and intensities.

Low-salt Diets. *See* Salt-free diets.

Lox. *See* Lax.

LSM. U.S. trade name for a low-sodium milk—contains 50 mg per litre, ordinary milk contains 500 mg sodium per litre.

Lucerne. *Medicago sativa* L. Essentially a forage crop but eaten by man to a small extent.

Lucozade. Trade name (Beecham Foods Ltd.) for a glucose beverage. $17 \cdot 9\%$ carbohydrate, 67 kcal per 100 g. (M&W.)

Lugol's Solution. 5% iodine in 10% potassium iodide. (Hawk.)

Lupeose. *See* Stachyose.

Lutein. Alternative name for xanthophyll.

Luteol. Alternative name for xanthophyll.

"Luxus Konsumption." A theory that normal people manage to keep their weight within reasonable limits by burning off any excess of food, while obese people suffer a failure of this mechanism. (DP.)

Lycine. Obsolete name for betaine.

Lychee. *See* Litchi.

Lycopene. Red pigment found in tomato, pink grapefruit and palm oil; straight chain derivative of carotene with no vitamin A activity. The synthetic material is sometimes used as a food colour.

Lymph. The fluid intermediate between the blood and the tissues; the medium in which oxygen and nutrients are conveyed from the blood directly to the tissues, and waste products back to the blood.

Chemically similar to blood plasma, contains salts, serum albumin and globulins, fibrinogen prothrombin and leucocytes (and can coagulate).

134

Part of the fat of the diet is absorbed without hydrolysis into the lymph, and transported to the thoracic lymph duct whence the fat is discharged into the blood-stream. The lymph, rich in emulsified fat, is milky due to the presence of fat droplets, called **chylomicrons;** the milky lymph is called **chyle.** Chyle and lymph differ only in their fat content. (Hawk.)

Lymphatics. Vessels through which the lymph flows.

Lyophilization. Expertise for freeze-drying, *which see.*

Lysergic Acid. *See* Ergot.

Lysine. An essential amino acid of special importance since it is the limiting amino acid in many cereals. Can be synthesized on the commercial scale, and when added to bread or rice or cereal-based animal feeds, it improves the nutritive value of the protein.

Is dibasic and can be produced as the free lysine, and the mono- and dihydrochlorides. Appears to occupy a special position in amino acid metabolism since it has a low "turn-over rate" in the body com-pared with other amino acids. Chemically diaminocaproic acid.

See also Amino acid, limiting. (BDS, DP.)

Lysozyme. An enzyme that digests certain high - molecular - weight carbohydrates. Bacteria that con-tain these carbohydrates as part of their cell wall structure disinte-grate or lyse under attack by lysozyme. Widely distributed, but particularly in egg-white, of which it comprises $2 \cdot 5\%$ of the total solids. (BDS.)

Lyxoflavin. Substance isolated from human heart muscle, similar to riboflavin but containing the sugar lyxose; function unknown. (Sebrell.)

M

Macaroni. *See* Alimentary pastes.

Macassar Gum. *See* Agar.

Maccaroncelli. *See* Alimentary pastes *and* Macaroni.

Mace. *See* Nutmeg.

Macedoine. Mixture of fruits or vegetables, diced, or cut into even-shaped pieces. (GH.)

Mackerel. *See* Fish, fatty.

Macon. Bacon made from mutton.

Macrocytes. Large red cells found in the blood in pernicious anaemia, due to disturbed development of the red blood cell. Hence macro-cytic anaemia. (BDS.)

Magma. Mixture of sugar syrup and sugar crystals produced dur-ing sugar refining.

Magnesium. An element that is essential to the diet although no deficiency has ever been shown in man. It is present in bone, and magnesium ions are necessary in many enzyme reactions.

Deficiency in cattle gives rise to grass tetany. Magnesium is part of the molecule of chlorophyll and is therefore present in all green foodstuffs. If the soil is deficient in this element the resultant deficiency in chlorophyll produces a pale plant suffering from "chlorosis". (Gil.)

Maillard Reaction. Two processes in foods can produce a brown colour. One is the enzymatic oxidation of phenolic substances, such as occurs at the cut surface of an apple. The other is a reaction between proteins or amino acids and sugars, and is variously known as the Maillard reaction, the browning reaction and non-enzymic browning.

It takes place on heating or on prolonged storage and is one of the deteriorative processes that take place in stored foods. It is accompanied by a loss in nutritive value since the part of the protein that reacts with the sugar is the free amino part of the lysine. This complex is not digested and there is thus a reduction in the biologically available lysine.

Maize. Grain of *Zea mays*, also called Indian corn. The starch prepared from maize is **cornflour; hominy, samp** and **cerealine** are maize preparations used in the southern states of America.

Maize is a staple article of the diet in many areas but its protein is of poor quality (lacking both lysine and tryptophan), and this, together with its low content of available nicotinic acid and the possible presence of a toxic factor can give rise to pellagra.

Composition: Protein 9·5%, fat 4·3%; Fe 2·3 mg, kcal 356 (1·56 MJ), vitamin A 140 μg, B_1 0.45 mg, B_2 0·1 mg, nicotinic acid 2 mg (not all available)—per 100 g.

Of all the varieties of maize two are of commercial importance, *Zea indurata* (**flint corn**) and *Zea dentata* (**dent corn**). Sweet corn, pod corn, popcorn and waxy corn are other varieties. (Matz 2, FAO.)

Maize, Flaked. Partly gelatinized maize used for animal feed. The grain is cracked to small pieces, moistened, cooked and flaked between rollers. (KJ.)

Maize Flour. Highly refined and very finely ground maize meal from which all bran and germ has been removed.

Maize Rice. Finely cut maize with bran and germ partly removed: also called **mealie rice.**

Malic Acid. Organic acid occurring in many fruits, particularly in apples, tomatoes and plums. Structure, $COOH.CH(OH).CH_2.COOH$ (i.e. hydroxysuccinic acid). (Cohen.)

Mallorizing. Application of high temperature to pasteurizing process—up to 265°F (129°C); named after inventor.

Malnutrition. Disturbance of form or function arising from a deficiency or excess of one or more nutrients.

Malpighia. *See* Cherry, West Indian.

Malt, Malt Extract. A mixture of starch breakdown products containing mainly maltose (malt sugar), prepared from barley or wheat.

The grain is allowed to sprout, when the enzyme diastase (or amylase) develops and hydrolyses the starch to maltose. The mixture is then extracted with hot water and this malt extract contains a solution of starch breakdown products together with diastase. Malt extract may be the concentrated solution or evaporated to dryness.

For brewing, a barley low in protein and rich in diastase is used and mixed with extra unmalted barley to provide more starch for the yeast fermentation.

136

See also Maltose *and* Diastatic activity.

Maltase. Enzyme that splits maltose (malt sugar) into two molecules of glucose; present in the pancreatic juice and intestinal juice. (BDS.)

Malted Barley. *See* Malt, Malt extract.

Malt Flour, Wheat Malt Flour. Germinated barley or wheat, dried and milled. Rich in diastase and added to flour of low diastatic content for bread-making, at 4 oz–2 lb per 280 lb sack, and also used to make a malt loaf. (KJ.)

Malthus. Author of an essay in 1798 postulating that any temporary or local improvement in living conditions will increase population faster than the food supply, and that disasters such as war and pestilence, which check population growth, are inescapable features of human society. (DP.)

Malting. *See* Beer.

Maltol. Substance with a fragrant, caramel-like odour and bitter-sweet taste used as flavour enhancer at 50–350 ppm; 3-hydroxy-2-methyl-4H-pyran-4-one.

Used in chocolate products, soft drinks, ice cream, table jellies.

Ethyl maltol enhances sweetness and allows a reduction of 5–15% of the sugar present.

Maltose. Malt sugar. A disaccharide composed of two molecules of glucose; these are liberated on acid hydrolysis or during digestion. Does not occur free in the tissues but is formed as an intermediate stage during the breakdown of starch to glucose.

33% sweetness of sucrose. *See also* Amylases. (BDS.)

Maltose Figure. *See* Diastatic activity.

Maltose Intolerance. *See* Disaccharide Intolerance.

Manganese. An element that is considered probably a dietary essential as it is necessary to activate certain enzymes such as arginase and alkaline phosphatase, although no deficiency has ever been observed in man.

Essential for animals and deficiency causes perosis (slipped tendon) in chicks, sterility in rats and bone malformations in rabbits. Also essential for plants.

Green foodstuffs and tea are rich sources of manganese. (Hawk, Gil., GMW.)

Mangelwurzel, mangoldwurzel. *Beta vulgaris rapa.* Cross between red and white beetroot, used as cattle food. Composition, water 75·4–94·3%, nitrogenous substances 0·47–3·65%, fat 0·02–0·45%, N-free extract 5·75–10·0%, fibre 0·39–2·14%, ash 0·59–2·77%, sucrose 3·5–8·7%.

Mango. *Mangifera indica*; fruit of Indo-Burmese origin extensively grown throughout the tropics, 3–6 inches diameter, orange-coloured edible flesh surrounding central stone, the depth of colour is an index of vitamin A activity which can be up to 700 μg per 100 g.

Composition per 100 g: 0·5 g protein, 15 g carbohydrate, 63 kcal (0·26 MJ), 0·5 mg iron, 200 μg vitamin A, 0·03 mg B_1, 0·04 mg B_2, 0·3 mg nicotinic acid, 30 mg C. (OF, Platt.)

Mangosteen. Fruit of Indian origin, the size of an orange with thick purple rind and sweet white pulp in segments, (*Garcinea mangostana*). Vitamin C content 9 mg per 100 g. (TND.)

Manihot Starch. *See* Cassava.

Manioc. *See* Cassava.

Manucol. Trade name (Alginate Industries Ltd.) for sodium alginate.

Manna. Dried exudate from the manna-ash Tamarisk tree (*Fraxinus ornus*). Abundant in Sicily and used as a mild laxative for children.

Composition 40–60% mannitol, 10–16% mannotetrose, 6–16% mannotriose, plus glucose, mucilage and fraxin.

This is thought to be the food eaten by the children of Israel in the wilderness.

Mannitol. Mannite or manna sugar. Formed by hydrogenation of the hexose sugar, mannose, when the terminal -CHO group is reduced to -CH₂OH. Also extracted commercially from seaweed (*Laminaria*). (AEB.)

Mannose. Hexose sugar related to glucose but of slightly different chemical configuration.

Mannotetrose. *See* Stachyose.

Maple Syrup. Sap of certain varieties of the maple tree, *Acer saccharum* (U.S.A. and Canada). Evaporated either to syrup or finally to sugar.

Maple syrup, 62·6% sucrose, 1·5% invert sugar. (Jacobs.)

Maple Syrup Urine Disease. An inborn error of metabolism in which unusually large amounts of the three amino acids, leucine, isoleucine and valine, are excreted in the urine; the urine smells like maple syrup. There is progressive cerebro-degeneration leading to early death. (AEB.)

Marasmus, Nutritional. Severe wasting of the body of infants because of gross dietary deficiency, also called total undernutrition.

Symptoms include atrophy of muscles and subcutaneous fat, a wizened and shrivelled face, but, unlike kwashiorkor, no oedema or fatty infiltration of the liver.

Together with kwashiorkor, marasmus is one of the major problems of infant nutrition in the developing countries. (TND.)

Margarine. Emulsion of fat and water flavoured with the butter aroma — diacetyl and acetyl methyl carbinol (or containing milk soured with selected organisms to develop the butter aroma).

The word is derived from the Greek 'margaros' meaning pearls and so pronounced with a hard 'g'.

Fats commonly used are a blend of several of the following; groundnut, cottonseed, whale, sunflower and soya (all hardened to some degree) and coconut palm and palm kernel.

Composition: not more than 16% water (by law), usually 1·5–2% salt, 82% fat, coloured with carotene, annatto or coal-tar dyes; not more than 10% butter fat may be added. In many countries margarine is fortified with vitamins A and D. In Gt. Britain the vitamin content is, A 230–280 μg and D, 2–2·5 μg per oz.

Also called oleomargarine (U.S.A.), butterine and lardine. (Bailey.)

Margarine, Kosher. Made only from vegetable fats since ordinary margarine can include animal fats that may not be kosher (*see* Kosher); also the margarine is fortified with carotene (which is derived from vegetable sources) instead of retinol (which can be obtained from non-kosher sources).

Marinade. Preparation of olive oil, lemon juice, vinegar and mixed herbs in which fish or meat is steeped before cooking.

Marinate. To pickle in salt, e.g. anchovy and Bismarck herrings.

Marjoram. Dried leaves of a number of aromatic plants of different species. The most widely accepted marjoram herb is *Origanum majorana* (perennial bush) and a sweet marjoram *majorana hortensis* (annual). Spanish wild marjoram is *Thymus mastichina*. The volatile oils contain terpenes and terpene alcohols. Used as seasoning for poultry and meats. (Jacobs.)

Marmalade. Originally a jam made from the Portuguese marmelo or quince. Now the name given to jam made from citrus fruits such as orange, lime, lemon, grapefruit.

Marmite. (1) The original form of pressure cooker used by Papin in 1681; it was an iron pot with a sealing lid.

(2) Cookery term for a stock.

(3) Trade name (Marmite Ltd.) for an extract of yeast flavoured with vegetable extract and used as a bread spread, beverage and flavouring agent.

Contains Ca 123 mg, Fe 7 mg, vitamin B_2 5·2 mg, nicotinic acid 59 mg—per 100 g.

Marrow. *See* Gourd.

Marshmallow. A soft sweetmeat made from an aerated mixture of gelatin or egg albumin with sugar or starch syrup. Differs from nougat in containing less glucose and more water.

Originally made from the root of the marshmallow plant (*Althaea*) which provides a mucilaginous substance as well as starch and sugar.

Marzipan. Sweetmeat or cake decoration composed of 25% ground almond paste and 75% sugar; also called **almond paste**.

Mashing. In the brewing of beer (*see* Beer) the malted barley is heated with water both to extract the soluble sugars and to continue enzymic reactions started during malting. (Matz.)

Mash Tun. Vessel used in brewing in which the malt is extracted from the sprouted barley with hot water.

Maslim or Mashlum. (1) Old term still used in Scotland, for mixed crop of beans and oats used as cattle food. (2) In Yorkshire and north of England it means a mixed crop of 2–3 parts of wheat and 1 part of rye which is used for bread.

Massecuite. The mixture of sugar crystals and syrup mother liquor obtained during the crystallization stage of sugar refining.

Mast. *See* Milks, fermented.

Maté. Also yerba maté, or Paraguay or Brazilian tea. Made from the dried leaves of *Ilex paraguayensis*. Contains caffeine and tannin. (Jacobs.)

Matoké. Cooked (steamed) green banana.

Maturation Factor. Substance in the liver which aids maturation

139

of red blood cells. May be vitamin B_{12} or combination of B_{12} with the intrinsic factor produced by the stomach. (WHSS.)

Matzka Process. Sterilization by combined use of silver ions (oligodynamic process) and limited heat—Katadyn process employs silver ions alone. In the presence of the silver the pasteurization temperature is only 8–11°C (15–20°F). Applied to fruit juices. (FM.)

Matzo, Motza. (Matzoth is the plural.) Unleavened bread or Passover bread made as thin, flat, round or square water biscuits, and, according to the injunction in Exodus, eaten by Jews during the eight days of Passover in place of leavened bread.

Maw. Fourth stomach of the ruminant.

Mawseed. Poppyseed.

Mayonnaise. See Salad cream.

Maysin. Coagulable globulin protein of maize.

Mazun. See Milks, fermented.

Mealie(s). Maize.

Mealie Rice. See Maize rice.

Meat. See separate headings for beef, mutton, pork, lamb. All meats are good sources of protein, although 70–80% water, and vitamins B_1, B_2 and nicotinic acid, iron and phosphate. Kidney and liver, but not carcass are rich in vitamin A. (FB.)

Meat Bar. Dehydrated cooked meat and fat; a modern form of pemmican. 7·5% water, 49% protein, 570 kcal (2·4 MJ), per 100 g.

Meat Content. See Meat factor.

Meat, Curing of. See Curing of Meat.

Meat Extract. The water-soluble part of meat that is mainly responsible for flavour. Commercially is made during the manufacture of corned beef; minced meat is immersed in boiling water, when the water-soluble extractives are partially leached out. This "soup" is concentrated and produces the meat extract (so-called No. 1 extract) of commerce. (Exhaustive extraction of the meat produces "Direct Extract", containing more gelatin.)

Rich in the B vitamins (particularly B_2, nicotinic acid and B_{12}), meat bases, and potassium. Shown by Pavlov that meat extract is the most powerful oral stimulant of gastric acid secretion.

Meat Factor. Factor used to determine the fat-free meat content of sausages and similar meat products from a nitrogen estimation: $100 \times N/3\cdot4$; applies to both pork and beef.

Meat Sugar. Obsolete name for inositol.

Medicinal Paraffin. A mineral oil of no nutritive value as it is not affected by digestive enzymes and passes through the intestine unchanged.

Used as a mild laxative because of its lubricant properties; if taken at the same time as the fat-soluble vitamins, these go into solution in the oil and pass through the digestive tract unabsorbed.

Medlar. *Mespilus germanica.* Can be eaten fresh from tree in Mediterranean areas but in colder climates, as Great Britain, does not become palatable until it is half rotten (bletted). (OF.)

140

Meeh Formula. *See* Surface area.

Melampyrin. Dulcitol, *which see.*

Melangeur. Mixing vessel consisting of rollers riding on a rotating horizontal bed. Used to mix substances of pasty consistency (hence melangeuring). (FM.)

Melangolo. Italian term for the bitter orange, *see* Orange, bitter.

Melezitose. Trisaccharide composed of two glucose and one fructose; hydrolysed to glucose plus the disaccharide turanose (3-α-D-glucosido-D-fructose).

Melibiose. Disaccharide, 6(αD galactoside)-D-glucose.

Melitose. *See* Raffinose.

Melitriose. *See* Raffinose.

Mellorine. U.S. term for ice-cream made from non-butter fat.

Melon. *See* Gourds.

Melting Point. Often characteristic of a particular chemical and used as a means of identification. Particularly valuable as an index of purity as impurities lower the melting point.

Membrane, Semi-permeable. One that allows the passage of small but not large molecules, e.g. pig's bladder is permeable to water but not salt, collodion is permeable to salt but not protein molecules.

The exchange of water and salts between tissues of the body and red blood cells is possible because of the semi-permeable nature of the walls. *See* Osmotic pressure *and* Isotonic. (BDS.)

Menadione. Obsolete term for vitamin K_3, 2-methyl-1,4-naphthoquinone. *See* Vitamin K.

Menaquinone. Generic descriptor for vitamin K, *which see.*

Menaquinone. 2-methyl-1,4-naphthoquinone, generic descriptor of substances with vitamin K activity; formerly called menadione.

Mercapturic Acid. Complex of cysteine with naphthalene or various halogenated aromatic hydrocarbons (such as bromobenzene) whereby the latter compounds are detoxicated and excreted in the urine. (Hawk.)

Meringues. Confections made by beating together a mixture of sugar and white of eggs. (FM.)

Meritene. Trade name (Doyle Pharmaceutical Co., U.S.A.) for a food concentrate based on skim milk powder. Composition: protein 33%, fat 0·2%, carbohydrate 58·4%; Ca 1 g, Fe 15 mg, kcal 365 (1·5 MJ), vitamin A 2 mg, B_1 2·4 mg, B_2 4·3 mg, nicotinic acid 22 mg, C 80 mg, D 14μg— per 100 g.

Mescal. *See* Tequila.

Mesocarp. *See* Albedo.

Mesomorph. Description given to a well-covered individual with well-developed muscles. (*See also* Ectomorph *and* Endomorph.)

Mesophiles. Micro-organisms that grow best at temperatures between 25 and 40°C; usually will not grow at temperatures below 5°C. (Tanner.)

Metabolic Rate. Rate of utilization of energy. *See also* Basal Metabolic Rate.

Metabolic Water. Produced in the body by the oxidation of foods.
100 g of fat produce 107·1 g of water.
100 g of starch produce 55·1 g of water.
100 g of protein produce 41·3 g of water. (BDS.)

Metabolism. The process of chemical change that goes on in living cells; growth of new tissues, breakdown of old tissue, production of energy. Anabolism is building up and catabolism is breaking down.

Intermediary metabolism describes the biochemical stages in the change of, for example, glucose to carbon dioxide and water. *See* Glucose metabolism. (BDS.)

Metabolism, Inborn Errors of. *See* Genetic disease.

Metalloproteins. Proteins linked to a metal, such as haemoglobin, cytochrome, peroxidase, ferritin, siderophilin, all of which contain iron, and chlorocruorin, which contains copper.

Metaproteins. Products of the action on proteins of dilute acids or alkalies; they are no longer soluble at their isoelectric points but are soluble in weak acid or alkali. (Hawk.)

Metercal. (U.S. product spelled Metrecal). Trade name (Mead Johnson Ltd.) for a "slimming" preparation comprising all the dietary essentials limited to 900 kcal (3·8 MJ), per day intake (in ½ lb)—in powder, liquid and biscuit form. Based on skimmed milk with added protein and full range of vitamins. (AEB.)

Methaemoglobin. Oxidized form of haemoglobin (unlike oxyhaemoglobin which is a loose and reversible combination with oxygen) which cannot transport oxygen to the tissues. Present in small quantities in normal blood, increased after certain drugs and after smoking; found rarely as a congenital abnormality.

Can be formed in blood of babies after consumption of the small amounts of nitrate found naturally in vegetables grown in certain areas and in some drinking water since the lack of acidity in the stomach does not prevent reduction of nitrate to nitrite. *See also* Nitrates.

Methionine. An essential amino acid; one of the three containing sulphur: cystine, cysteine and methionine.

Cystine is non-essential but can replace part of the methionine of the diet, hence the sulphur amino acids are always considered together. They occupy the outstanding position in protein nutrition, since not only are the sulphur amino acids the limiting factor in many proteins, but they are limiting in the total diet of most peoples that have been examined. In other words, the protein nutritive value of these diets can be improved by either adding more protein or more methionine (or cystine) but no other amino acid.

Methionine is available on the commercial scale and is added to animal feeds, where it is often, but not always, the limiting amino acid.

Chemically aminomethylthiol butyric acid. *See also* Amino acid, limiting. (BDS, DP.)

142

Methionine Sulphoximine. Substance formed by reaction between nitrogen trichloride ("agene") and the amino acid methionine when flour is treated with agene as a bleaching agent. Causes running fits in dogs and although it has never been shown to be toxic to man the use of agene as a bread improver was abandoned in Gt. Britain in 1955.

Methocel. Trade name (Dow Chemical Co.) for methyl cellulose.

Methofas. Trade name (Imperial Chemical Industries) for methyl hydroxypropyl cellulose.

Methyl Alcohol. The first member of the alcohol series. It is a highly toxic substance and leads to mental disturbance, blindness and death when consumed over a period. It is present in methylated spirits, to which it is added to denature the ethyl alcohol and render it undrinkable. Since methylated spirits is duty-free alcoholic addicts often drink this despite the presence of the toxic methyl alcohol. (Cohen.)

Methylated Spirits. Ethyl alcohol containing methyl alcohol, coloured with a dye and given a repulsive smell by the addition of pyridine. Its toxicity is due to the presence of the methyl alcohol.

Methyl Cellulose. *See under* Carboxymethylcellulose.

Methylene Blue. Blue dye that becomes colourless when reduced, the so-called leuco- form. Used in cell respiration experiments to indicate when oxygen is being consumed. *See also* Methylene blue dye-reduction test.

Methylene Blue Dye-reduction Test. When methylene blue or resazurin is added to milk the bacteria present take up oxygen and change the colour of the dye. Methylene blue goes colourless; resazurin changes blue-purple-pink–white.

The speed of the change indicates the bacterial content. Pasteurized milk must not reduce dye in half an hour. (Davis.)

Metmyoglobin. *See* Nitrosomyoglobin.

Meulengracht Diet. For peptic ulcer patients; sieved foods such as meat, chicken, vegetables, at 2-hourly intervals. Differs from Sippy and Lenhartz diets (*which see*) in being much richer in protein.

The intention is to neutralize the acid in the stomach by the buffering effect of the protein. (DP.)

Mevalonic Acid. Chemically, beta - delta - dihydroxy - beta - methyl-valeric acid; a growth promoting factor for *Lactobacillus acidophilus* distinct from lipoic acid, can replace acetate which is an essential factor for this organism.

It is an intermediate stage in the biosynthesis of sterols and terpenes (including possibly carotene). Isolated 1956 from distillers' dried solubles.

Michaelis Constant. A measure of the kinetics of enzyme reaction. Defined as the substrate concentration at which half the limiting velocity of the reaction is reached.

It is a characteristic of the enzyme and is useful as a means of following the stages of purification of an enzyme. (WHSS.)

Micro-aerophiles. Micro-organisms that can grow in extremely low concentrations of oxygen. Can thus spoil foodstuffs intended to be stored in the absence of air, if traces are left. (Tanner.)

Microbiological Assay. Biological assay using micro-organisms; used for vitamins and amino acids in particular.

The principle is that the organism is inoculated into a medium containing all the needed growth factors except the one under examination, the rate of growth is then proportional to the amount of this particular factor added in the test substance. Rate of growth determined by turbidity or by titrating the acid produced after 2–3 days' incubation.

Microgram. One thousandth part of a milligram, symbol μg.

Micron. One-thousandth of a millimetre; unit of measurement of bacterial size.

Micro-organisms. Term including bacteria, moulds and yeasts—classified as Fungi or Mycetes, a subdivision of *Thallophyta* or flowerless plants. (Baum.)

Middlings. *See* Wheatfeed.

Milk. The secretion of the mammary gland of a number of animals is used as food in different parts of the world, e.g. cow, buffalo, goat, ass, mare, ewe. The milks differ considerably in composition.

The most widely used is cow's milk; protein 3·3%, fat 3·6%, carbohydrate 4·7%; kcal 66 (0·28 MJ), Ca 120 mg, P 100 mg, Fe 0·03 mg, vitamin A 45μg, B_1 0·045 mg, B_2 0·15 mg, nicotinic acid 0·08 mg, vitamin C 2 mg, D 0·05 μg—per 100 g.

Legally milk is not considered genuine if the fat is less than 3% and the other solids less than 8·5%.

Jersey, Guernsey, South Devon and Channel Islands milk must contain not less than 4% fat. (Davis.)

Milk, Accredited. Term not used after October 1954. Referred to milk untreated by heat, from cows examined at specified intervals for freedom from disease.

Milk, Acidophilus. A preparation similar to cultured butter-milk but soured by *L. acidophilus* instead of acid-producing streptococci.

Milk-Alkali Syndrome. Weakness and lethargy caused by prolonged adherence to a diet rich in milk (more than 2 pints) per day and alkalis. (DP.)

Milk, Buddeized. Milk preserved by the addition of hydrogen peroxide. Not legally permitted. *See also* Hydrogen peroxide. (Davis.)

Milk, Citrated. Milk to which sodium citrate has been added to combine with the calcium and inhibit the curdling of caseinogen which would normally occur in the stomach. Claimed, with little evidence, to be of value in feeding infants and invalids. (DP.)

Milk, Designated. Legally milk may be designated pasteurized or sterilized and also Tuberculin Tested.

The special designation "accredited" has been abolished. (Bell.)

Milk, Dried. Milk that has been evaporated to dryness, usually by spray or roller-drying. May be whole or full-cream milk (26% fat), three-quarter cream (not less than 20% fat), half-cream (not less than 14% fat), quarter cream (not less than 8% fat), or skim milk (1% fat).

Milk, Dye-reduction Test. *See* Methylene blue dye-reduction test.

Milk, Evaporated. Concentrated to about 45% of its original volume by evaporation. Also called unsweetened, condensed milk.

Legally must contain not less than 7·8% fat and 25·5% total solids. First produced in 1883 by Meyenberg. (Bell, AEB.)

Milk Fat Test. *See* Gerber test.

Milk, Filled. Milk from which the natural fat has been removed and replaced with fat from another source. The reason may be economic, if the butter-fat can be replaced by a cheaper one, or, more recently, to replace a fat poor in the essential fatty acids with a vegetable fat rich in these factors.

Milk, Freezing-point Test. The sample of milk is cooled below its freezing point and seeded with a crystal of ice. The temperature rises to the F.P. of milk as the whole freezes—normally −0·530 to −0·560°C.

When milk has been adulterated the F.P. rises nearer to that of water. F.P.'s above −0·530°C are indicative of adulteration. (Davis.)

Milk, Frozen or Fresh Frozen. Milk is pasteurized, treated with an ultrasonic vibrator at 5 million cycles per second for 5 minutes and frozen to 10°F. It will keep for a year, and when thawed is indistinguishable from the original milk.

Milk, Half-cream. Usually refers to the dried product sometimes recommended for small and premature babies who are said by some paediatricians to be unable to digest the fat of whole milk. The fat is reduced by two methods (1) simple skimming of half the fat, when the protein content is proportionately increased from 26% to 29%, (2) by dilution with lactose when the protein is simultaneously diluted to 19%. Both types of half-cream milk are on the market for infant feeding.

Milk, Homogenized. After pasteurizing the milk is treated mechanically to break the fat globules into minute droplets which are evenly distributed throughout the milk. Homogenized milk therefore does not have a cream line.

Milk, Humanized. Cow's milk that has had its composition modified to resemble human milk. The main change is a reduction in protein content often achieved by dilution with carbohydrate and restoration of the fat content. (AEB.)

Milk, Irradiated. Milk that has been subjected to ultra-violet light, when the 7-dehydrocholesterol present naturally, is partly converted into vitamin D.

Milk, Long. A Scandinavian soured milk which is viscous because of "ropiness" caused by bacteria.

Milk, Long-life. Trade name (Express Dairy Co. Ltd.) for milk sterilized for a very short time (2 secs) at ultra-high temperature (137°C)—also called UHT milk.

Milk, Malted. A preparation of milk and the liquid separated from a mash of barley malt and wheat flour, evaporated to dryness. (Davis & Mac.)

Milk, Methylene Blue Test. *See* Methylene blue dye-reduction test.

Milk, Non-fat. U.S. term for skimmed milk.

Milk, Pasteurized. *See* Phosphatase test, Pasteurization *and* Methylene blue dye-reduction test.

Milk, Protein. *See* Protein milk.

Milk, Ropy. *See* Rope.

Milks, Fermented. In various countries milk, from the ass, mare, cow, goat and buffalo, is fermented with a mixture of bacteria and yeasts when the lactose is converted to lactic acid and, in some drinks, to alcohol. These fermented milks include busa (Turkestan), cieddu (Italy), dadhi (India), kefir (Balkans), kumiss (Steppes), leben (Egypt), mazun (Armenia), taette (N. Europe), skyr (Iceland), mast (Iran), crowdies (Scotland), kuban, and yoghurt. (Tanner, Davis.)

Milk, Sterilized. Legally milk that has been filtered, homogenized and maintained at a temperature not less than 100°C until it complies with the turbidity test, *see* Milk, turbidity test.

Milk-stone. Deposit of calcium and magnesium phosphates, protein, etc., produced when milk is heated to temperatures above 60°C.

Milk, Sweetened, Condensed. Evaporated to less than one-third volume and sugar added as preservative; may be full cream or skimmed. First patented in U.S.A. and U.K. by Borden 1856. (Hutch.)

Milk, Toned. Dried, skim milk added to a high fat milk such as buffalo milk, to reduce the fat content but maintain the total solids. If the fat were diluted simply by adding water the milk would not be "toned up".

Milk, TT. Tuberculin tested. Applied to milk from herd that has been attested free from tubercle by a veterinary inspector. (Davis.)

Milk, Turbidity Test. To distinguish sterilized milk from pasteurized. During sterilization, the milk is held at 104–116°C for 20–40 minutes, when all the albumin is precipitated. In the test the filtrate from an ammonium sulphate precipitation should remain clear on heating, indicating that no albumin was present in solution and the milk had therefore been sterilized. (Davis.)

Milk, Witches. *See* Witches' milk.

Millerator. Wheat-cleaning machine consisting of two sieves, the upper one retaining particles larger than wheat, the lower one rejecting particles smaller than wheat.

Miller's Offal. *See* Wheatfeed.

Millet. Cereal of a number of species of *Gramineae* smaller than wheat and rice and high in fibre content.

Common millet (*Panicum* and *Setaria* species) also known as China, Italian, Indian, French, hog, proso, panicled and broom corn millet; grows very rapidly, 2–2½ months from sowing to harvest.

Protein 10%, fat 2·5%, carbohydrate 73%.

Red, finger, South India millet or ragi is *Eleusine coracana*. Protein 6%, fat 1·5%, carbohydrate 75%.

Bulrush millet, pearl millet, bajoa or Kaffir manna corn is *Pennisetum typhoideum* or *americanum;* the staple food in poor parts of India. Protein 11%, fat 5%, carbohydrate 69%.

Other species are Kodo or haraka millet (*Paspalum scrobiculatum*) and Teff (*Eragrostis tef* or *abyssinica*) and jajeo millet (*Acroceras amplectens*). (TND, Platt.)

Milling. Usually applied to the process of converting wheat grains into flour. (KJ).

Millon's Test. For proteins; actually a test for the hydroxyphenyl group and therefore for tyrosine, but since every protein contains some tyrosine it is used as a general protein test.

The reagent consists of mercury in nitric acid and gives a white precipitate with proteins which turns red on heating. (Hawk.)

Mills. *See under various headings:* Ball mill, Hammer mill, Disc mill, Quern, Roller mill.

Milt. The soft roe of the male fish. Also the name given to the spleen of animals.

Minafen. Trade name (Trufood Ltd.) for food low in phenylalanine for treatment of phenylketonuria. (AEB.)

Minamata disease. Mercury poisoning from fish caught in Minamata Bay in Japan.

Mincemeat. Legally 30% dried fruit and peel, 30% sugar, 2·5% fat, 0·5% acetic acid, not less than 65% soluble solids.

In America a heavily spiced mixture of chopped meat, apples and raisins. (Bell.)

Mineralocorticoids. Obsolescent term for the steroid hormone of the adrenal cortex which controls the excretion of salt and water by the kidney. *See* Adrenal glands *and* Aldosterone. (BDS.)

Mineral Salts. The inorganic salts, including sodium, potassium, calcium, chloride, phosphate, sulphate, etc.

Minerals, Legal Claims. *See* Vitamins, legal claims.

Mineral Waters, Natural. Spring waters impregnated with carbon dioxide; some slightly alkaline; various minerals present in dilute solution. E.g. Apollinaris, Contrexéville, Evian, Perrier, Rosbach, Vichy, Vittel. (Hutch.)

Miners' Cramp. Cramp due to loss of salt from the body caused by excessive sweating; occurs in tropical climates and with severe exercise—mining often combines the two. Prevented by consuming salt, e.g., salt tablets in the tropics and for athletes.

Mint. Many varieties of the species *Mentha* — spearmint, *Mentha spicata;* peppermint, *Mentha piperita.* Used to flavour meat, fish, tobacco, etc.

Oil of peppermint is distilled from stem and leaves of *Mentha piperita* and used both pharmaceutically and as a flavour. (Merory.)

Miotin. Unidentified urinary excretion product of biotin, together with triotin and rhiotin. (Sebrell.)

Miracle Berry. *Richardella dulcifica* (also known as *Synsepalum dulcifium*); tropical fruit from west Africa containing a taste-modifying substance that causes sour foods to taste sweet. Hence the name miracle berry, and **miraculin** for the active principle, a glycoprotein.

Miraculin. *See* Miracle Berry.

Mirepoix. Bed of vegetables used to give flavour to braised meats and also soups and sauces.

147

Miso. Old Japanese food prepared by fermentation of mouldy rice or koji (Aspergillus) with soybean and salt.

Mixograph. An American instrument for measuring the physical properties of a dough similar in principle to the Farinograph, *which see*. (KJ.)

Molasses. Syrup produced by washing raw sugar. Is boiled and as much sugar as possible crystallized out. The syrupy residue, so rich in non-sugars that no more sucrose can be crystallized out, is molasses. (Ayl.)

Molisch Reaction. Test for carbohydrates. The reagent is a 5% solution of alpha-naphthol in alcohol; two drops added to the test solution and conc. sulphuric acid poured down the side of the tube to form a lower layer. Violet zone appears at the junction. (Hawk.)

Molybdenum. An element that is part of the enzyme xanthine oxidase and so may possibly be a dietary essential in small traces although there is no evidence for this. It is toxic in small doses and "teart" in cattle is associated with feeding on pastures containing molybdenum.
It is essential to plants. (Gil. GMW.)

Monellin. Active sweet principle from Serendipity Berry.

Monocalcium Phosphate. *See* Calcium acid phosphate.

Monoglycerides. *See* Superglycinerated fats.

Monophagia. Desire for one type of food.

Monosaccharides. Group name of the simplest sugars, including those composed of 3 carbon atoms (trioses), 4 (tetroses), 5 (pentoses), 6 (hexoses), and 7 (heptoses). Also known as monoses or monosaccharoses. (BDS.)

Monosaccharose. *See* Monosaccharides.

Monose. *See* Monosaccharides.

Monosodium Glutamate. *See* Glutamate, sodium.

Mortadella. *See* Sausage.

Moss, Irish. *See* Carageenan.

Mother of Vinegar. *See* Vinegar.

Mottled Teeth. In areas where the drinking water contains fluoride at a level of several parts per million, dull, chalky patches occur on the teeth known as mottling. These teeth are relatively free from decay, and lower levels of fluoride, about 1 ppm, reduce decay without causing mottling.

Mould Bran. A fungal amylase preparation produced by growing mould on moist wheat bran; used as source of starch-splitting enzymes.

Mould Inhibitors. *See* Antimycotics.

Moulds. Fungi that produce branched filaments, mycelia; reproduce by spores. Grow rapidly under good conditions and the reproductive cycle from spore to spore can be completed in 24 hours.
Include white *Mucor*, greygreen *Penicillium*, black *Aspergillus*, and also mushrooms and toadstools. Growth inhibited by propionates and sorbic acid.
Of technological use are *Aspergillus niger* for citric acid manufacture, various *Penicillia* for cheese ripening, and antibiotic production. (Baum, Tanner.)

148

M.P.F. *See* Multipurpose Food.

M.S.G. *See* Glutamate, sodium.

Mucin. Naturally occurring complexes of protein and carbohydrates; highly viscous.

Mucopolysaccharides. Complexes of sugars, sugar acids and aminohexoses, e.g. hyaluronic acid, heparin. Combined with protein they form mucoproteins.

Mucoproteins. Complexes of protein with mucopolysaccharides; they function as lubricants in the eye, respiratory tract and intestines.

Mucor. *See* Moulds.

Mucosa. Name given to the moist tissue lining, for example, the mouth (buccal mucosa) intestines and respiratory tract.

The intestinal wall has two sides, the inner or mucosal side, and the outer, or serosal side.

Muffins. *See* Dough Cakes.

Mulberry. *Morus nigra* (also white mulberry, *Morus alba*). Of little commercial importance.

Composition per 100 g: 14 g carbohydrate, 1·5 g protein, 60 kcal (0·24 MJ), 10 mg vitamin C. (OF, Platt.)

Multipurpose Food. Indian Multipurpose Food is made from peanut flour and chickpea flour with calcium carbonate, and vitamins A, B_1 and B_2 and contains 40% protein.

American Multipurpose Food is based on soya. (AEB.)

Muscarine. *See* Ptomaines.

Muscatels. Made by drying the large seed-containing grapes grown almost exclusively in Malaga (Spain). They are partially dried in the sun and drying completed indoors; they are left on the stalk and pressed flat for sale.

Muscatel is the name given to a sweet wine made from the same grape.

For analysis *see* Fruit, dried; *also* Raisins, Currants *and* Sultanas.

Muscle. The contractile cellular unit of skeletal muscle is the **fibre.** This is a long cylinder in shape and composed of many **myofibrils.** Chemically the muscle fibre is composed of three proteins, **myosin, actin** and **tropomyosin.**

The muscle fibre is surrounded by a thin membrane, the **sarcolemma.** Within the muscle fibre surrounding the myofibrils is the **sarcoplasm** or cytoplasm. Individual fibres are separated by a thin network of connective tissue, the **endomysium** and bound together in bundles by larger sheets of connective tissue, the **perimysium.**

Muscle tissue also contains structural elements, **collagen reticulin** and **elastin.** (Meat.)

Muscle Adenylic Acid. Adenosine-5-phosphoric acid; yeast adenylic acid is adenosine-3-phosphoric acid. (BDS.)

Muscovado. The impure sugar left after evaporating the juice from the sugar cane and draining off the molasses, moist and dark brown, often used in making wedding cakes.

Mushroom (*Agaricus campestris*). Composition (raw): water 91·5%, protein 1·8%, fat trace, carbohydrate nil; kcal 7 (0·03 MJ), Fe 1 mg, vitamin A nil, B_1 0·1 mg, B_2 0·4 mg, nicotinic acid 4 mg, C 3 mg—per 100 g. (M&W.)

Mushroom Sugar. α-α'-trehalose; found in most species of fungi,

149

yeasts, many bacteria and the blood of insects.

Mussel (*Mytilus edulis*). Bivalve, cultivated at 25–50 tons per acre, yield 5–10 tons wet weight of meat per acre; take 4 years to reach marketable size—5 cm; 20% of weight is meat.

Boiled: Water 79%, protein 16·8%, fat 2%, carbohydrate trace only; kcal 87 (0·36 MJ), Ca 200 mg, Fe 13·5 mg—per 100 g.

Mustard. Powdered seed of black or brown mustard (*Brassica nigra* or *juncea*) mixed with yellow or white (*Sinapsis alba*). Active principles are glycosides—sinigrin in black, sinalbin in white. When moistened the enzyme myrosinase liberates the characteristically-flavoured oil. Legally (U.K.) mustard condiment must yield not less than 0·35% allyl isothiocyanate after maceration with water for 2 hours at 37°C.

Still referred to in parts of England as **Durham mustard** after Mrs Clements of Durham who made the first commercial preparations of ground mustard seed, wheat flour and turmeric (1711).

English mustard: contains not more than 10% wheat flour and water.

Dijon mustard: made exclusively from *B. nigra* or *juncea* with vinegar, grape juice or wine and not coloured.

Violet mustard: coloured with grape jiuce.

French mustard: white mustard, vinegar, salt, turmeric, cayenne pepper, cloves, pimento.

Mustard leaves eaten raw in salads (**mustard and cress**) are seed leaves of *Sinapsis alba*; much of the commercial product is a strain of rape (*Brassica napus*), a different strain from that used for edible oil. (*See* Rape).

Composition of mustard and cress per 100 g: 1·6 g protein, 0·9 g carbohydrate, 10 kcal (0·04 MJ), 66 mg calcium, 4·5 mg iron, 80 μg vitamin A, 80 mg vitamin C. (OF, M&W.)

Mustard Oil. Used as cooking fat in Bengal and Bihar. The seeds are often contaminated with seeds of epidemic dropsy since the *san-mexicana* which contains an alkaloid, sanguinarine. The contaminated mustard oil is the cause of epidemic dropsy as the sanguinarine inhibits the oxidation of pyruvic acid which accumulates in the blood. (DP.)

Mutachrome. *See* Citroxanthin.

Mutton. Meat of sheep older than one year. Protein 11·9%, fat 21·1%; kcal 241 (1·0 MJ), Ca 7 mg, Fe 1·4 mg, vitamin A nil, B_1 0·11 mg, B_2 0·14 mg, nicotinic acid 3·6 mg, vitamin C nil—per 100 g. (FAO.)

Mycelia. *See* Moulds.

Mycoderma aceti. *See* Acetobacter.

Mycotoxin. A toxin of fungal origin.

Myoacets. Trade name (Distillation Products, U.S.A.) for a range of distilled monoglycerides, *see* Superglycinerated fats.

Myofibril. *See* Muscle.

Myogen. Protein of muscle, about 20% of the total; an albumin, not present in the muscle fibrils but only in the sarcoplasm in which the fibrils are embedded. (Hawk.)

Myoglobin. A complex protein in muscle, similar to the haemoglobin of the blood (but one fourth of its molecular weight), composed of the iron-containing pigment, haem and the protein, globin. It serves as a storage mechanism for oxygen for the cells as it can reversibly add oxygen to form oxymyoglobin.

The globin is denatured by heat to a brown pigment, hence the change from the red colour of raw meat to brown on cooking.

When meat is cured with nitrite the myoglobin is converted into bright red nitric oxide-myoglobin or nitrosomyoglobin. (Meat.)

Myosin. Major fraction, about two-fifths, of muscle protein. A globulin, insoluble in water but soluble in salt solution. Combines with the protein actin, to form actomyosin; the complex dissociates in the presence of ATP. (Hawk.)

Myristic Acid. One of the long chain saturated fatty acids, $CH_3(CH_2)_{12}COOH$. Occurs as triglyceride in nutmeg butter, coconut, butter, lard, spermaceti and wool wax.

Myrosinase. Glycosidase enzyme in mustard seed that hydrolyses myrosin or sinigrin to glucose and allyl isothiocyanate (mustard oil). *See also* Mustard *and* Horse radish.

Mysore Flour. A blend of 75% tapioca flour and 25% peanut flour, used as a partial substitute for cereals in large-scale feeding trials in Madras State, India.

Myxoedema. Underactivity of the thyroid gland (hypothyroidism). *See also* Cretinism, Goitre *and* Thyroid gland. (BDS.)

Myxoxanthin. Carotenoid pigment in algae with vitamin A activity.

N

NAD (and NADP). *See* Nicotinamide adenine dinucleotide (and nicotinamide adenine dinucleotide phosphate).

Naphthoquinone. Basic part of the molecule of vitamin K; the various forms of vitamin K are referred to as substituted naphthoquinones.

Naringin. Glucoside found in the pith of the grapefruit, especially when unripe, but no other citrus fruit. Often crystallizes in tiny beads from canned grapefruit segments and concentrated juice, particularly if the fruit was not fully ripe.

Very bitter, stronger than quinine and can be detected at dilution of 1:50,000. Complex of glucose, rhamnose and naringenin.

Hydrolysed by the enzyme naringinase to the glucoside—**prunin,** which is less bitter, and to naringenin, which is not bitter. Bitter grapefruit and juice can be debittered thus. (Brav.)

National Flour. *See* Wheatmeal, national.

Natto. Fermented soy bean (Japan.)

Natural Waters. *See* Mineral waters, natural.

NDGA *See* Nordihydroguaiaretic acid.

NDpCal. *See* Net Dietary protein Energy Ratio.

Neats Foot. Ox or calf's foot used for making soups and jellies. Now called cow's heels.

Neat's-foot Oil. Oil obtained from the knuckle bones of cattle; used in leather working and for canning sardines.

N.E.F.A. *See* Non-esterified fatty acids.

Neohesperidin Dihydrochalcone. 1,000 times as sweet as sucrose; formed by hydrogenation of naturally-occuring flavonoid, neohesperidin.

Neomycin. Antibiotic isolated 1949 from *Streptomyces fradii*, used to some extent in controlling infections in food processing.

Neroli Oil. Prepared from blossoms of the bitter orange by steam distillation (Southern France, Spain, Italy, South America). Yellowish oil with intense odour of orange blossom. (Merory.)

Nescafé. Trade name (Nestlés Ltd.) for a dried, instant coffee. Contains more potassium than any other food—5·5%. (M&W.)

Nessler Reagent. Alkaline solution of the double iodide of mercury and potassium. Gives an orange-brown with ammonia and used for quantitative estimation. (Hawk.)

Net Dietary protein Calories. *See* Net Dietary protein Energy Ratio.

Net Dietary protein Energy Ratio. The protein content of a diet or food expressed as protein energy multiplied by net protein utilization (*which see*) divided by total energy.

Before the change from calories to joules this was termed net dietary protein calories per cent, NDpCal%. (AEB.)

Net Protein Utilization. Measure of quality of protein in terms of the amount of dietary protein retained in the body under specified experimental conditions. Previously expressed as a percentage, i.e. egg protein and human milk had NPU 100; wheat protein 50; now expressed as ratio, 1·0 and 0·5 respectively.

By convention measured at 10% dietary protein level, NPU_{10}, at which level the protein synthetic mechanism in the growing animal can utilize all the protein so long as the balance of amino acids is correct. When fed at 4% dietary protein level, said to be that level which the NPU is maximum, the value is termed NPU standardized. If the food or diet is fed as it is, i.e. not incorporated into a diet with other ingredients, the value is NPU operative (NPU_{op}). (AEB.)

Net Protein Value. Product of net protein utilization and protein content per cent.

Neuberg Ester. Name given to fructose-6-phosphate, one of the intermediates in glucose metabolism, *which see*.

Neuraminic Acid. *See* Sialic acid.

Neurine. *See* Ptomaines.

New Zealand Process. Drying process applied to meat. It is immersed in hot oil under vacuum, when it dries to 3% moisture in about 4 hours. The fat is removed from the dry meat in a hydro-extractor.

NFE Nitrogen-free extract. In the analysis of foods and animal feedingstuffs this fraction contains the sugars and starches plus small amounts of other materials.

Niacin. Generic descriptor for pyridine-3-carboxylic acid and derivatives exhibiting qualitatively the biological activity of nicotinamide. The term nicotinic acid refers specifically to pyridine-3-carboxylic acid; its amide is nicotinamide.

In the old, obsolete nomenclature niacin was synonymous with nicotinic acid and niacinamide with nicotinamide. Earlier designation was **PP-factor,** pellagra-preventative. *See* Nicotinic acid.

Niacinamide. Obsolete term for nicotinamide. *See* Nicotinic acid.

Niacytin. The vitamin nicotinic acid occurs in some foods partly in a bound form as niacytin, which is not available to the body (nor to bacteria) until it has been hydrolysed. It is a complex of nicotinic acid with glucose, xylose, arabinose, and cinnamic acid derivatives.

Nib. *See* Cocoa.

Nickel. Present in foods and in animal and human tissues. Not shown to be essential for plants or animals but improves growth of many plants.

Metallic nickel used as catalyst in hydrogenation of fats. (GMW.)

Nicol Prism. *See* Polarimeter.

Nicotinamide. *See* Nicotinic acid.

Nicotinamide Adenine Dinucleotide (NAD). Complex of nicotinamide with adenine, two molecules of ribose and two molecules of phosphate. Also known as **Coenzyme I, diphosphopyridine nucleotide (DPN) cozymase** and as **Euler's yeast coenzyme.**

Essential part of the mechanism of oxidation in the tissues. (WHSS.)

Nicotinamide Adenine Dinucleotide Phosphate (NADP). Complex of nicotinamide with two molecules of ribose, adenine, and three molecules of phosphate. Also known as **triphosphopyridine nucleotide (TPN), Coenzyme II** and **Warburg and Christian's coenzyme.**

Essential part, along with NAD, of the mechanism of oxidation in the tissues. (WHSS.)

Nicotinate, Sodium. Sodium salt of nicotinic acid; used, among other purposes, to preserve the red colour in fresh and processed meats.

Nicotinic Acid. Vitamin of the B complex with no numerical designation; sometimes called **vitamin PP** (pellagra-preventative). The amide, **nicotinamide,** has the same biological function and both are known according to internationally agreed nomenclature as niacin. (In the U.S.A. the old designations niacin and niacinamide for nicotinic acid and its amide are still used.)

Functions as a coenzyme in the oxidation of carbohydrates as nicotinamide adenine dinucleotide. Deficiency leads to pellagra—mental disorder, intestinal disorders and dermatitis. Can be formed in the body from the amino acid tryptophan at the rate of 1 mg from 60 mg tryptophan, hence niacin content of foods often recorded as **niacin equivalents,** being the sum of preformed niacin plus one-sixtieth of the tryptophan.

Pellagra occurs particularly in maize-eating areas because the niacin in maize is not available and maize protein is low in tryptophan.

Recommended daily intake 10 mg; found in meat, liver and yeast; that present in cereals often largely unavailable; added to flour in many countries. *See also* Pellagra. (Sebrell.)

Nicotinic Acid, bound form. *See* Niacytin.

Night Blindness or Nyctalopia. Inability to see in dim light through deficiency of vitamin A. Dark-adaptation test is used as an index of vitamin A deficiency as night blindness is the first symptom. *See* Dark adaptation. (Sebrell.)

Ninhydrin Test. For proteins and amino acids (actually for the amino group). Pink, purple or blue colour is developed on reacting the amino acid or peptide with ninhydrin (triketohydrindene hydrate). (Hawk.)

Nioigome. Perfumed rice.

Nisin. Antibiotic isolated 1944 from lactic streptococci group N. Nontoxic, polypeptide, inhibits some but not all clostridia; not used medically.

The only antibiotic permitted in Great Britain in food preservation (in certain foods). It is naturally present in cheese, being produced by a number of strains of cheese starter organisms. Useful to prolong storage life of cheese, milk, cream, soups, canned fruits and vegetables, canned fish and milk puddings. Used at 2–4 micrograms per g of processed cheese and 1–5 micrograms per g of canned peas. It also lowers the resistance of many thermophilic bacteria to heat and so permits a reduction in the time and/or temperature of heating in the processing of canned vegetables. (Bell.)

Nitrates. Occur naturally in many foods; used sometimes in combination with nitrites to cure meat such as bacon, ham and luncheon meat. During pickling process nitrate is partly reduced to nitrite which combines with meat pigment, myoglobin, to form red nitrosomyoglobin. Nitrite and its breakdown products inhibit growth of pathogens.

Nitrites can react with amines in foods to form nitrosamines, many of which are carcinogenic. Permitted content in cured meats in U.K. restricted to 500 ppm sodium or potassium nitrate and 200 ppm nitrite. *See also* Methaemoglobin.

Nitrites. *See* Nitrates.

Nitrogen. This is, of course, a gas, comprising about 80% of the atmosphere, but in nutrition the term "nitrogen" is used to refer to ammonium salts and nitrates as plant fertilizers, to proteins and amino acids as animal nutrients, and to urea and ammonium salts as excretory products. In other words all nitrogen-containing substances are loosely referred to as "nitrogen".

Nitrogen Balance. Condition in which intake equals output, as in the normal adult. In negative balance the excretion exceeds the intake; positive balance is the reverse.

Growing children and convalescents are in positive nitrogen balance; patients with wasting diseases are in negative balance. Alternatively known as **nitrogen equilibrium.** (BDS.)

Nitrogen Equilibrium. *See* Nitrogen balance.

154

Nitrogen, Metabolic. Nitrogen of the faeces derived from internal or endogenous sources, as distinct from nitrogen residues from dietary sources (exogenous nitrogen). This nitrogen consists of unabsorbed digestive juices, the shed lining of the gastro-intestinal tract and bacteria from the intestine, and continues to be excreted on a protein-free diet.

Nitrogen Trichloride. As bread "improver", *see* Aging.

Nitrosamines. *See* Nitrates.

Nitrosomyoglobin. The red colour of cured meat. It is formed by the reaction of nitric oxide from the pickling salts (saltpetre) with the muscle pigment, myoglobin.

Fades in light to yellow-brown metmyoglobin.

Nitrous Oxide. A gas used as a propellant in pressurized containers, e.g. to eject cream or salad dressing from containers.

Noggin. Used as a measure of liquor$=\frac{1}{4}$ pint; also known as a quartern.

Non-enzymic Browning. *See* Maillard reaction.

Non-essential Amino Acids. *See* Amino acid.

Non-esterified Fatty Acids. Free fatty acids in the blood, about 10% of the total blood fatty acids, usually $0\cdot5-1\cdot0$ micromole per litre.

They have a rapid turnover rate and may be the primary fuel of working muscles. The fuel for sudden bursts of hard exercise is glycogen, but for long-continued work the free fatty acids are said to be the source of energy. Also known as **unesterified fatty acids,** or **U.F.A.** or **N.E.F.A.**

Non-pareils. The silver beads used to decorate confectionery, made from sugar coated with silver foil or aluminium-copper alloy.

Non-saponifiable Fraction. *See* Saponification.

Noodles. *See* Alimentary Pastes.

Nor–. Chemical prefix to the name of a compound indicating one methyl group less, e.g. noradrenalin contains a methyl less than adrenalin, similarly norleucine, norvaline.

Noradrenaline. Hormone secreted by the adrenal medulla together with adrenaline (*which see*); also known as **norepinephrine.** Physiological effects similar to adrenaline, chemically differs only by the loss of a methyl group.

The nerve endings in certain parts of the nervous system liberate noradrenaline as a chemical stimulator of the muscles. (BDS.)

Norconidendrin. *See* Conidrendrin.

Nordihydroguaiaretic Acid. Or NDGA; substance of plant origin (the creosote bush) used as an antioxidant for fats.

Norepinephrine. *See* Noradrenaline.

Norite. Activated carbon used to decolorize solutions.

Norite Eluate Factor. Early name given to folic acid.

Normocytes. Red blood cells.

Notatin. Enzyme glucose oxidase isolated from the mould *Penicillium notatum*. Oxidizes glucose to gluconic acid and at the same time forms hydrogen peroxide; specific for glucose and used for quantitative estimation of this sugar and for removing traces of glucose from foodstuffs.

155

Its property of using free oxygen is made use of by adding the enzyme as a stabilizer, e.g. $\frac{1}{2}$ g added to a barrel of beer after fermentation.

Nougat. Sweetmeat made from a mixture of gelatin or egg albumin with sugar and starch syrup, and the whole thoroughly aerated.

Novadelox. Trade name for benzoyl peroxide used for treating flour. *See* Aging.

Novain. Old name for carnitine.

No. 1 Extract. *See* Meat extract.

NPU. Net protein utilization.

NPV. Net Protein Value.

Nubbing. Term used in the canning industry for "topping and tailing" of gooseberries.

Nucellar Layer. Of wheat, the layer of cells that surrounds the endosperm and protects it from the entry of moisture. (KJ.)

Nucleic Acids. Combined with proteins they form the nucleoproteins of cell nuclei.

There are two main types of nucleic acid: ribonucleic acid (RNA) consisting of phosphoric acid, two purines (adenine and guanine), two pyrimidines (cytosine and uracil), and the sugar ribose; and desoxyribonucleic acid (DNA) which differs in containing desoxyribose as the sugar, and thymine in place of uracil.

RNA and DNA are believed to play a key role in the synthesis of proteins in the body and in the transmission of hereditary characteristics.

Nucleoproteins are present in some foods such as fish roe and are useful as a source of protein, but they are not essential to the diet and the nucleic acids are readily synthesized in the body. (BDS.)

Nucleo-Albuminate, Iron. A preparation of iron and casein, also called iron caseinate.

Nucleoproteins. Specific type of proteins found in cell nuclei of both plants and animals. *See* Nucleic acids (BDS.)

Nucleosides. Compound of purine or pyrimidine base with a sugar. E.g. adenine plus ribose forms adenosine—the nucleoside. With the addition of phosphoric acid a nucleotide is formed. (BDS.)

Nucleotides. Compound of purine or pyrimidine base with sugar and phosphoric acid. (BDS.)

Nuoc Mam. Fermented fish sauce from Vietnam and Cambodia. The fish is digested by autolytic enzymes in the presence of added salt to inhibit bacteria.

Nutmeg. Dried ripe seed of *Myristica fragrans;* mace is the seed coat (arillus) of the same species. Both contain fixed oils and their volatile oils are similar but not identical. Both mace and nutmeg are used as flavourings in meat products and bakery goods. (Jacobs, Merory.)

Nutrient Enemata. Rectal feeding can be carried out with nutrient solutions as the colon can absorb 1–2 litres of solution per day; maximum daily amount of glucose that can be given is 75 g, and of nitrogen, in the form of hydrolysed protein, 1 g. (Clark.)

Nutrients. Essential dietary factors such as vitamins, minerals, amino acids and fats. Sources of energy are not termed nutrients so that a commonly used phrase is "energy and nutrients" (calories and nutrients).

Nutrition. The study of foods in relation to the needs of living organisms.

Nutritionist. According to the United States Department of Labour, Dictionary of Occupational Titles—one who applies the science of nutrition to the promotion of health and control of disease; instructs auxiliary medical personnel; participates in surveys. *See also* Dietitian.

Nutritive Ratio. Measure of the value of a feeding ration for growth (or milk production) compared with its fattening value. It is the sum of the digestible carbohydrate, protein and 2·3 × fat, divided by digestible protein. (Calorie value of fat is 2·3 times carbohydrate and protein.) Ratio 4–5 for growth, 7–8 for fattening. (Davis.)

Nutritive Value Index. Term used in animal feeding; intake of digestible energy expressed as energy digestibility multiplied by voluntary intake of dry matter of a particular feed divided by metabolic weight (weight to the power of 0·75), compared with standard feed.

Nutro-biscuit. A biscuit baked from a mixture of 60% wheat flour and 40% peanut flour—contains 16–17% protein; developed in India. (AEB.)

Nutro-macaroni. A mixture of 80 parts wheat flour, 20 parts defatted peanut meal (total 19% protein); developed in India. (AEB.)

Nuts. Hard-shelled fruit of a wide variety of trees, e.g. almonds (*Prunus amygdalis*), Brazil nut (*Bertholletsia excelsa*), cashew nuts (*Anacardium occidentale*), walnut (*Juglans regia*)—all have high fat content, 45–60%, high protein content 15–20%, 15–20% carbohydrate, much of which is in the form of pentosans and other indigestible forms.

The chestnut (*Castanea sativa*) is something of an exception with 3% fat and 3% protein, being largely carbohydrate 37%.

A number of nuts are grown specially for their fat content, such as groundnuts, coconut, and palm, *which see*. (FB, OF.)

Nyctalopia. *See* Night blindness.

O

Oats. Grain from species of *Avena*, the three best known being *A. sativa, steritis* and *strigosa*.

Composition: Protein 13%, fat 7·5%; kcal 385 (1·62 MJ), calcium 56 mg, iron 4 mg, vitamin B_1 0·6 mg, B_2 0·1 mg, nicotinic acid 0·9 mg—per 100 g.

Contains large amounts of phytic acid which can prevent the absorption of calcium from the diet and so induce rickets unless extra calcium and vitamin D are consumed.

Oatmeal—ground oats; **oat flour**—ground, and bran removed; **groats**—husked oats; **Embden groats** — crushed groats; **Scotch oats**—groats cut into granules of various sizes; **Sussex ground oats**—very finely ground oats; **rolled oats**—crushed by rollers and partially precooked. (Hutch, KJ, FAO.)

157

Obesity Drugs. *See* Anorectic agents.

Odoratism. Disease experimentally produced by feeding sweet-pea seeds, *Lathyrus odoratus*, to rats. Damage to the spine and aorta, caused by the presence of a toxic substance, BAPN (beta-amino propion nitrile). This is present both in the sweet pea and the Singletary pea (*L. pusillus*), but not in the chick pea, *L. sativus*, which causes lathyrism in man. *See also* Lathyrism.

Oedema. Excess fluid in the body indicated by pitting of the subcutaneous tissues when pressure is applied with the finger. May be caused by cardiac, renal or hepatic failure and by starvation (famine oedema). (DP.)

Oenin. An anthocyanidin from the skin of purple grapes.

Oestradiol. *See* Oestrogens.

Oestriol. Urinary excretion product of the female hormones oestrone and oestradiol. *See* Oestrogens.

Oestrogens. Female sex hormones. There are two groups, oestrone and oestradiol, that stimulate the ovaries, and progesterone, produced by the corpus luteum, that stimulates the uterus.

Synthetic hormones include ethinyl oestradiol, stilboestrol and hexoestrol. The latter two are used in chemical caponization of cockerels, by implantation under the skin, and to increase the growth rate of cattle, by implantation during the last three months before slaughter.

Oestrogenic substances are also found in spring grass. (BDS.)

Oestrone. One of the female sex hormones. *See* Oestrogens.

Offal. A corruption of off-fall. In reference to meat originally meant only the entrails; now used for all parts that are cut away when a carcass is dressed, including heart, liver, kidney, brain, spleen, pancreas, thymus, tripe, tongue.

In reference to flour-milling means the bran and germ that are removed in the milling of white flour.

Oilseed. A wide variety of seeds are grown as a source of oils, e.g. cottonseed, sesame, groundnut, sunflower, soya, palm, etc. After extraction of the oil the residue is a valuable source of protein, the so-called seed cake.

Oils, Essential. *See* Essential oils.

Oils, Fixed. Refers to the triglycerides, the edible oils, as distinct from the volatile or essential oils, *which see*.

Okra. Also known as **Gumbo, Bamya, Bamies** and **Ladies' Fingers** (*Hibiscus esculentus*). Small ridged mucilaginous pods resembling a small cucumber, grown in South America, West Indies and India; used in soups and stews.

Carbohydrate 6%, protein 2%; iron 1 mg, vitamin A 250 μg, B_1 0·1 mg, B_2 0·1 mg, nicotinic acid 0·8 mg, vitamin C 25 mg—per 100 g. (TND.)

Oleandomycin. An antibiotic used as an addition to chick feed to stimulate growth and improve feed efficiency. Used in U.S.A. at 1–2 g per ton but not permitted for laying hens. The tolerance limit in uncooked edible tissues of chicken or turkey is zero.

Oleic Acid. Long-chain fatty acid with total of 18 carbon atoms; unsaturated with one double bond, 9-octadecenoic acid; found

158

in most fats; high percentage in human fat, and butter. By far the most abundant of the unsaturated acids. (Cohen.)

Oleomargarine. *See* Margarine.

Oleo Oil. *See* Premier jus *and* Tallow, rendered.

Oleoresins. In the preparation of some spices such as pepper, ginger and capsicum, the aromatic material is extracted with solvents which are evaporated off leaving behind thick oily products known as oleoresins.

Oleostearin. *See* Premier jus *and* Tallow, rendered.

Oligodynamic. Sterilizing effect of traces of certain metals. E.g. silver in concentration of 1 in 5 million will kill *Escherichia coli* and staphylococci in 3 hours.

Electrolytic method of getting silver into water is Katadyn process. Suggestions have been made for its use for the treatment of water, fruit juices and various foods. (Tanner, GMW.)

Olive. Fruit of evergreen tree, *Oleo europea*; picked unripe when green or ripe when they have turned dark blue or purplish and usually pickled in brine. Olives have been known since ancient times; tree continues to fruit for many years and there are claims that trees are still fruiting after 1,000 years.

Composition per 100 g: 0·9 g protein, 11 g fat, trace carbohydrate, 106 kcal (0·45 MJ), 60 mg Ca, 1 mg iron. Little or no vitamins when pickled.

Olive oil, obtained by pressing the ripe fruits, is used in cooking, as salad oil and for canning sardines. It is one of the few vegetable oils to contain only small amounts of polyunsaturated fatty acids. (OF, M&W.)

Omasum. *See* Rumen.

Omophagia. Eating of raw or uncooked food.

Oncotic Pressure. The osmotic pressure of colloids. Blood plasma has an oncotic pressure of 28 mm of mercury.

Onions. Bulb of *Allium cepa*. Protein 1·3%, fat 0·2%; kcal 37 (0·16 MJ), Ca 30 mg, Fe 0·5 mg, vitamin A 15 μg, B₁ 0·03 mg, B₂ 0·04 mg, nicotinic acid 0·2 mg, vitamin C 8 mg—per 100 g (FAO.)

Oolong Tea. *See* Tea.

Ophthalamin. Obsolete name for vitamin A.

Opsomania. Craving for special food.

Optical Activity. Certain substances such as sugars and acids, possess the ability to rotate polarized light (*which see*) and are thus said to exhibit optical activity.

If the rotation is to the right the substance is dextrorotatory, designated (+), if to the left it is laevorotatory (−). (The old nomenclature used to be d and l, not to be confused with capital D- and L-, *see* D-.)

Optical activity depends upon the molecule being non-symmetrical. A mixture of the (+) and (−) forms, which results when the compound is prepared by synthesis, is optically inactive and is termed **racemic.**

The degree of rotation under standard conditions, measured in a polarimeter, can serve as a measure of the quantity or purity of an optically active compound.

Sucrose is dextrorotatory and yields on hydrolysis glucose, which is (+) and fructose which is more strongly (−). Thus on hydrolysis the dextrorotation changes to laevo and the hydrolysis of sucrose is termed "inversion" and the mixture of glucose and fructose are the **"invert sugars"**.

Optical Rotation. *See* Optical activity.

Opuntia. *See* Pear, prickly.

Orange. Fruit of *Citrus sinensis*. Of nutritive value mainly because of its vitamin C content. The juice has the same composition. Protein 0·6%, fat 0·1%, Calories 32, Ca 24 mg, Fe 0·3 mg, vitamin A 120 i.u., B_1 0·06 mg, B_2 0·02 mg, nicotinic acid 0·1 mg, vitamin C 36 mg—per 100 g. (FAO.)

Blood oranges are coloured by the presence of anthocyanins (cyanidin-3-glucoside and delphinidin-3-glucoside) in the juice vesicles.

Orange, Bitter. *Citrus aurantium;* known as **Seville orange** in Spain, **bigaradier** in France, **melangol** in Italy, and **khushkhash** in Israel.

Used mainly as root stock because of its resistance to the gummosis disease of citrus. Fruit is too acid to be edible, used in manufacture of marmalade; the peel oil is used in the liqueur curaçao; the peel and flower oils (neroli oil) and the oils from the green twigs (petit-grain oils) are used in perfumery. (Brav.)

Orange Butter. Chopped whole orange is cooked, sweetened and homogenized.

Orange Colours. Orange G—disodium salt of 1-phenylazo-2-naphthol-6:8-disulphonic acid. Stable to reducing agents.

Orange RN—sodium salt of 1 - sulpylazo - 2 - naphthol - 6 - phenhonic acid.

Orange-flower Water. Neroli oil is made from the flowers of the bitter orange by steam distillation. The condensed water layer from the distillation is orange-flower water. (Brav.)

Orange Juice. A classical source of vitamin C. Commercially the juice is concentrated sixfold for export and this is the concentrate distributed as a Welfare food in Great Britain for infants. For composition *see* Orange.

Orange Oil. The peel oil, 90% limonene, main odoriferous constituent *n*-decylic aldehyde (decanal), also linalool and nonylic alcohol.

Oil of bitter orange is similar but contains a glucoside that confers the bitterness. *See also* Terpenes. (Brav.)

Orange Pekoe. *See* Tea.

Orcanella. *See* Alkannet.

Orchil. Red colour obtained from lichens of the *Roccella* species; legally permitted in food in most countries. Colouring principle is orcin (dihydroxy toluene) and orcein, slightly soluble in water to give wine-red solution, yellower with acid, blue with alkalies. (Jacobs.)

Oreganum. Or Mexican sage. *See* Marjoram.

Organic. When used appertaining to chemicals means those that contain carbon in the molecule (with the exception of carbonates and cyanides).

Substances of animal and vegetable origin are organic, minerals are inorganic.

160

Organoleptic. Technical term for taste and smell. Only four tastes can be distinguished on the tongue, bitter, sweet, acid and salt, all others are detected only by smell. (BDS.)

Ornithine. Amino acid that is part of the urea cycle, *which see*; not of nutritional importance since it is not found in protein foodstuffs.

Ornithine-Arginine Cycle. *See* Urea cycle.

Orotic Acid. Uracil-4-carboxylic acid; an intermediate in the biosynthesis of pyrimidines; a growth factor for certain micro-organisms and called vitamin B_{13}.

Ortanique. Citrus fruit; cross between orange and tangerine.

Orthophenyl Phenol. *See* Diphenyl.

Oryzanin. Obsolete name for thiamin (vitamin B_1).

Oryzenin. The major protein of rice; classed as one of the glutelins.

Osazones. Derivatives formed by reaction of aldehydes and ketones with phenylhydrazone. Used to distinguish between sugars since the corresponding osazones of the different sugars have different crystal shape (glucose and fructose form the same osazone). (BDS.)

Oslo Breakfast. Introduced into Oslo, Norway, 1929, for school children before classes started: requires no preparation.
  Rye-biscuit, bread made of high extraction flour, butter or vitaminised margarine, whey cheese and cod liver oil paste, ⅓ litre of milk, raw carrot, apple, half orange.

Osmazome. Old (obsolete) name given to an aqueous extract of meat that is soluble in alcohol—regarded as the pure essence of meat.

Osmophilic Yeasts. Few organisms can grow in high concentrations of sugar or salts, e.g. in jams or brine pickles, due to the high osmotic pressure. Those few yeasts that are able to grow under these conditions are termed osmophilic.
  Zygosaccharomyces can tolerate up to 80% sugar and cause spoilage in honey, chocolate centres, sugar products. (Baum.)

Osmosis. Passage through a semi-permeable membrane. *See* Membrane, semi-permeable, *and* Osmotic pressure.

Osmotic Pressure. The attractive power exerted by a solution for water molecules.
  Usually demonstrated by placing a solution of a salt in a vessel separated by a semi-permeable membrane (e.g. pig's bladder) from pure water. Water passes across the membrane to dilute the salt solution until the hydrostatic pressure of the solution counterbalances the attractive power of the solution for the water, i.e. its osmotic pressure.
  See Membrane, semi-permeable. (BDS.)

Ossein. Organic structure of the bone left behind when the mineral salts are removed by solution in dilute acid. Chemically similar to collagen and hydrolysed by boiling water to gelatin, hence the manufacture of glue from bones—known as ossein gelatin. (Jacobs.)

Osseomucoid. A mucoid substance forming part of the structure of bone.

Osteomalacia. Bone disorder in adults equivalent to rickets in

161

children; due to shortage of vitamin D leading to inadequate absorption of calcium and loss of calcium from the bones. (DP.)

Ostermilk. Trade name (Glaxo Laboratories) for dried milk for infant feeding. Ostermilk No. 1 is half-cream; No. 2 is normal.

Ovalbumin. The albumin of egg-white, comprises 55% of the total solids.

Ovaltine. Trade name (A. Wander Ltd.) for a preparation of malt extract, milk, eggs, cocoa and soya, for consumption as a beverage when added to milk. Fortified with vitamins B_1, D and nicotinic acid.

Oven Spring. The sudden increases in the volume of a dough during the first 10–12 minutes of baking —due to increase rate of fermentation and to expansion of gases.

Overrun. Term used in ice-cream manufacture—the percentage increase in the volume of the mix caused by the beating-in of air. Optimum overrun, 70–100%.

To prevent excessive aeration United States regulations state that ice-cream must weigh 4·5 lb per gallon. (Davis.)

Ovoflavin. Name given to substance isolated from eggs, shown to be identical with riboflavin.

Ovomucin. A carbohydrate-protein complex in egg-white, 1–3% of the total solids. Responsible for the firmness of egg-white.

Ovomucoid. A protein of egg-white, 12% of the total solids. Acts as a specific inhibitor of the digestive enzyme trypsin, but is destroyed by the stomach enzyme pepsin.

Oxalated Blood. See Blood, oxalated.

Oxalic Acid. Lowest member of the dicarboxylic acid series, COOH.COOH. Poisonous, but not in small doses; present in spinach, chocolate and rhubarb. The toxicity of rhubarb leaves is due to their high content of oxalic acid.

Oxalic acid is normally excreted in human urine, 15–20 mg per day, increased in diabetes and liver disease. (Hawk.)

Oxidase, Glucose. See Notatin.

Oxidase, Phenol. See Phenol oxidases.

Oxidases. Enzymes that oxidize compounds by removing hydrogen and adding it to oxygen to form water. They thus differ from dehydrogenases since the latter cannot pass the hydrogen directly on to oxygen, but only to an intermediate.

See also Intermediate hydrogen carrier.

Oxidation. Gain in oxygen, or loss of hydrogen or (covering all cases such as oxidation of ferrous chloride to ferric chloride when neither oxygen nor hydrogen is involved) loss of electrons. See Oxidases and Intermediate hydrogen carrier.

Oximetry. The continuous measurement of the amount of oxygen in the circulating blood. (BDS.)

Oxo. Trade name (Oxo Ltd.) for a dried preparation of hydrolysed meat, meat extract, salt and cereal in cube form, used as a drink or a gravy.

Protein 9·5%, fat 3·4%, carbohydrate 12·0%; Ca 180 mg, Fe 25 mg, kcal 116 (0·49 MJ)—per 100 g. (M&W.)

Oxycalorimeter. Instrument for measuring the oxygen used and carbon dioxide produced when a food is burned (as distinct from the bomb calorimeter which measures the heat produced).

Oxyhaemoglobin. Form in which oxygen is transported from the lungs to the tissues; a loose combination of oxygen with the haemoglobin, which is readily decomposed. (BDS.)

Oxymyoglobin. Myoglobin is the coloured protein in muscle that serves as a store of oxygen; it takes up oxygen to form oxymyoglobin which is bright red, while myoglobin itself is purplish-red. The surface of fresh meat which is exposed to oxygen is bright red from the oxymyoglobin, while the interior of the meat is darker in colour where the myoglobin is not oxygenated. (Meat.)

Oxyntic Cells. Or parietal cells; glands in the stomach that produce hydrochloric acid of the gastric juice. (BDS.)

Oyster. *Ostrea edulis*, bivalve, only 10–15% of weight is meat; cultivated at 100 per square yard yields 25 tons to the acre or $2 \cdot 5$–$3 \cdot 7$ tons wet weight of meat; take 5 years to reach marketable size.

(Raw)—Water 86%, protein 10%, fat 1%, carbohydrate trace only, kcal 50 ($0 \cdot 21$ MJ), Ca 190 mg, Fe 6 mg, vitamin A 75 μg, B_1 $0 \cdot 1$ mg, B_2 $0 \cdot 2$ mg, nicotinic acid $1 \cdot 5$ mg—per 100 g.

Ozone. Chemically composed of three atoms of oxygen, O_3. Powerful germicide, used to sterilize water, in antiseptic ice for preserving fish, few ppm in the atmosphere to preserve eggs, etc.

P

PABA. Abbreviation for *para*-amino benzoic acid, *which see*.

Paddy. Rice in the husk after threshing; also known as **rough rice.** *See* Rice.

Palestine Bee. *See* Bee wine.

Palmitic Acid. One of the long chain saturated fatty acids, $CH_3(CH_2)_{14}COOH$. Occurs as triglyceride in many animal and vegetable fats including spermaceti and beeswax. (Cohen.)

Palm Kernel Oil. Oil extracted from the kernel of the nut of *Elaeis guineensis*. The oil from the pulp is termed palm oil, *which see*. Used for margarine and cooking fat.

Palm, Oil. *Elaeis guineensis*; one of the most important sources of oil, greater yield per acre than any other vegetable oil.

Fruit is produced as bunches of nuts; beneath the outer skin is a layer of fibrous pulp, the mesocarp or pericarp which is rich in oil called (red) **palm oil.**

Inside is the seed from the inner kernel from which is obtained **palm kernel oil.**

The palm oil is red in colour from the high content of beta-carotene (up to 10 mg retinol equivalent) together with other carotenoids.

Both palm oil and palm kernel oil are used for margarine and cooking fats. (OF, Platt.)

Palm, Wild date. *Phoenix sylvestris*, relative of the true date palm, *P. dactylifera*, grown in India as a

163

source of sugar obtained from the sap. (OF.)

Panada. A mixture of fat, flour and liquid (such as stock or milk) mixed to a thick paste; used to bind mixtures such as chopped meat and also as the basis of soufflés and choux pastry.

Panary Fermentation. Yeast fermentation of dough in bread-making.

Pancreas. A gland in the abdomen with two functions; it secretes (a) the hormone insulin, (b) the pancreatic juice.

Known by the butcher as sweetbread, or gut sweetbread in distinction from chest sweet-bread which is thymus. (BDS.)

Pancreatic Juice. Digestive juice produced by the pancreas and secreted into the duodenum; slightly alkaline, contains the enzymes trypsinogen, chymotrypsinogen, carboxypeptidase, aminopeptidase, lipase, amylase, maltase, sucrase, lactase and nucleases. (BDS.)

Pancreatin. A preparation made from the pancreas of animals and therefore containing the enzymes of pancreatic juice. Used as an aid to digestion.

Pancreozymin. Hormone produced by the intestinal mucosa that stimulates the pancreas to secrete enzymes. *See also* Secretin. (Hawk.)

Panettone. Italian, half bread-half cake.

Pangamic Acid. N-diisopropyl derivative of glucuronic acid. Powerful methylating agent concerned with respiratory enzymes in cells. Also termed vitamin B_{15}

but no evidence that it is a dietary essential.

Pantothenic Acid. A vitamin with no numerical designation; chemically beta-alanine plus pantoic acid. Is part of the structure of Coenzyme A, needed for the transfer of acetyl groups and therefore essential for the metabolism of fats and carbohydrates.

Dietary shortage never arises; universally distributed in all living cells, best sources are liver, kidney, yeast, bees' royal jelly and fresh vegetables.

Deficiency symptoms in rats include greying of the hair, dermatitis, adrenal damage; in chicks, dermatitis; in dogs, gastro-intestinal symptoms; but no definite pathological lesions in man.

Based on the needs of animals, human requirements would be 6–8 mg per day.

Also known as **filtrate factor.** (Sebrell.)

Pantoyltaurine. Similar to pantothenic acid but with the carboxyl group replaced by a sulphonic acid group; acts as an antagonist to the vitamin.

When given to man leads to dizziness, postural hypotension, tachycardia, drowsiness and anorexia. Also called **thiopanic acid.** (Hawk.)

Papain. Proteolytic enzyme from the juice of the papaya (*Carica papaya*) used in tenderizing meat; sometimes called **vegetable pepsin.** Rate of reaction slow at room temperature, increased at 55–75°C, maximum activity at 80°C and rapidly inactivated at temperatures higher than this, hence papain continues to tenderize the meat during the early stages of cooking. (Meat.)

Papaya. *See* Pawpaw.

Papin's Digester. Early version of the pressure cooker. Named after Papin, French physicist 1647–1712; originally invented for the purpose of softening bones for the preparation of gelatin.

Paprika. *See* Pepper.

Para-amino Benzoic Acid. Essential growth factor for micro-organisms and therefore classed as a vitamin. No deficiency symptoms in higher animals except greying of the hair (achromotrichia) in rats.

Is part of the molecule of folic acid and it is assumed that one of the functions of *p*-amino benzoic acid is the formation of folic acid.

Sulphanilamide is chemically very similar and kills bacteria by blocking access to the vitamin.

Occurs in yeast, wheat germ; smaller amounts in meat, liver, vegetables. Also called the **anti-grey hair factor.** (Sebrell.)

Paraben, methyl and propyl. Methyl and propyl parahydroxy-benzoates—used as preservatives at a concentration of $0 \cdot 1\%$.

Paracasein. *See* Caseinogen.

Paraffin, Medicinal. *See* Medicinal paraffin.

Paraflow. Trade name (APV Co. Ltd.) for a plate heat exchanger used for pasteurizing liquids.

Parakeratosis. Disease of swine characterized by cessation of growth, erythema, seborrhoea and hyperkeratosis of the skin; due to zinc deficiency, and essential fatty acids may be involved.

Paralactic Acid. *See* Sarcolactic acid.

Parathormone. *See* Parathyroid glands.

Parathyroid Glands. Four glands situated in the neck near to the thyroid gland but not connected with its function. They secrete the parathyroid hormone (parathormone) which controls the level of the calcium in the blood and the excretion of phosphate in the urine. An overactive parathyroid causes withdrawal of calcium from the bones, so raising the blood level and causing excretion in the urine. When there is a fall in serum calcium, the parathyroid responds by reducing blood phosphate by excreting it in the urine. (BDS.)

Parboil. Partially cook. Of special interest in nutrition is the parboiling of brown rice, that is steaming of the rice in the husk before milling. The water-soluble B vitamins diffuse from the husk into the grain. When the rice is then polished the white rice contains far more of these vitamins than polished raw rice. (FB.)

Parchita. *See* Passion fruit.

Parietal Cells. *See* Oxyntic cells.

Parillin. Highly toxic glycoside from sarsaparilla root; consists of glucose, rhamnose and parigenin. Also known as **smilacin.**

Parsley. A culinary herb, *Petroselinum crispum*, widely used in sauces, soups and salads and to decorate other dishes. Described in textbooks as a rich source of iron, vitamin C and carotene but as the amounts eaten (in U.K.) are insignificant its nutritive value cannot be taken seriously.

Parsnips (*Pastinaca sativa*). Protein $1 \cdot 0\%$, fat $0 \cdot 3\%$; kcal 49 ($0 \cdot 21$ MJ); Ca 37 mg, Fe $0 \cdot 5$ mg; vitamin A nil, B_1 $0 \cdot 05$ mg, B_2 $0 \cdot 08$ mg, nicotinic acid $0 \cdot 1$ mg, vitamin C 12 mg—per 100 g. (FAO.)

Parts Per Million. Or **ppm.** Method of describing small concentrations and means exactly what the term says. Mgm per kg is also ppm.

Usually used with regard to traces of metallic impurities and food additives, e.g. jam must not contain more than 40 ppm of sulphur dioxide.

Passion Fruit. Also known as **parchita, granadilla** and **water lemon**; fruit of the tropical American vine, *Passiflora* species. Purple or greenish-yellow when ripe, watery pulp containing small seeds; used in fruit drinks.

Carbohydrate 16%, protein 1·2%; vitamin A 60 μg, C 20 mg—per 100 g. (TND.)

Pasta. *See* Alimentary pastes.

Pasteurization. Vegetative forms of many bacteria can be killed by mild heat treatment, pasteurization, whereas total destruction of all bacteria and spores, sterilization, requires higher temperatures for longer periods, often spoiling the product in the process. Pasteurization will prolong the storage life of foods but usually only for a limited period.

Pasteurization of milk destroys all the pathogens, and although the milk will sour within a day or two it is not a source of disease.

Legally, pasteurization of milk means maintaining at 145–150°F (63–66°C) for 30 minutes, followed by immediate cooling, or so-called "high-temperature short-time process", 161°F (72°C) for 15 seconds. *See also* Phosphatase test, Flash-pasteurization *and* Methylene blue dye-reduction test. (Tanner.)

Pasteurizer. Equipment used to pasteurize liquids such as milk, fruit juices, etc. They function, in effect, as heat-exchangers. The material to be pasteurized is passed continuously over heated plates, or through pipes, where it is heated to the required temperature, maintained at that temperature for the required time, then immediately cooled.

Patent Flour. *See* Extraction rate.

Pathogens. Disease-causing bacteria as distinct from those that are harmless.

Pavlov Pouch. Surgical technique, introduced by Pavlov, in which a portion of the stomach is brought to the body wall. It is then possible to take a sample of the stomach contents directly from this pouch, as the secretion into the pouch is identical with that into the main part of the stomach. (BDS.)

Pawpaw. Or **papaya.** Large green or yellow melon-like fruit of the *Carica papaya*, a tree similar to the palm. It is the commonest tropical fruit second to the banana and is a rich source of vitamin A and C. Water 89%, carbohydrate 9%; kcal 38 (0·16 MJ), vitamin A 800 μg, vitaim C 80 mg—per 100 g.

The proteolytic enzyme, **papain,** is obtained as the dried latex of the skin of the fruit by scratching it while still on the tree, and collecting the flow. In the tropics meat is often tenderized by wrapping in pawpaw leaves. (TND, OF.)

Pea, Garden. Seed of the legume, *Pisum sativum*.

Fresh: Protein 2·9%, fat 0·2%, kcal 36 (0·15 MJ), Ca 11 mg, Fe 0·9 mg, vitamin A 78 μg, B₁ 0·15 mg, B₂ 0·08 mg, nicotinic acid

1·1 mg, vitamin C 11 mg—per 100 g. For sizes, see Petit pois. (FAO.)

Pea, Processed. Refers to peas that have been dried as distinct from fresh, garden, green, canned and frozen peas.

Peanut. Also known as **groundnut, earth nut** and **monkey nut.** Seed of the legume, *Arachis hypogaea*; Spanish and Virginia types have 2 kernels per pod, Valencia has 3–4.

The nuts serve as an important source of protein in many tropical diets. The oil, known as **arachis oil**, is used for cooking, as salad oil, for canning sardines and for margarine manufacture. The residue after oil extraction is a valuable source of protein for animal feed.

Composition per 100 g: 25·6 g protein, 43 g fat, 550 kcal (2·3 MJ), 1·9 mg iron, 9 μg vitamin A, 0·84 mg B_1, 0·12 mg B_2, 16 mg nicotinic acid. *See also* Bombarra groundnut. (FAO, OF.)

Peanut Butter. Ground, roasted peanuts; commonly prepared from a mixture of Spanish and Virginia peanuts since the first alone is too oily and the second is too dry. Separation of the oil is prevented by partial hydrogenation of the oil and the addition of emulsifiers. (Matz.)

Pear. Fruit of many species of *Pyrus*, cultivated varieties all descended from *P. communis*.

Composition per 100 g: 0·4 g protein, 0·3 g fat, 50 kcal (0·2 MJ), very small amounts of carotenoids, B vitamins and C. (FAO, OF.)

Pear, Prickly. Fruit of the cactus *Opuntia*, also called **Indian fig, barberry fig,** and **tuna**—an important part of the diet in certain areas of Mexico.

Composition: Water 81%, protein 1%, carbohydrate 26%, vitamin C 15 mg, kcal 68 (0·29 MJ)—per 100 g. (TND.)

Peas. A wide variety of leguminous seeds classed with beans and lentils; good source of protein (20–30%), moderate source of iron and vitamins B_1, B_2 and nicotinic acid. Form vitamin C on germination.

Pigeon pea or **red gram** (*Cajanus indicus*); **Chick pea** or **Bengal gram** (*Cicer arietinum*); **garden pea** (*Pisum sativum*). *See also* Pulses *and* Beans. (TND. FB.)

Pectase. Enzyme in the pith of citrus fruits that removes the methoxyl groups from pectin to form water-insoluble pectic acid. The intermediate compounds with varying numbers of methoxy groups are pectinic acids.

Also known as **pectin esterase, pectin methyl esterase** and **pectin methoxylase.**

Pectin. Plant tissues contain **protopectins** (which are chemically hemicelluloses) cementing the cell walls together. As fruit ripens, there is maximum protopectin present, thereafter it breaks down to pectin, pectinic acid and finally pectic acid under the influence of enzymes, and the fruit loses its firmness and becomes soft as the adhesive between the cells breaks down.

Pectin is the setting agent in jam. Soft fruits, as strawberry, raspberry and cherry, are low in pectin; plum, apple and bitter orange are rich. Apple pulp and orange pith are the commercial source of pectin. Used to add to jams, confectionery, chocolate; added to ice-cream as an emulsifier and stabilizer instead of agar; in making jellies; and as anti-staling agent in cakes. See Jam *and* Firming Agents. (Jacobs.)

Pectinase. Enzyme present in the pith (albedo) of citrus fruits, that hydrolyses pectins or pectic acids into smaller polygalacturonic acids, and finally galacturonic acid and its methyl ester.

Also known as pectolase and polygalacturonase. (Brav.)

Pectinesterase. Alternative name for pectase, *which see.*

Pectin Methoxylase. See Pectase.

Pectins, Low-methoxyl. Partially de-esterified pectins which can form gels with little or no sugar and therefore used in low-calorie jellies.

Pectolase. Alternative name for pectinase, *which see.*

Pectosase. See Protopectinase.

Pectosinase. Alternative name for protopectinase, *which see.*

Pekar Test. A comparative test of flour colour. The flour is pressed on a board with a smooth applicator and colour comparisons are made immersed in water. (KJ.)

Pekoe. See Tea.

Pelagic Fish. Oily fish containing up to 20% fat; swim near the surface; include herring, mackerel, pilchards. *See also* Demersal fish.

Pellagra. Disease due to deficiency of nicotinic acid. Symptoms include characteristic symmetrical dermatitis on exposed surfaces such as face and back of hands, mental disturbances and digestive disorders. (Students' mnemonic

—dermatitis, dementia and diarrhoea—arising from diet of meat, maize and molasses.) (DP.)

Pemmican. Mixture of dried, powdered meat and fat; 3% water, 40% protein, 45% fat, 560 kcal (2·4 MJ), per 100 g.

Used as concentrated food source, e.g. on expeditions. (M&W.)

Penicillin. The first of the antibiotics, isolated from the culture fluid of the mould *Penicillium notatum*, 1929. Active against a wide range of bacteria and of great value clinically. Not used as food preservative in case repeated small doses cause penicillin resistance.

Penicillium. See Moulds.

Pentosans. Complex carbohydrates widely distributed in plants, e.g. fruit, wood, corncobs, oat hulls. Not digested in the body but broken down by acid to yield the 5-carbon sugars or pentoses.

Pentose. Simple sugar with 5 carbon atoms. The most important is ribose. (BDS.)

P-enzyme. Potato phosphorylase, specific for 1:4 alpha links. (WHSS.)

Pepper. Three types. (1) Sweet pepper, **paprika,** bell pepper, bullnose pepper, Spanish name **pimiento** (not the same as pimento or allspice); fruits of the annual plant *Capsicum annum*. Red, yellow or brown fruits, often eaten raw in salads when green and unripe; very variable size and shape; some varieties can be spicy but mostly non-pungent.

Composition per 100 g: 2 g protein, 0·5 g fat, 6 g carbohydrate, 37 kcal (0·16 MJ), 1 mg iron (green peppers 40 μg vitamin A, red peppers 300 μg), 0·06 mg B_1, 0·08 mg B_2, 1 mg nicotinic acid, 150 mg C (range 50–289).

(2) Red pepper, **chilli** (or chili), small red fruit of *Capsicum frutescens*, bushy, perennial plant. Usually sun-dried therefore wrinkled; very pungent, ingredient of curry powder, pickles and tabasco sauce. **Cayenne pepper** is made from the powdered dried fruits.

Composition per 100 g (dried): 15 g protein, 11 g fat, 33 g carbohydrate, 25 g fibre, 290 kcal (1·2 MJ), 9 mg iron, 300 μg vitamin A, 0·6 mg B_1, 0·5 mg B_2, 12 mg nicotinic acid, 10 mg C.

(3) Black and white pepper, fruit of climbing vine, *Piper nigrum*, grows in wet tropical conditions; fruits are **peppercorns**. **Black pepper** is made from sun-dried unripe peppercorns when red outer skin turns black. **White pepper** made by soaking ripe berries and rubbing off outer skin. Pungency due to alkaloids piperine, piperdine and chavicine.

Composition per 100 g: 12 g protein, 7 g fat, 59 g carbohydrate, 5 g fibre, 347 kcal (1·48 MJ), 0·04 mg B_1, 0·2 mg B_2, 1 mg nicotinic acid. (Merory, OF, Platt.)

Pepperoni. *See* Sausage.

Pepsi-Cola. Trade name (Pepsicola Co. Ltd.) of a soft drink composed of sugar, vanilla, essential oils, spices and extract of cola nut coloured with caramel. Originally made in 1896 in U.S.A. by Caleb Bradham, druggist.

Pepsin. Proteolytic enzyme in the gastric juice which hydrolyses certain of the linkages of proteins to produce peptones. Functions only at acid pH, 1·5–2·5. Secreted as the inactive precursor pepsinogen, which is activated by acid. (BDS.)

Peptidases. Old name for exopeptidases, *which see.*

Peptides. Compounds formed when amino acids are linked together through the —CO—NH— linkage. Two amino acids so linked form a dipeptide, three a tripeptide, etc. Long chains are polypeptides.

Proteins are composed of multiple bundles of long chains of polypeptides joined by cross-linkages. (BDS.)

Peptones. Partial degradation product of protein, in the chain protein–proteoses–peptones–polypeptides–amino acids. Distinguished from proteoses since they are not precipitated by ammonium sulphate.

The name peptone is often given to a partial hydrolysate of protein of any type; thus bacteriological peptone is a bacterial medium produced by partial acid hydrolysis of protein. (BDS, Hawk.)

Pericarp. In reference to cereal grain this consists of two to four fibrous layers next to the outer husk and outside the testa; of low digestibility and removed from grain during milling. It is the major constituent of bran. (KJ.)

Perillartine. Non-nutritive sweetening agent derived from perillaldehyde, extracted from shiso oil (commercially available in Japan); 2,000 times as sweet as sucrose.

Perimysium. *See* Muscle.

Peristalsis. Method of movement along the intestine, peristaltic waves, caused by contraction of a ring of muscle, preceded by a wave of relaxation. (BDS.)

169

Pernicious Anaemia. *See* Anaemia *and* Intrinsic factor.

Peroxidase. Plant enzyme that splits hydrogen peroxide into water and oxygen, only when there is a substance present to accept the oxygen (unlike catalase that splits peroxide into water and gaseous oxygen).

Contains haematin in the molecule, and blood itself has a peroxidase-like activity that is used in the benzidine test for blood. (WHSS.)

Peroxide. *See* Hydrogen peroxide.

Peroxide Number. Or peroxide value; measure of the oxidative rancidity of fats by determination of the peroxides present. Measured by the amount of iodine liberated from potassium iodide: peroxide value is the ml. of $0.002 N$ sodium thiosulphate per gram of sample. (FM.)

Perrier Water. Mildly alkaline, well-aerated natural water, containing sodium bicarbonate. Obtained mainly from Les Bouillens, Vergèze, France. (Hutch.)

Perry. Fermented pear juice analogous to cider from apples.

Persian Berry. Yellow colour obtained from the berries of the buckthorn (*Rhamnus*) family; legally permitted in food in most countries. Contains the glucosides of two colouring matters, rhamnetin and rhamnazin. (Jacobs.)

Persimmon. Fruit of the tree *Diospyros virginiana* (a variety of ebony).

Egg-shaped fruit 1–2 inches in diameter: yellow in colour; astringency decreases as it ripens, also known as date plum.

Water 80%, protein 0.5%, carbohydrate 18%; kcal 73 (0.3 MJ), Fe 0.4 mg, vitamin A 700 μg, B_1 0.02 mg, B_2 0.02 mg, nicotinic acid 0.2 mg, C 10 mg— per 100 g. (Platt.)

Peruvita. Protein-rich baby food developed in Peru. Sweet version, 30% protein, made from quinua and cotton-seed flour, with skim-milk powder, sugar, spices, vitamins A, B_1 and B_2 and calcium carbonate.

Savoury version, 35% protein, contains salt in place of sugar.

Pervaporation. Evaporation from a colloidal suspension by heating in a collodion bag. If there are any crystalloids present they pass through the membrane and are deposited on the outside of the bag.

Petechiae, Petechial haemorrhages. Small, pin-point bleedings in the skin; one of the symptoms of scurvy. (BDS.)

Petit-grain Oils. Prepared from twigs and leaves of the bitter orange by steam distillation; similar to neroli oil but less fragrant.

Petitgrain Portugal prepared from leaves of sweet orange, Mandarin petitgrain from tangerine tree leaves, and lemon petitgrain. (Merory.)

Petit Pois. Small peas; according to the code of practice for canned fruits and vegetables, up to and including 11/32 inch in diameter; medium, up to 13/32 inch; large or standard, greater than 13/32 inch.

PGA. Pteroyl glutamic acid. *See* Folic acid.

pH. Abbreviation of potential hydrogen, used to denote the degree of acidity of a substance.

Defined as the negative logarithm of the hydrogen-ion concentration in gram-atoms per litre. The scale runs from 0 (1 gram of H ion per litre), extremely strongly acid, to 14 (one hundred million millionth of a gram of H ions) extremely strongly alkaline.

Pure water is pH 7, which is neutral; below 7 is acid, above is alkaline. (Hawk.)

Phaeophytin. Formed from chlorophyll by the removal of the magnesium; occurs in acid medium. It is brownish-green in colour and accounts for the colour change when green vegetables are cooked. (Griswold.)

Phage. See Bacteriophage.

Phagomania. Morbid obsession with food, also sitomania.

Phagophobia. Fear of food, also sitophobia.

Phase Inversion. Milk is an emulsion of fat in water; butter is an emulsion of water in fat. The change from cream to butter is termed phase inversion. (Davis.)

Phaseolin. Globulin protein in kidney bean.

Phaseolunatin. A cyanogenetic glucoside found in certain legumes (such as lima bean, chick pea, common vetch), which hydrolyses to produce glucose, acetone and hydrocyanic acid; not proved harmful when present in the diet.

PHB Ester. p-Hydroxybenzoic acid—ethyl and propyl esters and their sodium salts. Used as preservative in some countries.

Phenetylurea. See Dulcin.

Phenol Oxidases. Enzymes that oxidize phenolic compounds to quinones. E.g. monophenol oxidase in mushrooms; polyphenol oxidases in potato and apple that are responsible for the development of the brown colour when the cut surface is exposed to air; tyrosinase in plants and animals that is responsible for brown and black pigmentation. (WHSS.)

Phenylalanine. An essential amino acid. The non-essential tyrosine can partially replace phenylalanine in the diet.

It is rarely, if ever, the limiting amino acid in any food.

Inability to metabolize phenylalanine is an inherited disease and causes mental disorder, phenylketonuria, which see. (BDS.)

Phenylketonuria. Inherited metabolic defect wherein the essential amino acid, phenylalanine, is incompletely metabolized and the end-product, phenylpyruvic acid, is excreted in the urine. The product affects the brain and causes imbecility. The effect can be moderated by strict limitation of the phenylalanine intake. (AEB.)

Phitosite. High calorie food.

Phloridzin. See Phlorrhizin.

Phlorrhizin. Also spelled phloridzin and phlorhizin. A glycoside of plant origin; abolishes the renal threshold for glucose, which therefore appears in the urine (glycosuria). This is known as renal diabetes or phlorhizin diabetes. Used to examine the formation of glucose from other ingredients of the diet. (BDS.)

Phosphatase Test. For adequate pasteurization of milk. Depends on the fact that the enzyme phosphatase, normally present in milk, is destroyed at a temperature slightly greater than that required to destroy the tubercle bacillus and other pathogens. This enzyme liberates inorganic phosphate from phenyl phosphate and its activity can be measured by either the phenol or the phosphate.

In the tintometer (see Lovibond comparator) more than $2 \cdot 3$ Lovibond blue units (phosphate estimation), under the conditions of the test, indicates inefficient pasteurization. Can detect $0 \cdot 2\%$ raw milk in pasteurized milk. (Davis.)

Phosphate. Salt of phosphoric acid, which see, also Phosphate bond, energy-rich, Phosphorus and Polyphosphates.

Phosphate Additives. See Polyphosphates.

Phosphate Bond, Energy-rich. Phosphates of organic compounds fall into two groups depending on the amount of energy released when the phosphate portion is hydrolysed. (a) Low energy potential, the ordinary phosphates that liberate $1 \cdot 2$—$1 \cdot 5$ kcal (e.g. phospho-sugars, phospho-glycerols, phosphoglyceric acids, phosphocholine); (b) high-energy potential, or energy-rich phosphates, that liberate about 8—10 kcal (e.g. anhydrides, where phosphate is linked to phosphate, acidic enols such as phosphoenolpyruvic acid, acetyl phosphate and nitrogen linked to phosphate).

Phosphate-bond energy is the only form of energy that can be used by any living cell (muscular activity, osmotic work, the shock produced by the electric eel).

Adenosine triphosphate (ATP) is the key compound because it acts as a store of the energy-rich phosphate bonds. (WHSS.)

Phosphatides. Also phospholipins or phospholipids. Fatty substances including phosphoric acid and a nitrogenous base in the molecule. Include lecithins, cephalins, sphingomyelins, and cerebrosides. Part of the structure of the brain and nervous tissue and involved in fat transport.

Also combined with proteins as lipoproteins.

Are partly soluble in water as well as in fats and used in food technology as emulsifiers. From the dietary point of view they may be regarded as simple fats. (BDS.)

Phosphokinases. Enzymes that transfer the phosphate radical, together with its energy, to or from adenosine di- or tri-phosphate. Various other molecules can be involved but one of the pair of reactants is adenosine di- or tri-phosphate. (WHSS.)

Phospholipins. See Phosphatides.

Phosphoproteins. Conjugated proteins containing phosphate other than as nucleic acid (nucleoproteins) or lecithin (lipoproteins), e.g. casein from milk, ovovitellin from egg yolk. (Hawk.)

Phosphoric Acid. May be one of three types—orthophosphoric acid (H_3PO_4) metaphosphoric acid (HPO_3) or pyrophosphoric acid ($H_4P_2O_7$).

Used in acid-fruit flavoured beverages such as lemonade. See also Phosphorus.

Phosphorolysis. Hydrolysis in which the elements of phosphoric acid are added at the broken linkage, e.g. the enzyme phosphorylase hydrolyses glycogen not to glucose but to glucose phosphate. (WHSS.)

Phosphorus. This element occurs in all biological tissues as phosphate, i.e. salts of phosphoric acid. In the body most of it (80%) is present in the skeleton and teeth as calcium phosphate $(Ca_3PO_4)_2$, about 10% in the muscles and 1% in the nervous system. It is of vital importance in metabolism as many compounds (such as vitamins B_1, B_2, glucose, adenosine, etc.) function as phosphates.

The parathyroid glands control the level of phosphate in the blood.

Human dietary needs (about $1 \cdot 3$ g per day) are always met, a deficiency never occurs in man. Phosphate deficiency, however, is one of the commonest deficiencies in livestock and gives rise to osteomalacia (also known as sweeny or creeping sickness).

Phosphate is also essential for plant growth, hence the use of bone meal as fertilizer. Bone meal (calcium phosphate), is often used as a supplement in human foods but as a source of calcium rather than phosphate.

In calculating the amount of phosphate in foodstuffs text-books vary in expressing the value as phosphorus (P) or phosphate (P_2O_5); 31 parts of P are equivalent to 142 parts of P_2O_5.

See also Phytic acid, Phosphate bond, energy-rich, Polyphosphates, Calcium-phosphorus ratio *and* Phosphoric acid. (DP, Gil.)

Photosynthesis. Manufacture by plants of complex foods from simple salts and carbon dioxide, with the aid of chlorophyll (*which see*) and energy from sunlight. This is the ultimate source of all food and the truth of the sentence "all flesh is grass".

Phthiocol. *See* Vitamin K.

Phrynoderma. A follicular hyperkeratosis of the skin (blocked pores or toad-skin) often encountered in malnourished people.
Originally thought to be due to vitamin A deficiency but possibly due to other deficiencies, and occurs mildly in well-nourished people. (DP.)

Phylloquinone. *See* Vitamin K.

Physalin. Zeaxanthin dipalmitate; a carotenoid pigment found in the fruits of the Chinese lantern, *Physalis.*

Physin. Growth factor needed by rats and occurring in liver; probably vitamin B_{12}.

Phytase. Phosphatase enzyme that hydrolyses phytin to inositol and phosphoric acid. Present in yeast, liver, blood, malt and seeds. If a high level of yeast is used in baking with high-extraction flours, some of the phytin is broken down. *See also* Phytic acid. (FB.)

Phytic Acid. Inositol hexaphosphoric acid; present in the husk of cereals, dried peas and beans and some nuts.

The phosphate is insoluble and not digested. Part of the phytic acid may be present as the calcium salt (**phytin**), but this is also unavailable to the consumer. Moreover, phytic acid can combine with calcium and also iron from other foods in the diet and render them insoluble and unavailable. For this reason it has been held responsible for rickets and iron-deficiency anaemia among people eating large amounts of whole-grain cereals.

However, phytic acid is partially hydrolysed by the enzymes of yeast (e.g. in bread baking), and that present in peas and beans is partially hydrolysed if these are soaked in water so the rôle of phytic acid in preventing the absorption of iron and calcium is not clear.

It is not present in highly milled cereals since it is contained in the outer branny layers. (DP, FB.)

Phytin. *See* Phytic Acid.

Phytosterol. General name given to sterols occurring in plants, the chief of which is sitosterol (structurally closely related to cholesterol).

Phytylmenaquinone. *See* Vitamin K.

Pica. Perverted appetite (eating of earth, sand, clay, paper, etc.).

Piccalilli. Mixture of chopped, brine-preserved vegetables in mustard sauce (mustard and vinegar, thickened with tapioca starch, plus other spices, coloured with tartrazine).

Pickles, Dill. Pickles that are fermented in a mixture of brine, cured dill weed, mixed spices and vinegar. (Jacobs.)

Pickling. (*See* Halophilic bacteria *and* Curing of meat.) Also called brining. Vegetables immersed in 5–10% brine undergo lactic acid fermentation, while the salt prevents the growth of undesirables. The sugars in the vegetables are broken down to lactic acid; at 25°C the process takes a few weeks, finishing at 1% acidity. (Jacobs.)

Pidan. *See* Chinese eggs.

Pikelets. *See* Dough Cakes.

Pilchard. Fatty fish, *Sardina* (*clupea*) *pilchardus*; young is the **sardine.**

Composition per 100 g: 21·9 g protein, 10·8 g fat, 191 kcal (0·8 MJ), 230 mg calcium, 3 mg iron. (M&W.)

Pimento. *See* Allspice.

Pimiento. *See* Pepper.

Pineapple. Fruit of the tropical 0·3%, fat 0·1%; kcal 30 (0·13 MJ), Ca 12 mg, Fe 0·3 mg vitamin A 18 μg, B_1 0·05 mg, B_2 0·02 mg, nicotinic acid 0·1 mg, vitamin C 26 mg—per 100 g. (FAO.)

Pineapple Oil. *See* Flavours, synthetic.

Pint, Reputed. 13⅓ fluid oz. *See* Quart, reputed.

Pipe. Cask for wine of volume that varies with the type of wine, e.g. port, 115 gallons; Teneriffe, 100; Marsala, 93.

Pipecolic Acid. Chemically piperidine-2-carboxylic acid. Occurs in fresh green beans, potatoes and mushrooms, in fresh fruit and the dried seeds of legumes. Its pharmacological effects are unknown.

Pith. *See* Albedo.

Pits. Stones from cherries, plums, peaches, apricots. The oil is extracted from these pits and used in cosmetics, pharmaceuticals, canning sardines and as table oil. The press cake left behind contains the bitter principle, amygdalin.

Plansifter. A nest of sieves mounted together so that material being sieved is divided into a number of fractions of different size. Widely used in flour milling. (KJ.)

Plantain. Variety of banana with higher starch and lower sugar content than dessert bananas, picked when flesh is too hard to be eaten raw and used for cooking. Some varieties become sweet if left to ripen, others never develop a high sugar content.

Composition per 100 g: 1 g protein, 0·2 g fat, 32 g carbohydrate, 128 kcal (0·05 MJ), 0·05 mg iron, 30 μg vitamin A, 0·05 mg B_1, 0·05 mg B_2, 0·7 mg nicotinic acid, 20 mg C. (OF, Platt.)

Plasma, Blood. Blood consists of red cells, white cells and platelets, suspended in a clear protein solution, the plasma. Plasma proteins include fibrinogen, albumins and globulins. Of the 9% total plasma solids, 7% are proteins. (BDS.)

Plasmapheresis. Experimental method of reducing the serum proteins to a low level by removing part of the blood and returning only the red cells to the blood stream. (BDS.)

Plasma Proteins. In solution in the blood plasma—three main types, fibrinogen (0·2–0·4 g per 100 ml), albumin (4·4–5·3) and globulin (1·9–2·8). (BDS.)

Plate Count. To estimate the number of bacteria in a sample it is poured on to an agar plate when each bacterial cell or group of cells multiplies to produce a colony which is visible to the naked eye. A count of the number of colonies gives the number of bacteria in that portion of the sample that was taken.

Pasteurized milk contains about 100,000 bacteria per ml., good-quality raw milk contains less than 500,000 per ml.

Plato. *See* Balling.

PLJ—Pure Lemon Juice. Trade name (Beecham Foods Ltd.). Lemon juice containing 53 mg vitamin C per 100 g.

Pluck. Butchers' term for heart, liver and lungs of an animal.

Plum. Numerous species of *Prunus.* Common European plums are *P. domestica*; blackthorn or sloe is *P. spinosa*; bullace is *P. insititia*; damson is *P. damascena*; gages are

P. italica. Small amounts of protein, carbohydrate and fat.

Composition per 100 g: 60 kcal (0·24 MJ), 100 µg vitamin A, 0·5 mg nicotinic acid, 5 mg C. (FAO, OF.)

Pneumatic Conveying. Transfer of material in powder form by means of air currents. Applied to flour, sugar, cement, etc.

Pneumatic Dryer. The material is dried almost instantaneously in a turbulent stream of hot air, which also acts as a conveyor system. Applicable to powdered, granular and flaky materials. (RJC.)

Pneumatic Ring Dryer. A pneumatic dryer (*which see*) in which the product travels several times through a ring duct, impelled by hot air, and the drying time, temperature and rate of flow of the material can be controlled.

Used for starch, mashed potatoes, cereals, flour, powdered soups.

Poach. To cook for a short time in a shallow layer of liquid kept at a temperature just below the boiling point.

P.O.E.M.S. Polyoxyethylene monostearate, *see* Polyoxyethylene.

Poikilotherms. Cold-blooded animals, those whose temperature varies with their environment.

Poisoning, Food. *See* Food poisoning.

Polarimeter. Instrument used to determine the degree of rotation of polarized light. Consists of two Nicol prisms (calcite), the first of which polarizes the light and the second is used after the light has passed through the test solution to determine the rotation.

All optically active substances such as sugars and amino acids, rotate polarized light and the degree of rotation is used as a quantitative measure of the substance.
See also Optical activity. (Hawk.)

Polariscope. Alternative name for polarimeter, *which see*.

Polarized Light. Ordinary light vibrates in many planes; after passing through a crystal of quartz or "polaroid", it vibrates in only one plane, i.e., it is polarized. Many naturally-occurring compounds in solution possess the ability to rotate the plane of polarized light, i.e. they are optically active. *See* Optical activity.

Polarogram. *See* Polarograph.

Polarograph. Instrument used to measure traces of metallic ions by change in electric current.

The test solution is the electrolyte between two mercury electrodes; a continuously increasing negative potential is applied to the cathode and the change in current with voltage is recorded—the polarogram. The rise in current at a particular voltage is a measure of the concentration of the metal ion present.

Polenta. Kind of porridge made from maize meal, common dish in Italy often with cheese added.

Polished Rice. *See* Rice, polished.

Pollards. *See* Wheatfeed.

Polycythaemia. Increase in the number of red blood cells; results from strenuous physical exercise, residence at high altitudes, administration of drugs or cobalt, and certain diseases. (BDS.)

Polymorphism. The ability to crystallize in two or more different forms. For example, depending on the conditions under which it is solidified, the fat tristearin can form three kinds of crystals each of which has a different melting point, namely, 54, 65 and 71°C.

Polymyxin. Antibiotic isolated 1947 from *Bacillus polymyxin* (*Bacillus aerosporin*). There are several polymyxins, of which polymyxin A is aerosporin. They are polypeptides, active against coliform bacteria; apart from clinical use they are of value in controlling infection in brewing.

Polyols. Sugar alcohols such as glycerol, sorbitol, inositol, etc.

Polyose. Polysaccharide.

Polyoxyethylene. Monoglycerides are soluble in fat, but by reacting with ethylene oxide the resulting polyoxyethylene derivatives become water-soluble to whatever degree is required. These compounds are polyoxyethylene esters, ethers, sorbitol esters, etc. They are valuable as emulsifying agents in bakery.

One of the best known is **polyoxyethylene stearate,** used as a crumb-softener. (Bailey.)

Polypeptides. *See* Peptides.

Polyphagia. Excessive or continuous eating.

Polyphosphates. Complex phosphates added to foods, in particular to meat products; they prevent sausage discoloration, aid mixing of the fat, speed penetration of the brine in curing, cause protein fibres of meat to retain more water and swell (so improving texture).

Include pyrophosphate ($Na_4P_2O_7$), tripolyphosphate ($Na_5P_3O_{10}$), and longer phosphate chains of 100 phosphate units, polyphosphate glasses prepared by rapid quenching of Na_2O-P_2O_5 melts '(e.g. Calgon, 12 unit chain length), etc.

Polysaccharides. Complex carbohydrates formed by the condensation of large numbers of monosaccharide units, e.g. starch, glycogen, cellulose, dextrins, inulin. On hydrolysis the simple sugar is liberated. (BDS.)

Polysaccharose. Polysaccharide.

Pomace. Residue of crushed apple pulp after expressing juice; also applied to any pressed fruit pulp and to fish from which oil has been expressed.

Pombé. African beer prepared from millet seed. The seed is sprouted to break down the starch to fermentable sugar, a process similar to malting in beer manufacture, and then allowed to ferment spontaneously. (Loes.)

Pome. Botanical term for type of fruit represented by apple, pear and quince.

Pomegranate. (*Punica granatum*). Juice contained in a pulpy sac surrounding each of a mass of seeds—outer skin contains tannin and therefore bitter.

Sweet juice used to prepare grenadine syrup for alcoholic and fruit drinks.

Water 80%, protein 1%, carbohydrate 18%; kcal 77 (0·32 MJ), Fe 0·7 mg, vitamin A nil, B_1 0·02 mg, B_2 0·03 mg, nicotinic acid 0·2 mg, C 8 mg—per 100 g. (Platt.)

Pomelo. Also spelled pomeloe and pummelo; alternative name shaddock; *Citrus grandis* from which the grapefruit is descended.

Pomes. Botanical name for fruit formed by the enlargement of the receptacle which becomes fleshy and surrounds the carpels, e.g. apple, pear.

Ponceau Colours. A series of strawberry red colours. Ponceau MX—disodium salt of 1-(2:4- or mixed xylylazo)-2-naphthol-3:6-disulphonic acid; also called Ponceau R and 2R and RS.

Ponceau 4R—trisodium salt of 1-(4-sulpho-1-naphthylazo)-2-naphthol-6:8-disulphonic acid; also called Cochineal red A.

Ponceau SX—disodium salt of 2-(5-sulpho-2:4-xylylazo)-1-naphthol-4-sulphonic acid; called Red No. 4 in U.S.A.

Ponceau 3R—disodium salt of 1-pseudocumylazo-2-naphthol-3:6-disulphonic acid, called Red No. 1 in U.S.A.; Marachino cherry red colour.

Ponceau 6R—tetra sodium salt of 2-(6'-sulpho-1'-m-xylylazo)-1-naphthol-5-sulphonic acid. (Bell.)

Ponderal Index. An index of adipose tissue; height divided by the cube root of the body weight; high for thin people, low for fat people.

Ponderocrescive. Foods tending to increase weight: easily gaining weight; opposite to pondoperditive—stimulating weight loss.

Poonac. The residue of coconut after the extraction of the oil.

Popcorn. Variety of maize, *Zea mays*, that expands on heating.

Pork Carcass. Fat: protein 8·8%, fat 49%; kcal 480 (2·0 MJ); Fe 1·1 mg; vitamin A nil, B_1 0·31 mg, vitamin C nil—per 100 g.

Medium: protein 10·4%, fat 39%; kcal 396 (1·65 MJ), Fe 1·2 mg; vitamin A nil, B_1 0·36 mg,

B_2 0·10 mg, nicotinic acid 2·4 mg, vitamin C nil—per 100 g.

Lean: protein 11·8%, fat 29%; kcal 312 (1·32 MJ), Fe 1·4 mg; vitamin A nil, B_1 0·41 mg, B_2 0·12 mg, nicotinic acid 2·7 mg, vitamin C nil—per 100 g. (FAO.)

Porphyra. Red alga cultivated in Japan to make "Komba". In Gt. Britain it is collected from the sea to make laverbread, *which see*.

Porphyrins. Ring system of four joined pyrrol nuclei, formed when the iron is removed from haem. Combine with metals, thus haemoglobin is an iron porphyrin, chlorophyll is a magnesium porphyrin. (BDS.)

Porphyropsin. Photosensitive pigment in the retinas of the eyes of fresh-water fish, containing dehydro retinol—analogous to rhodopsin in the eyes of marine fish, mammals, birds and amphibians. (WHSS.)

Porter. *See* Beer.

Posset. Drink made of hot milk curdled with ale or wine, sometimes thickened with breadcrumbs and spiced. Formerly used as remedy for colds.

Postum, Instant. Trade name (General Foods Corp., U.S.A.) for a preparation of bran, wheat and molasses consumed as a beverage.

Potassium. An element present in the body in considerable amounts, about 250 grams, mostly inside the cells. It is not of dietary importance since there are adequate amounts in almost all foods

It is essential in the body to maintain acid-base balance, the osmotic pressure and the irritability of nerves and muscle. *See also* Acid-base balance, Acid foods, Sodium-potassium ratio *and* Water balance.

It is one of the most important of the plant nutrients. (Gil.)

Potassium Nitrate. *See* Saltpetre, Nitrates *and* Nitrites.

Potassium Sorbate. *See* Sorbic acid.

Potato, Irish. Tuber of *Solanum tuberosum.* Although commonly classed as a carbohydrate food, potato contains 80% water; its main contribution to the diet is vitamin C, and in winter potatoes provide as much as a third of the intake of this vitamin in the United Kingdom. The high vitamin C content of new potatoes falls during storage.

Protein 1·7%, fat 0·1%, Ca 7 mg, Fe 0·6 mg, kcal 70 (0·29 MJ), vitamin A nil, B_1 0·08 mg, B_2 0·03 mg, nicotinic acid 1·2 mg, vitamin C 8 mg—per 100 g. (FAO.)

Potato Flour. Dried potato tuber. Protein 8·5%, fat 0·4%, kcal 349 (1·47 MJ), Ca 30 mg, Fe 3 mg, vitamin A nil, B_1 0·21 mg, B_2 0·1 mg, nicotinic acid 5 mg, vitamin C 20 mg—per 100 g. (FAO.)

Potato Starch. Also called **farina.** Prepared from potato tuber and widely used as a stabilizing agent when gelatinized. Large grains gelatinize very easily when heated.

Potato, Sweet. Tubers of herbaceous climbing plant *Ipomoea batatas.* The flesh may be white, yellow or pink (if carotene is present); the leaves are edible.

Protein 1·1%, fat 0·3%, kcal 97 (0·41 MJ), Fe 0·8 mg, vitamin A 150 μg, B_1 0·08 mg, B_2 0·04 mg, nicotinic acid 0·5 mg, vitamin C 19 mg—per 100 g. (FAO.)

Pot-au-Feu. Traditional French dish made by stewing meat with vegetables. Soup is made from the liquor. (GH.)

Potential Energy. *See* Energy.

Pottle. English wine measure of half a gallon.

Pound Cake. Rich cake containing a pound, or equal quantities, of each of the major ingredients.

P.P. Factor. *See* Nicotinic acid.

PPM. Parts per million.

P.P. Vitamin. *See* Nicotinic acid.

Praline. Rich paste of ground nuts and sugar used as chocolate centres.

Prawn, Dublin Bay. *See* Lobster.

Prawns. Shellfish of various tribes of suborder *Macrura*.

Large fish of species of *Palaemonidae*, *Penaeidae* and *Pandalidae* are prawns, smaller fish are **shrimps.**

In addition Deepwater Prawn is *Pandalus borealis*; common pink shrimp is *Pandalus montagui*, brown shrimp is species of *Crangon*.

Dublin Bay Prawn is **Lobster,** *which see.*

Composition per 100 g: 21 g protein, 1·8 g fat, 104 kcal (0·42 MJ), 145 mg calcium, 1·1 mg iron.

Precursor, Enzyme. Some enzymes are secreted as an inactive precursor that has to undergo a reaction before it shows normal activity. Thus trypsin is secreted as inactive trypsinogen that must react with enterokinase before it becomes active; similarly pepsinogen and chymotrypsinogen. (WHSS.)

Premier Jus. Best-quality suet prepared from oxen and sheep kidneys. The fat is chilled, shredded and heated at moderate temperature.

When pressed, premier jus, like rendered tallow, separates into a liquid fraction (oleo oil or liquid oleo) and a solid fraction (oleo-stearin or solid tallow). (Hilditch.)

Preservation. During storage food can deteriorate under the influence of micro-organisms, its own enzymes and chemically by oxidation. Preservation must stop these reactions, and the normally practised methods, such as refrigeration, sterilization, dehydration and addition of chemicals, control them to varying extents. Short-term preservation is achieved by pasteurization, salting, smoking and pickling.

Some destruction of the vitamins, a small degree of leaching out of the minerals and vitamins, and under conditions of severe heating, some small degree of damage to proteins, can occur during preservation. In general, refrigeration and dehydration under vacuum or by freeze-drying, cause no nutritional loss.

See also Sterile, Sterilization, cold, Irradiation *and* Preservatives.

Preservatives. Defined as any substance capable of retarding or arresting the process of fermentation, acidification or other decomposition of food, or masking putrefaction.

The only permitted preservatives in U.K. are sulphur dioxide and benzoic acid, and, in specified cases, methyl or propyl *p*-hydroxybenzoate, sorbic acid and the antibiotic, nisin.

The following are excluded from the regulations: salt, saltpetre, sugar, lactic and acetic acids, glycerine, alcohol, spices, essential oils and herbs.

179

See also Tetracyclines, Hydrogen peroxide, Boric acid, Sterile, Irradiation, Nitrate *and* Diacetate, sodium. (Baum., Bell.)

Pressure Cooking. *See* Autoclave.

Pressure, Oncotic. *See* Oncotic pressure.

Pressure, Osmotic. *See* Osmotic pressure.

Pretzels. Hard brittle German biscuits made from flour, water, shortening, yeast and salt. The dough is fermented and chopped into lengths and shaped; they are boiled in 0.3% sodium hydroxide, salted, baked and dried.

Originally called bretzels and still made in the shape of the letter B. (Loes.)

Procea. Trade name (Procea Ltd.) of a white loaf with slightly increased protein content.

Protein 10.7%, fat 2.4%, carbohydrate 50.3%; Ca 140 mg, Fe 1·8 mg, kcal 255 (1·07 MJ) —per 100 g. (M&W.)

Proenzymes. Inactive precursors to enzymes, also called Zymogens.

Profiteroles. Tiny rounds of choux pastry used to decorate cakes.

Proflo. Trade name (Trader Oil Mill Co., U.S.A.) for partially defatted, cooked, cottonseed flour.

Progesterone. *See* Oestrogens.

Prolamins. Proteins insoluble in water, neutral solvents and absolute alcohol, but soluble in 70–80% alcohol; e.g. wheat gliadin, corn zein, barley hordein, malt bynin.

Low in lysine, rich in proline and glutamic acid. (Hawk.)

Proline. A non-essential amino acid. Chemically pyrrolidine carboxylic acid. (BDS.)

Prolo. Protein-rich baby food (49% protein) made in Great Britain from soya flour with methionine, minerals and vitamins A, B_1, B_2 and nicotinic acid.

Pronutro. Protein-rich baby food (22% protein) developed in South Africa; made from maize, skimmilk powder, groundnut flour, soya flour and fish protein concentrate with yeast, wheat germ, vitamins A, B_1, B_2 and nicotinic acid, iodized salt and sugar.

Proof Spirit. A method of describing the alcohol content of spirits. Proof spirit contains 57.07% alcohol by volume and 49.24% by weight in Gt. Britain. In U.S.A. it contain 50% alcohol by volume.

Thus absolute alcohol is 175·25 degrees proof U.K. and 200 degrees proof U.S.A.

Spirits are described as under or over proof. A mixture 30 degrees over proof contains in 100 volumes as much alcohol as 130 volumes of proof spirit; 30 degrees under proof means that 100 volumes contain as much alcohol as 70 volumes of proof spirit.

In Germany per cent alcohol by weight is used, in Italy and France it is per cent by volume.

Proof spirit is a solution of alcohol of such strength that it will ignite when mixed with gunpowder; specifically at 10°C it weighs $\frac{12}{13}$ parts of an equal volume of distilled water. (Cruess.)

Propionates. Salts of propionic acid, CH_3CH_2COOH. The free acid and its sodium and calcium salts are used as mould inhibitors, e.g. on cheese surfaces; also to inhibit rope in bread.

Propionic acid is formed in the

rumen of cattle together with acetic and butyric acids, and all three are converted into milk constituents.

In the body it is metabolized to pyruvic acid, which is normally formed in the body, and thus considered harmless.

Propyl Gallate. *See* Antioxidants.

Prosparol. Trade name (Duncan and Flockhart, Edinburgh) for an emulsion containing 50% vegetable fat—405 kcal (1·7 MJ) per 100 g; used as a concentrated source of energy.

Prosthetic Group. With reference to enzymes, the non-protein fraction of certain enzymes. They are therefore conjugated proteins, and are firmly attached to and part of the enzyme, unlike activators and coenzymes.

Certain oxidizing enzymes have a prosthetic group that functions as a built-in hydrogen acceptor. Example, peroxidase contains haematin as its prosthetic group. *See also* Coenzymes. (WHSS.)

Protamines. The simplest natural proteins containing only a limited number of amino acids, chiefly the basic ones, especially arginine. Soluble in water, not coagulated by heat, so basic that they form salts with strong mineral acids, e.g. salmine from salmon sperm, sturine from sturgeon sperm, clupeine from herring sperm, scombrine from mackerel sperm. (Hawk.)

Proteans. Slightly altered proteins, probably an early stage of denaturation, which have become insoluble. (Hawk.)

Protein, Alpha. Trade name for a protein isolated from soya-bean, used for paper coating, water-miscible paints, leather finishing, adhesives. 88·7% protein, 8·5% water.

Proteinases. Old name for endopeptidases, *which see*.

Protein, Bence-Jones. Unusual protein excreted in the urine in multiple myelomatosis, leukaemia and eczema; coagulates at 55°C and redissolves on boiling. (Hawk.)

Protein, Beta. Trade name for a protein isolated from soya-bean, mainly used to prepare adhesives for plywood.

Protein-bound Iodine. *See* Thyroglobulin.

Protein calories per cent. *See* Protein-energy Ratio.

Protein, Crude. Total nitrogen multiplied by the factor 6·25 (=100 divided by 16). The nitrogen content of most pure proteins is 16% and determination of crude protein, in effect, assumes that all the nitrogen present is protein. The error involved in this assumption is not usually large unless there is an abundance of purine nitrogen present.

For milk protein the factor is 6·38, for cereals 5·7. *See* Kjeldahl determination. (BDS, DP.)

Protein Efficiency Ratio. A measure of the nutritive value of proteins carried out on young growing animals. Is defined as the gain in weight per gram of protein eaten. The maximum values, e.g. egg protein, are about 4·4.

Zero values are obtained for those proteins which, when fed alone, do not permit growth, but may still have some limited value.

Protein-energy Ratio. Protein content of a food or diet expressed as ratio of energy from protein to total energy. Previously termed protein calories per cent, being expressed as a percentage of total calories supplied by protein.

Protein Equivalent. A measure of the digestible nitrogen of an animal feeding stuff in terms of protein. It is measured by direct feeding or calculated from the digestible pure protein plus half the digestible non-protein nitrogen. (KJ.)

Protein Factor. *See* Protein, crude *and* Meat factor.

Protein, First Class. First and second class proteins are obsolete terms indicating those of high or low nutritive value, generally, but not invariably, animal and plant protein respectively.

Protein Milk. Partially skimmed lactic acid milk plus milk curd (prepared from whole milk by rennet precipitation); richer in protein and poorer in fat than ordinary milk—supposed to be better tolerated in digestive disorders. Also known as **Albumin milk** *and* **Eiweiss Milch.**

Protein Rating. Term used in Canadian Food Regulations to assess overall protein quality of a food. Protein efficiency ratio multiplied by protein content of food (per cent) multiplied by the amount of food that is reasonably consumed.

Foods with rating above 40 may be designated excellent dietary sources; foods with rating below 20 are considered to be insignificant sources; 20–40 may be described as good sources. (AEB.)

Protein, Reference. *See* Reference Protein.

Proteins. Essential constituents of all living cells; distinguished from fats and carbohydrates in containing nitrogen; basically composed of carbon, hydrogen, oxygen, nitrogen, sulphur and sometimes phosphorus.

All proteins are composed of large combinations of 20 amino acids (some bacterial proteins contain additional unusual amino acids). Meat, fish, eggs, cheese, hair, leather, fur, and many hormones are proteins. (DP.)

Proteins, Conjugated. The molecule contains protein and a non-protein prosthetic group; e.g. nucleoproteins, glycoproteins, phosphoproteins, chromoproteins, lipoproteins, *which see.* (Hawk.)

Protein Score. A chemical method of defining the nutritional value of proteins; the ratio of the amount of the limiting essential amino acid in the protein, to the target value. *See also* Chemical Score.

Protein Shift. Name applied in flour milling to the phenomenon in which the protein content of the smaller particles of flour (up to 15 microns) is higher, namely 15–20%, than the flour as a whole, 8–14%, while particles of intermediate size, 15–35 microns, have a lower protein content than the flour as a whole.

Protenum. Trade name (Mead, Johnson Ltd., U.S.A.) of a concentrated food preparation containing 42% protein, 46% carbohydrate and 2% fat.

Proteolysis. The hydrolysis of proteins to amino acids by alkali, acid or enzymes.

Proteoses. Partial degradation products of proteins; soluble in water. The stages of breakdown are protein–proteoses–peptones–polypeptides–amino acids. The proteoses are distinguished from peptones in that they are precipitated from solution by ammonium sulphate whereas peptones are not.

Primary proteoses precipitated with half saturated ammonium sulphate, secondary proteoses require full saturation. (Hawk.)

Prothrombin. Protein of the plasma involved in coagulation of the blood, *which see*.

Protogen. *See* Lipoic Acid.

Protone. Protein-rich baby food (24% protein), made in Great Britain and Congo from maize, skim-milk powder, yeast with added vitamins and minerals.

Protopectin. *See* Pectin.

Protopectinase. The enzyme in the pith of citrus fruits that converts protopectin into pectin with the resultant separation of the plant cells from one another. Also known as pectosinase and pectosase. (Brav.)

Proving. In bread-making this is the fermentation of the dough at the stage just before it goes into the oven. (KJ.)

Provitamin. A substance that is converted into a vitamin such as 7-dehydrocholesterol which is converted into vitamin D. In the old nomenclature carotene was termed provitamin A.

Proximate Analysis. Nearly complete analysis comprising protein, fat and ash, and, by subtracting these from the total, calculating "carbohydrate by difference". The last value may be corrected for crude fibre.

Prunes, Dried. *See* Dried fruit.

Prunin. *See* Naringin.

Pseudoglobulin. Water-soluble globulin which is not precipitated from salt solutions by dialysis against distilled water. Pseudoglobulin fractions occur in blood serum, in animal tissues, and in milk. *See also* Euglobulin.

Pseudokeratins. *See* Keratin.

Psychrophilic Bacteria. Prefer temperatures 15–20°C (59–68°F) and will still grow at and below 0°C (32°F), that is, in cold stores. Bacteria of the genera *Achromobacter, Flavobacterium, Pseudomonas,* and *Micrococcus. Torulopsis* yeasts, and moulds of the genera *Penicillium, Cladosporium, Mucor* and *Thamnidium* can all develop at low temperatures.

Temperatures must be reduced to about −10°C (13°F) before growth stops, but the organisms are not killed and will regrow when the temperature rises. (Baum.)

Psyllium. A vegetable mucilage preparation used to increase the bulk of the intestinal contents.

Pteroyl Glutamic Acid. *See* Folic acid.

Ptomaines. Compounds produced during the decomposition of proteins; some are poisonous, hence ptomaine poisoning.

Cadaverine (diaminopentane) formed by decarboxylation of lysine; muscarine (hydroxyethyl trimethylammonium hydroxide); putrescine (tetra methylene diamine) formed by the decarboxylation of arginine; and neurine (trimethyl vinyl ammonium hydroxide). (Cohen.)

Ptyalin. Old name for salivary amylase.

Pudding, Black. Sausage made of suet, pearl barley, and oatmeal and sometimes including pig's blood.

Pudding, Hasty. Old dish made from oatmeal boiled with water for only 2–3 minutes; the finished dish is very low in water content.

PUFA. Polyunsaturated fatty acids. *See* Essential Fatty Acids.

Puff Pastry. During preparation continuous layers of fat are formed between layers of dough; upon baking steam accumulates between the dough layers and causes them to expand forming large spaces between thin layers of pastry. (KJ.)

Pulque. Sourish beer produced by the rapid natural fermentation of aquamiel, the sweet mucilaginous sap of the Agave (American aloe or century plant). Contains 6% alcohol by volume, common in Central and South America. (Jacobs.)

Pulses. Seeds of the leguminosa family which consists of peas, beans and lentils. Fresh peas and beans are 65–90% water but the mature seeds are only 10–13% water. Their protein content is higher than that of cereals (20% of dry weight); they are a good source of thiamin and nicotinic acid; although they do not contain any vitamin C this vitamin is formed during germination so that sprouted pulses are a valuable source.

Pulses constitute a valuable part of tropical and subtropical diets as an important source of protein. *See also* Peas, Beans, Dhals *and* Grams. (DP.)

Pumpernickel. Bread made wholly from rye, baked at rather low temperature for up to 12 hours in steam. It is brownish-black and has no crust. (KJ.)

Pumpkin. *See* Gourds.

Purines. Compounds containing the structure

$$N{=}CH$$
$$HC \quad C{-}NH$$
$$\qquad \qquad {>}CH$$
$$N{-}C{-}N$$

adenine—amino derivative,
guanine—amino oxy derivative,
hypoxanthine—oxypurine,
xanthine—dioxypurine,
uric acid—trioxypurine.

They occur in nucleic acids, *which see*. Caffeine and theobromine are purines. When taken in the diet purines are excreted as uric acid. Sweetbread (pancreas) is rich in purines, followed by sardines and anchovies, then meat and fish, with little in vegetables, none in fruits and cereals. (BDS, Hawk.)

Purothionine. A sulphur-containing protein found in wheat flour; kills yeast at a concentration of $0 \cdot 0001$–$0 \cdot 005$ mg per ml and may be the "yeast-poisonous" principle that has long been known by bakers and brewers to be present in wheat flour.

Putrescine. *See* Ptomaines.

Pyrexia. Rise in body temperature.

Pyridine Nucleotides. *See* Nicotinamide adenine dinucleotide.

Pyridoxal. *See* Vitamin B_6.

Pyridoxamine. *See* Vitamin B_6.

Pyrocarbonate. *See* Diethyl Pyrocarbonate.

184

Pyridoxine. *See* Vitamin B_6.

Pyrimidines. Compounds containing the structure

$$N=CH$$
$$| \quad |$$
$$HC \quad CH$$
$$\| \quad \|$$
$$N—CH$$

cytosine—oxyamino pyrimidine,

uracil—dioxypyrimidine,

thymine—dioxymethylpyrimidine.

They occur in nucleic acids, *which see*. (BDS.)

Pyrithiamine. Pyridine analogue of thiamin; antagonistic to the vitamin. (Hawk.)

Pyrogens. Substances produced by living bacteria (not yeasts or moulds) that cause a rise in body temperature on injection. Thus any material that has been infected may, despite subsequent sterilization, contain pyrogens and be unsuitable for injection. Pyrogens are not destroyed by heat and water supplies can be pyrogenic.

Pyruvate Oxidation Factor. *See* Lipoic acid.

Pyruvic Acid. $CH_3CO.COOH$. Occupies a central position in the metabolism of carbohydrate. The anaerobic breakdown of glucose produces pyruvic acid, which is then oxidized via the tricarboxylic acid cycle to carbon dioxide and water.

It accumulates in the blood in vitamin B_1 deficiency; it is reduced to lactic acid. (Cohen.)

P.4000. A class of synthetic sweetening agents, chemically nitro amino alkoxybenzenes. One member of the group, propoxy amino nitrobenzene is 4,100 times as sweet as sugar and 8 times as sweet as saccharine but these compounds are not considered harmless and are not permitted in foods.

Dutch name is Aros.

Q

Q-enzyme. Factor isolated from potatoes that catalyses the formation of branching linkages of the 1:6-alpha-type in starches; the reaction appears to be irreversible, i.e. the Q-enzyme cannot hydrolyse these 1:6-alpha-linkages. (WHSS.)

Q_{O_2}. Symbol used in measuring cell respiration in the Warburg manometer; the number of microlitres of oxygen consumed (or carbon dioxide or other gas produced) per mg dry weight of tissue per hour. (Hawk.)

Quart, Reputed. Customary measure in relation to bottled wine and spirits is a "bottle" known as a reputed quart, approx. two thirds of an imperial quart, or $26\frac{2}{3}$ fl. oz.

Reputed pint is $13\frac{1}{3}$ fl. oz.

Quebracho. Or aspidosperma; obtained from the bark of *Aspidosperma quebrachoblanco*; used as source of tannins and alkaloids.

Queen Substance. The material secreted by the queen bee which inhibits the ovaries of the worker bees and stops them constructing queen cells. Thought to be chemically 10-hydroxy delta-2-decenoic acid.

Quenelle. A ball of chopped, spiced meat or fish.

Quercetin. A flavone found in onion skins, tea, hops, horse chestnuts; the disaccharide derivative containing rhamnose and glucose is rutin.

Quercitol. *See* Acorn Sugar.

Quercitron. *See* Flavin.

Querns. Pair of stones used for pulverizing grain (about 4000 B.C. to 2000 B.C.). The lower stone was slightly hollowed and the upper stone was rolled by hand on the lower one. (KJ.)

Quetelet's Index. Weight times 100 divided by height squared; index of adiposity.

Quick Breads. Term for baked goods such as biscuits, muffins, popovers, griddles, cakes, waffles and dumplings in which no yeast is used, but the raising carried out quickly with baking powder or other chemical agents. (Griswold.)

Quick Freezing. As the term implies, a rapid freezing of food by exposure to a blast of air at a very low temperature. Unlike slow freezing, small crystals of ice are formed which do not rupture the cells of the food and so the structure is relatively undamaged.

A quick-frozen food is commonly defined as one that has been cooled from a temperature of 0°C to −5°C or lower, in a period of not more than 2 hours, and then cooled to −18°C. (FB.)

Quillaja. Or soapbark; the dried bark of *Quillaja saponaria* which contains sapotoxin, tannin and quillaja. Used to produce foam in soft drinks and shampoos and fire extinguishers.

Quince. Pear-shaped sour fruit of *Cydonia* species, with flesh similar to that of the apple; rich in pectin and used chiefly in jams and jellies; used to be known as the apple and the vine.

Water 83%, protein 0·4%, fat trace, carbohydrate 6%; kcal 25 (0·1 MJ), vitamin C 15 mg—per 100 g.

Quinoa. Glutinous seeds of a plant (*Chenopodium album*) grown in Chile and Peru; made into bread.

Protein 12%, fat 5%, carbohydrate 63%, fibre 5%; calcium 120 mg, iron 7 mg, vitamin B_1 0·5 mg, B_2 0·3 mg, nicotinic acid 1·5 mg—per 100g. (Platt.)

R

Rabbit. Protein 17%, fat 5%; kcal 118 (0·5 MJ); Ca 14 mg, Fe 1 mg; vitamin A nil, B_1 0·06 mg, B_2 0·05 mg, nicotinic acid 6 mg, vitamin C nil—per 100 g. (FAO.)

Racemic. *See* Optical activity.

Racemic Compounds. A mixture of two isomers which cancel their optical activity, *which see*.

Radappertization. Treatment of food by radiation in doses suffi-cient to reduce the number of organisms below detectable levels, i.e. "commercial sterility".—*see* Appertisation.

Radiation. *See* Irradiation.

Radiation Sterilization. *See* Irradiation.

Radicidation. Treatment of food by radiation in doses sufficient to reduce the number of viable specific non-spore-forming pathogens below detectable levels, i.e.

doses lower than radappertization, *which see*.

The term radiation pasteurization has recently been differentiated into radicidation and radurization (*which see*).

Radioactivity. Isotopes of various elements break down with the emission of ionizing radiation. Advantage is taken of this property to prepare substances of physiological interest with radioactive carbon or hydrogen or other element in the compound. When these are administered to the subject their metabolic fate can be observed.

Also used therapeutically, e.g. radioactive iodine accumulates in the thyroid gland and is used to depress an overactive thyroid. Radioactive materials are also used to inhibit enzymes and micro-organisms in foodstuffs and so effect a **"cold sterilization"**. *See also* Isotopes *and* Irradiation.

Radio Frequency Heating. *See* High frequency heating.

Radiopasteurization. Sterilization of foods by ionizing radiation often confers unpleasant flavours on the food. This can be avoided by using a combination of heat with a lower dose of radiation (radiopasteurization). Doses of 200,000–300,000 rads plus heat can lengthen the shelf life of meat 5–10 times.

Radishes. Root of *Raphanus* genus. Protein $0 \cdot 6\%$, fat $0 \cdot 2\%$; kcal 11 $(0 \cdot 05$ MJ$)$, Ca 21 mg, Fe $0 \cdot 6$ mg, vitamin A 6 μg, B_1 $0 \cdot 02$ mg, B_2 $0 \cdot 01$ mg, nicotinic acid $0 \cdot 2$ mg, vitamin C 13 mg—per 100 g. (FAO.)

Radurization. Treatment of food by radiation in doses sufficient to enhance its keeping properties by reducing the number of spoilage organisms. The term radiation pasteurization has recently been differentiated into radicidation and radurization. *See also* Radappertization.

Radyne. Trade name (Radyne Ltd.) for high frequency heater (*which see*).

Raffinade. Best quality refined sugar.

Raffinose. A trisaccharide found in cotton seed, sugar-beet molasses and Australian manna; also known as **melitose** or **melitriose**; hydrolyses to fructose and melibiose, which in turn hydrolyses to glucose and galactose. 23% sweetness of sucrose. (Hawk.)

Raising Powder. *See* Baking powder.

Raisin Oil. Obtained from seeds of Muscat grapes, which are removed before drying the grapes for raisins. The oil is used primarily to coat the raisins to prevent them sticking together, and render them soft and pliable and less subject to insect infestation. (Merory.)

Raisins. Dried seedless grapes of several kinds. **Valencia raisins** from Spanish grapes; fruit dipped in potash lye and dried on cane trays in the sun.

Thompson seedless raisins produced mainly in California from the sultanina grape (the skins are coarser than the sultana). Raisins are also produced in Australia, S. Africa and U.S.A.

For analysis *see* Fruit, dried; *see also* Currants, Sultanas *and* Muscatels.

Ralston. American breakfast cereal; whole wheat plus added wheat germ.

Ramekin. (1) Porcelain or earthenware mould in which mixture is baked and then brought to the table. Paper soufflé cases nowadays called ramekin cases.

(2) Formerly the name given to toasted cheese: now tarts filled with cream cheese are called ramekins.

Randomization. As used of fats is the same as interesterification, *which see.*

Rape. *Brassica napus,* closely related to garden swede. Also known as **cole** or **coleseed.** Seed used as source of edible oil although its content of erucic acid has raised problems. Residual oilcake used for animal feed although it contains goitrogens.

Raspberry. Fruit of *Rubus idaeus.* Protein 1·3%, fat 1·3%, kcal 66 (0·28 MJ), Ca 40 mg, Fe 0·9 mg, vitamin A 39 μg, B_1 0·02 mg, B_2 0·07 mg, nicotinic acid 0·3 mg, vitamin C 24 mg—per 100 g. (FAO.)

Rastrello. Sharp-edged spoon used to cut out the pulp from halved oranges or other citrus fruit. (Brav.)

Ratafia. Flavouring essence made from bitter almonds; also a small light macaroon biscuit used in trifles; also a liqueur made from plum, peach and apricot kernels and bitter almonds.

Ravioli. Square envelope of pasta stuffed with minced meat.

Raw Sugar. Brown unrefined sugar, 96–98% pure, as imported for refining. Contaminated with mould spores, bacteria, cane fibre, and dirt. (Ayl.)

Reciprocal Ponderal Index. Height divided by cube root of weight; index of adiposity.

Recknagel's Phenomenon. Slight rise in specific gravity of milk that may continue for up to 12 hours after milking; total effect may be equivalent to 0·15% solids-not-fat in the milk. The cause has not been explained. (Davis & Mac.)

Recommended Intake. As applied to nutrients this is the amount thought to be needed to maintain health, and excludes any additional needs arising from disease, stress, etc. *See tables at end of book.*

Rectal Feeding. *See* Nutrient enemata.

Rectifying Column. A distillation column so arranged that the vapour condenses and redistils many times before it is finally condenses to form the distillate, and so is purified to a greater degree than in simple distillation.

Red Blood Cell. *See* Blood, red cell.

Red Colours. Red 10 B—disodium salt of 8-amino-2-phenylazo-1-naphthol-3 : 6-disulphonic acid.

Red 2G—disodium salt of 8-acetamido-2-phenylazo-1-naphthol-3:6-disulphonic acid.

Red 6B—disodium salt of 8-acetamido-2-p- acetamido-phenylazo-1-naphthol-3:6-disulphonic acid.

Red FB—disodium salt of 2-(4-(1-hydroxy-4-sulpho-2-naphthylazo) - 3 - sulphophenyl) - 6 - methylbenzothiazole.

Fast Red E—disodium salt of 1-(4-sulpho-1-naphthylazo)-2-hydroxynaphthalene-6-sulphonic acid.

See also Ponceau colours, Carmoisine, Amaranth *and* Erythrosine.

Red Herrings. Herrings that have been well salted and smoked for about 10 days. **Bloaters** are salted less and smoked for a shorter time; kippers lightly salted and smoked overnight. Also called **Yarmouth bloaters.**

Red Pepper. *See* Pepper.

Reducing Sugars. Sugars that contain the aldehydic or ketonic reducing group, e.g. glucose, fructose, lactose, pentoses. They are tested for by their ability to reduce reagents such as Fehling's, Benedict's.

Reductinic Acid. *See* Reductones.

Reduction. Loss of oxygen, or gain in hydrogen, or (in more general terms to cover reactions such as the reduction of ferric chloride to ferrous chloride) gain of electrons.

Reductones. Enediols which may be formed from sugars carrying a free carboxyl group by heating in alkaline solution. The simplest is hydroxyglycolaldehyde. Reductones may be formed in carbohydrate foods during heat processing, and as they have similar properties to vitamin C they interfere with its estimation.

Similar interfering substances are the reductinic acids formed by acid treatment of pentoses.

Reference Man. An arbitrary physiological standard; defined as a man of 25 years, healthy, weight 65 kg, living in a temperate zone at a mean annual temperature of 10°C, assumed to require an average daily intake of 3,200 kcal (13·5 MJ). (DP.)

Reference Protein. A theoretical concept of the perfect protein which is used with 100% efficiency at whatever level it is fed in the diet. Used as a means of expressing recommended intakes.

The nearest approach to this theoretical protein are egg and human milk proteins which are used with 90–100% efficiency when fed at low levels in the diet (4%) but not when fed at high levels (10–15%). (AEB.)

Reference Woman. An arbitrary physiological standard; defined as 25 years of age, 55 kg weight, engaged in general household duties or light industry, using 2,300 kcal (9·7 MJ) per day, and, as reference man, living in a temperate zone at a mean annual temperature of 10°C.

Refractive Index. A measure of the bending or refraction of a beam of light on entering a denser medium; the ratio of the sine of the angle of incidence of the ray of light to the sine of the angle of refraction. It is constant for pure substances under standard conditions.

Used as a measure of sugar or total solids in solution, purity of oils, etc.

Refractometer. Optical instrument used to measure the refractive index (*which see*).

The **Abbé refractometer** consists of two prisms between which is spread the substance under examination (jam, fruit juice, sugar syrup, etc.) and light is reflected through the solution.

The **immersion refractometer** dips into the solution. (Ayl.)

Refrigeration. *See* Psychrophilic bacteria *and* Preservation.

Rehfuss Tube. Instrument for removing samples of food from the stomach after a test meal. It is a small-diameter tube with a slotted metal tip. Another type is the Ryle tube, *which see*. (Hawk.)

Reichert-Meissl Value. Measure of the volatile fatty acids in fats. Defined as ml of N/10 NaOH required to neutralize the distillate from 5 g of fat; = Reichert-Meissl number. (Bailey.)

Relative Humidity. Important in food preservation as micro-organisms require moisture to live, but under some moist conditions, e.g. in a high concentration of sugar solution, the moisture is not available. Moulds will not grow on jam, 30% water, but will grow on cereals, 10% water. Available moisture conveniently expressed as Relative Humidity.

Bacteria need more moisture than yeasts, therefore less of a hazard. Minimum R.H. for yeasts 75–95%, increasing as temperature decreases. *See* Osmophilic yeasts. (Baum.)

Release Agents. Substances applied to tinned or enamelled surfaces or plastic films to prevent the food adhering; e.g. fatty acid amides, microcrystalline waxes, petrolatums, starch, methylcellulose.

Renal Threshold. Blood level of a particular substance at which it is excreted through the kidney. E.g. renal threshold of glucose is about 180 mg per 100 ml, and diabetics excrete glucose because this level is exceeded.

Various drugs can reduce the renal threshold. (BDS.)

Rendering. The process of liberating the fat from the fat cells that constitute the adipose tissue. Dry rendering, heating the fat dry, or wet rendering, when water is present.

Rennet. Extract of calf stomach; contains the enzyme rennin which clots milk. Used in cheese-making and for junkets. (Hutch.)

Rennet, Vegetable. Name given to proteolytic enzymes derived from plants, such as bromelin (from the pineapple) and ficin (from the fig).

Rennin. Digestive enzyme that clots milk. Found in the stomach juices of young mammals; secreted as the precursor prorennin, activated by hydrochloric acid. Is the active principle of commercial preparations of rennet.

Converts the soluble milk casein into paracasein, the calcium salt of which is insoluble so that a clot or curd is formed. (BDS.)

Rentschlerizing. Sterilizing by treatment with ultra-violet light; named after Dr. H. C. Rentschler, who developed the lamp.

R-enzyme. Enzyme present in beans and potatoes that splits the 1:6 linkage between the chains in starches; similar to the amylo-1:6-glucosidase found in muscle. Also known as the "de-branching" factor. (WHSS.)

Resazurin Test. *See* Methylene blue test.

Resins, Ion-exchange. *See* Ion-exchange resins.

Respiration. Although commonly used to mean breathing, more specifically relates to the consumption of oxygen and the production of carbon dioxide. Thus respiratory enzymes are those involved in cell oxidations.

Respiratory Quotient. Ratio of the volume of carbon dioxide produced when a substance is oxidized, to the volume of oxygen used.

In respiration in man the oxidation of carbohydrate results in R.Q. of 1·0; of fat, 0·71; and of protein, 0·8. (BDS.)

Retardin. Substance from the pancreas claimed to regulate fat metabolism.

Reticulin. One of the structural elements (together with elastin and collagen) of skeletal muscle. Chemically it is identical with collagen but histologically it stains black with silver while collagen stains yellow or brown; it is thought to be a precursor or a degraded form of collagen. (Meat.)

Reticulocyte. Young form of the red blood cell (normocyte or erythrocyte) in which the remains of the nucleus is visible as a reticulum. Very few are seen in the normal blood, they are retained in the marrow until mature, but on remission of anaemia, when there is a high rate of production, reticulocytes appear in the bloodstream (reticulocytosis). (BDS.)

Reticulo-endothelial System. A "system" of cells distributed throughout the body, with phagocytic properties. Present in spleen, bone marrow, liver, and lymph nodes, and are also mobile in the tissues and blood stream. They act as scavengers of tissue débris and bacteria.

The reticulo-endothelial system also removes red blood cells when they have completed their life of 120 days. The iron is recovered for further use, the rest of the haemoglobin is converted to bile pigments, stercobilin in the faeces and urobilin in the urine. (BDS.)

Reticulum. *See* Rumen.

Retinal. Aldehyde of retinol, formerly termed A aldehyde.

Retinene. Obsolete name for retinal.

Retinoic Acid. Acid derived from retinol, formerly vitamin A acid.

Retinol. Formerly termed vitamin A alcohol, *see* Vitamin A.

Retort. In connection with food technology, an autoclave.

Retrogradation. A change in gelatinized starch occurring on storage which results in reduced solubility and a change of texture. It is important in products such as dehydrated potatoes and baked products.

In ungelatinized (raw) starch the granules are in a definite pattern, which is lost when the starch is heated and gelatinized. On storage the granules slowly associate with each other to reform a pattern—the gel is destroyed and amylose is precipitated as an insoluble floc. This "crystallization" is retrogradation.

It is involved in the staling of bread crumb (not crust) and crumb-softeners such as polyoxyethylene and monoglyceride derivatives of the fatty acids function by slowing retrogradation. (Matz.)

RF Heating. *See* High frequency heating.

Rhamnose. A methyl pentose sugar; 33% sweetness of sucrose.

Rheology. Science of deformation and flow of matter. In food technology it involves brittleness and plasticity of fats, doughs, milk curds, grains, etc.

Rhiotin. Unidentified urinary excretion product of biotin, together with miotin and triotin. (Sebrell.)

Rhizopterin. *See* Folic acid.

191

Rhodamine B. Hydrochloride of diethyl-*m*-amino phenol phthalein —until recently used as a red colour in meat paste and mint rock, but not now permitted in U.K. and most other countries.

Rhodopsin. *See* Visual purple *and* Vitamin A.

Rhubarb. Leaf-stalks of perennial plant, *Rheum rhaponticum*; contains only traces of protein and carbohydrate; 6 kcal (0·02 MJ) per 100g, 10 mg vitamin C raw, 7 mg cooked. High content of oxalate, leaves are toxic for this reason. (M&W.)

Ribena. Trade name (Beecham Foods Ltd.) for a preparation of black currant juice and sugar syrup plus added vitamin C. Very rich source of vitamin C 206 mg per 100 g, 61% sugar, 229 kcal (0·97 MJ), per 100 g. (M&W.)

Riboflavin. Vitamin B_2.

Ribonucleic Acid. *See* Nucleic acids.

Ribose. A pentose sugar of outstanding physiological importance; it is part of vitamin B_2, of coenzyme I and II, of adenylic acid, and in the nucleoproteins either as ribose or desoxyribose. (BDS.)

Ribosomes. Particles found in animal cells, plants, yeasts, and as a major constituent of bacterial cytoplasm—believed to be the site of protein synthesis; composed of ribonucleic acid. (BDS.)

Ribotide. Trade name (Takeda Chemical Industries, Japan) for a mixture of disodium inosinate and disodium guanylate used as a flavour enhancer for savoury dishes.

Rice. Grain of *Oryza sativa;* major food in many countries. Rice when threshed is known as **paddy,** and is covered with a fibrous husk comprising nearly 40% of the grain. When the husk has been removed **brown rice** is left. When the outer bran layers up to the endosperm and germ are removed the ordinary **white rice** of commerce or **polished rice** is obtained (usually polished with glucose and talc).

Brown rice, including the germ, consists of protein 7·5%, fat 1·8%; calcium 15 mg, iron 1·4 mg, kcal 357 (1·5 MJ), vitamin B_1 0·3 mg, B_2 0·05 mg, nicotinic acid 4·6 mg—per 100 g.

In conversion to polished rice there is considerable loss of vitamin B_1 (and nicotinic acid), hence the widespread occurrence of beriberi among rice-eating peoples.

White rice: Protein 6·7%, fat 0·7%: calcium 10 mg, iron 1 mg, Calories 360, vitamin B_1 0·08 mg, B_2 0·03 mg, nicotinic acid 1·6 mg—per 100 g. (FAO, TND.)

Rice, American. Bulgur, *which see.*

Rice Crispies. Trade name (Kellogg's Ltd.) for a breakfast cereal made from rice.

Composition per 100 g: 6 g protein, 87 g carbohydrate, 360 kcal (1·5 MJ), 0·7 mg iron, 1 mg B_1, 1·4 mg B_2, 16 mg niacin.

Rice Diet. *See* Kempner diet.

Rice, Glutinous. For most purposes separate rice grains are wanted that do not stick together in a glutinous mass. Glutinous rice is rich in soluble starch, dextrin and maltose and on boiling the grains adhere in a sticky mass; this rice is used for sweetmeats and cakes. (TND.)

Rice Grass, Indian. *See* Indian rice grass.

Rice, hungry. A variety of millet, *Digitaria exilis*, important in west Africa.

Rice Krispies. Trade name (Kellogg Co.) for a breakfast cereal prepared from rice grains by heating under pressure and then rapidly reducing the pressure so that the superheated steam in the grain suddenly expands and "puffs" the grain.

Protein 5·7%, fat 1·1%, carbohydrate 85·1%; Ca 6 mg, Fe 0·7 mg, Calories 351—per 100 g. (M&W.)

Rice Paper. Smooth white paper made from the pith of a tree peculiar to Formosa. It is edible and macaroons and similar biscuits are baked on it and the paper can be eaten with the biscuit.

Rice, Parboiled. The rice is soaked in water and boiled for a short time before removing the husk so that considerably more of of the thiamine and nicotinic acid remains with the rice compared with raw dehusked rice. (TND.)

Rice, red. West African species, *Oryza glaberrima*, with red bran layer.

Rice, Synthetic. *See* Tapioca-macaroni.

Rice, Unpolished. Rice which has been undermilled in that the husk, germ and bran layers have been partially removed. Term used in the United States. (TND.)

Rice, wild. Also known as **zizanie, Tuscarora rice, Indian rice** and **American wild rice** (American rice is bulgur); *Zizania aquatica*. Native to eastern N. America, grows 12 feet high; long, thin, greenish grain; little is grown and difficult to harvest so is strictly a gourmet food.

Higher in protein content than ordinary rice at 14%, fat 7·0%, carbohydrate 74%, fibre 1·5%. (Matz 2.)

Rice Wine. *See* Saké.

Ricing. A culinary term meaning cutting into small pieces about the size of rice grains.

Rickets. Malformation of the bone in growing children due to shortage of vitamin D leading to poor absorption of calcium. In adults the equivalent is osteomalacia. *See* Vitamin D. (DP.)

Rickets, Refractory. Rickets that does not respond to normal doses of vitamin D but requires massive doses; it is suggested that refractory rickets is a congenital abnormality.

Riffle Flumes. Washing equipment consisting of stepped channels along which the product being washed is carried in a flow of water; stones and grit are retained on the steps.

Rigor Mortis. Stiffening of muscle that occurs after death. At death muscle is soft and pliable, the cessation of blood flow causes the remaining metabolism of the tissue to be anaerobic, with formation of lactic acid and a fall in pH. As the concentration of adenosine triphosphate decreases the muscles harden—this is rigor mortis and meat eaten at this stage would be tough. After hanging for a few days in a cooler the muscles soften by some undefined mechanism and the meat becomes edible.

Meat that has been kept in this way ("conditioned") is preferable to freshly killed meat with regard to texture. (Meat.)

Ringer's Solution. Solution of the chlorides of sodium, potassium and calcium in which isolated tissues will continue to survive (960 ml of 0.154M NaCl, 20 ml. 0.154M KCl, and 20 ml 0.11M CaCl$_2$.) (Hawk.)

Ripening of Fruit. *See* Pectin.

RNA. Ribonucleic acid, *see* Nucleic acids.

Roasting. Essentially baking in a closed oven. Meat shrinks and squeezes out juices, but some of the juice evaporates before it has time to drip away. This leaves some of the meat extractives on the surface, improving the flavour and reducing the losses. Only 20% of the extractive is lost in roasting compared to 50% in steaming or boiling.

Losses of vitamin B$_1$ greater than boiling, amounting to 35–50%; 10–20% loss of B$_2$ and nicotinic acid—same as boiling. Roasting suitable only for prime cuts as tough connective tissue is not broken down during roasting. *See also* Connective tissue. (Johnson.)

Robison Ester. Name given to a mixture of glucose-6-phosphate and fructose-1 phosphate, which are intermediary stages in glucose metabolism, *which see*.

Rocambole. Similar to garlic.

Rochelle Salt. Potassium sodium tartrate; used to combine with the copper in Fehling's test for reducing sugars.

Roe. Hard roe is the eggs of the female fish; soft roe is from the male fish, also known as **milt**.

Rokelax. Scandinavian term for smoked salmon.

Roller Dryer. The material to be dried is spread over the surface of internally heated rollers and dry-ing is complete in a few seconds. The rollers rotate against a knife that scrapes off the dried film as soon as it forms.

There is little damage by this method; for example, roller-dried milk is not scorched, but there is some loss of vitamins B$_1$ and C, more than in spray drying. (RJC.)

Roller Mill. Pairs of horizontal cylindrical rollers, separated by only a small gap and revolving at different speeds. The material is thus ground and crushed in the one operation. Used in flour milling. (KJ.)

Roll-on Closure (R.O.). Aluminium or lacquered tin plate cap for sealing on to narrow-necked bottles with a threaded neck. The unthreaded cap is moulded on to the neck of the bottle and forms an air-tight seal. (Baum.)

Root Beer. Non-alcoholic carbonated beverage flavoured with oil of sassafras and oil of wintergreen.

Rope. Bacteria of the type *B. mesentericus* and *B. subtilis* occur on wheat and thence in flour. These organisms form spores that can survive baking and then are present in the bread. Under the right conditions of warmth and moisture the spores will germinate and the mass of bacteria convert the bread into sticky, yellowish patches which can be pulled out into rope-like threads—hence the term ropy bread. The bacterial growth is inhibited by acid substances.

Can also occur in milk and carbonated beverages.

Rose-Gottlieb Test. For fat in milk; accurate gravimetric method, by extracting the fat with solvent. (Davis.)

Rose Hips. The fruit of the rose; a rich source of vitamin C from which rose-hip syrup is prepared.

Rose Hip Syrup. Extract of rose hip with added sugar, used as source of vitamin C—150 mg per 100 g.

Rosemary. A bushy shrub, *Rosmarinus officinalis*, cultivated commercially for its essential oil, used in medicine and perfumery. The dried leaves are used to flavour soups, sauces and meat. (Merory.)

Rotary Louvre Dryer. Hot air passes through a moving bed of the solid inside a rotating drum. (RJC.)

Roth-Benedict Spirometer. *See* Spirometer.

Roughage. Undigestible carbohydrate material in plant foodstuffs, e.g. cellulose (flesh, skin and seeds), bran (in cereals). As the material is not digested it passes through the intestine unchanged, but absorbs and holds water and acts as a laxative.

Roux. A preparation of flour and butter for thickening gravies and sauces.

Rovimix. Trade name (Hoffman La Roche Ltd.) for retinol stabilized in beadlet form in a gelatin-sugar-starch base. (AEB.)

Royal Jelly. The food on which bee larvae are fed and which causes them to develop into queen bees. Richest known source of pantothenic acid (500 micrograms per g dry weight): also contains vitamin B_6 and 2% of its dry weight is 10-hydroxy-delta-2-decenoic acid.

Claimed without foundation, to have rejuvenating virtues for human beings.

R.Q. Respiratory Quotient, *which see.*

Rubble Reel. Machine for cleaning materials such as wheat. The material is fed into a long inclined reel made of perforated metal that rotates inside a frame. The perforations become larger nearer the bottom so that there is a graded sieving of the material as it passes down the reel.

Rubner Factors. Factors used to calculate the energy content of foods in kilocalories after allowing for losses of urinary nitrogen but not allowing for incomplete absorption, therefore greater than Atwater factors; protein 4·1, fat 9·3, carbohydrates 4·1. *See also* Energy. (DP.)

Rum. A spirit distilled from fermented molasses. There are three main categories, Cuban, Jamaican and Dutch East Indies.

Rumen. Ruminating animals such as the cow, sheep and goat, possess four stomachs in distinction from monogastric animals such as man, pig, dog and rat. These four are: the rumen, or first stomach, where bacterial fermentation produces lower fatty acids, and from whence the food is returned to the mouth for further mastication (chewing the cud); the reticulum, where further bacterial fermentation produces lower fatty acids; the omasum; and the abomasum or true stomach.

The bacterial fermentation allows ruminants to obtain nourishment from grass and hay which cannot be digested by monogastric animals. (Abrams.)

Ruminant. *See* Rumen.

Rutabaga. American name for swede.

Rutin. A disaccharide (rhamnose and glucose) derivative of quercetin; found in grains, tomato stalk, elderberry blossom. *See* Vitamin P.

Rye. Grain of cereal *Secale cereale*, the predominant cereal in some parts of Europe; very hardy and withstands adverse conditions better than wheat.

Rye flour is dark and the dough lacks elasticity; rye bread is usually made with sour dough or leaven rather than yeast. *See also* Pumpernickel *and* Crispbreads.

Protein 8%, fat 1·5%; kcal 350 (1·47 MJ), calcium 25 mg, iron 3·5 mg, vitamin B_1 0·27 mg, B_2 0·1 mg, nicotinic acid 1·2 mg —per 100 g. (KJ, OF.)

Ryle Tube. Instrument for removing samples of the contents from the stomach at intervals after a test meal. It is a narrow rubber tube with a blind end containing a lead weight, with holes above this level. Another type is the Rehfuss tube, *which see*. (Hawk.)

Ryvita. Trade name (Ryvita Co. Ltd.) for a crisp bread (*which see*).

Protein 7·1%, fat 2·1% carbohydrate 76·8%; Ca. 41 mg, Fe 3·7 mg, kcal 345 (1·45 MJ)—per 100 g. Phytic acid phosphorus 54% of total P (295 mg/100 g). (M&W.)

S

Saccharases. A group of enzymes that attack sugars to liberate glucose or fructose depending on the type of saccharase. *See* Invertase.

Saccharic Acid. Dibasic acid derived from glucose.

Saccharimeter. Polarimeter used to determine the purity of sugar; graduated on the International Sugar Scale—degrees sugar.

26% solution of pure sucrose reads 100° sugar in a 200-mm tube. *See also* Optical Activity. (Ayl.)

Saccharin. A chemical, benzoic sulphimide, 550 times as sweet as cane sugar. Soluble saccharin is the sodium salt. Has no food value; useful as a sweetening agent for diabetics and slimmers. Discovered in U.S.A. in 1879.

Saccharometer. Floating device used to determine the specific gravity of sugar solutions (distinct from saccharimeter).

Saffron. Dried stigma of *Crocus sativus* (related to garden crocus). Contains glycoside picrocrocin, and colouring principles crocin and crocetin. Used as natural dyestuff (permitted food colour) and spice. Very soluble in water. (Jacobs.)

Sage. Dried leaf of the Dalmatian sage, *Salvia officinalis*, of the mint family; fragrant and spicy and is the most important herb used in the kitchen for flavouring meat and fish dishes and in poultry stuffing. Other sages (Greek, Spanish, English) differ in flavour from the Dalmatian variety. Also sage oil from the same source by steam distillation. Contains the essential oil thujone together with alpha-pinene, cineol, borneol and d-camphor. (Merory.)

Sago. Starchy grains prepared from the pith of the sago palm (*Metroxylon sago*); almost pure starch free from protein.

Composition, protein 0·5%, fat negligible, carbohydrate 88%, trace of B vitamins.

Saithe. *Polachius virens.* Also known as **coley** and **coal fish.** Apart from being eaten cooked, it is smoked, salted and dyed red, when it is similar to smoked salmon.

Saké. Japanese beer made from rice. Cooked whole rice grains are fermented with a yeast-like fungus culture for 10–14 days and stored in wooden barrels. Contains about 17% alcohol, by volume. Also known as **rice wine.** (Jacobs.)

Salad Cream. Oil-in-water emulsion made from vegetable oil, vinegar, salt, spices, emulsified with egg yolk and thickened.

Legally, in U.K., must contain not less than 25% by weight of vegetable oil and not less than 1·35% egg-yolk solids. Mayonnaise usually contains more oil, less carbohydrate and water.

By U.S.A. regulations salad dressing contains 30% vegetable oil and 4% egg yolk; mayonnaise contains 65% oil plus egg yolk.

Salad Dressing. *See* French dressing.

Salamagundi. Old English dish consisting of diced fresh and salt meats mixed with hard-boiled eggs, pickled vegetables and spices, dressed on a bed of salad.

Salinometer. Or salimeter or salometer. Hydrometer to measure concentration of salt solutions.

Salisbury Cure. Exclusive protein diet, supposed to cure or alleviate a number of diseases. (Hutch.)

Salisbury Steak. Similar to hamburger—minced lean beef mixed with bread, eggs, milk and seasoning, shaped into cakes and fried.

Saliva. Secretion of the salivary glands in the mouth. There are three pairs of glands, parotid, submandibular and submaxillary. Dilute solution of the protein, mucin, and the enzyme, amylase, with small quantities of urea, potassium thiocyanate, sodium chloride and bicarbonate.

One to 1·5 litres per day secreted of solution of 0·5% solids. The mucin lubricates the food, and the amylase hydrolyses starch to maltose. (BDS.)

Salivary Glands. *See* Saliva.

Sally Lunn. A sweet, spongy, yeast cake, named after a girl of that name who sold her tea cakes in the streets of Bath 1788.

Salmon. *See* Fish, fatty.

Salmonellae. Genus of bacteria of family *Enterobacteriaceae.* Common cause of food poisoning, *which see.* Found in eggs from infected hens, sausages, etc.; can survive in brine and in the refrigerator, destroyed by adequate heating. (Tanner.)

Salt. Usually refers to sodium chloride, i.e. common salt or table salt (although any compound of acid and alkali is a salt). *See* Sodium *and* Salt-free diets.

Salt Content. *See* Salt-free diets.

Salt-free Diets. More correctly these are diets low in (never completely free from) sodium, but as most of the sodium of the diet is consumed as sodium chloride or salt, they are referred to as low-salt diets. It is the sodium and not the chloride that is of importance.

Sodium controls the retention of fluid in the body and reduced retention, aided by low-sodium diets, is required in cardiac insufficiency accompanied by oedema, in certain kidney diseases, toxaemias of pregnancy and hypertension.

The average sodium intake is 1,000–2,000 mg per day and restricted diets are usually about 500 mg and can be as low as 150 mg.

To improve the palatability of such diets "salt" mixtures are available containing potassium and ammonium chlorides together with citrates, formates, phosphates, glutamates, as well as herbs and spices.

Foods low in salt (0–20 mg/ 100 g):—sugar, flour, fruit, green vegetables, macaroni, nuts; medium salt—(50–100 mg/100 g) chicken, fish, eggs, meat, milk; high salt (500–2,000 mg/100 g), corned beef, bread, ham, bacon, kippers, sausages, cheese. (Hutch, AEB.)

Saltlicks. An adequate intake of sodium chloride is necessary to all animals. Grass is relatively poor in sodium, and its high potassium content induces excretion of sodium in the urine. This loss causes a craving for sodium which is satisfied by natural or artificial salt-licks.

Saltpetre or Bengal Saltpetre. Potassium nitrate, used together with salt in the curing of meat. The salt restrains the growth of unwanted organisms; the nitrate is converted to nitrite which combines with muscle pigment to give the red colour of pickled meat. *See also* Nitrates.

Salts, Bile. *See* Bile.

Salts, Indian. Greek and Roman name for sugar.

Sambol. Name given to a curry of fairly solid consistency in India and other parts of the East. (TND.)

Sami. Socially acceptable monitoring instrument. A small, heart-rate counting apparatus used to estimate energy expenditure of human subjects. (BDS.)

Samna. *See* Ghee.

Samp. Coarsely cut portions of maize with bran and germ partly removed.

Sanatogen. Trade name (Genatosan Ltd.) for a preparation of casein and sodium glycerophosphate for consumption as a beverage when added to milk.

Sanka. Trade name (Maxwell House Ltd.) for a decaffeinated instant coffee.

Sapodilla. Fruit of the sapodilla tree (*Achras sapota*); size of a small apple, rough grained, yellow to greyish pulp.

Water 75%, protein 0·4%, fat 1%, carbohydrate 22%; kcal 97 (0·41 MJ), Fe 0·8 mg, vitamin B_2 0·03 mg, nicotinic acid 0·2 mg, vitamin C 15 mg—per 100 g.

Chicle, the basis of chewing gum, is made from the latex of the same tree. (Platt.)

Saponification. Splitting of fat into its constituent glycerol and fatty acids by boiling with alkali. The fatty acids will be present as the sodium salts, also called the sodium soaps.

Method of concentrating vitamin A from oils, because the vitamin does not saponify and can then be separated from the rest of the fat in the so-called non-saponifiable fraction. The latter also contains mineral oils and higher alcohols such as cholesterol. (Hawk.)

Saponification Value. Used with reference to fats as an indication of the nature (molecular weight) of the fatty acids present.

Defined as the number of milligrams of potassium hydroxide required to saponify 1 g of fat. Values greater than 200 are short chain fatty acids, below 190 are of high molecular weight. (Bailey.)

Saponins. Group of substances that occur in plants and can produce a soapy lather with water. Extracted commercially from soapwort or soapbark and used as foam producer in beverages, fire extinguishers, as detergent and for emulsifying oils. Bitter in flavour.

There is a second group, the steroid saponins, that are cardiac active and are used as a starting material for the synthesis of sex hormones.

Saracen Corn. See Buckwheat.

Saran. Generic name for thermoplastic materials made from polymers of vinylidine chloride and vinyl chloride. They are clear transparent films used for wrapping food, resistant to oils and chemicals, can be heat-shrunk on to the product.

Sarcolactic Acid. Old name for the form of lactic acid which turns the plane of polarized light to the right, i.e. (+) lactic acid; found in muscle, as distinct from the inactive lactic acid (mixture of + and −) found in sour milk. Also known as **paralactic** acid.

Sarcolemma. See Muscle.

Sarcoplasm. See Muscle.

Sardine. Young pilchard, *Sardina* (*Clupea*) *pilchardus*.

Composition of canned product per 100 g: 20·4 g protein, 22·6 g fat, 294 kcal (1·23 MJ), 400 mg calcium, 4 mg iron, 30 μg vitamin A, 8 μg vitamin D, 0·2 mg B_2, 5 mg nicotinic acid. (M&W.)

Saridele. Protein-rich baby food (26–30% protein) developed in Indonesia; extract of soya bean with sugar, calcium carbonate, vitamins B_1, B_{12} and C.

Sarsaparilla. Flavour prepared from oil of sassafras and oil of wintergreen or oil of sweet birch; used in a carbonated beverage.

Sassafras Oil. Used to flavour root beer and similar beverages. Main component is safrole, believed to be a weak hepatic carcinogen and banned in some countries.

Sauerkraut. Prepared by lactic fermentation of shredded cabbage. In the presence of 2–3% salt, acid-forming bacteria thrive and convert sugars in the cabbage into acetic and lactic acids which then act as preservatives. (Tanner.)

Sauerteig. See Black bread.

Sausage. Chopped meat, mostly beef or pork, seasoned with salt and spices, mixed with cereal (usually wheat rusk prepared from crumbed unleavened biscuits) and packed into casings made from the connective tissue of animal intestines or cellulose.

There are six main types, fresh, smoked, cooked, smoked and cooked, semi-dry and dry. Frankfurts, Bologna, Polish and Berliner sausages are made from cured meat and are smoked and cooked.

Thuringer, soft salami, morta-

199

della and soft cervelat are semi-dry sausages. Pepperoni, chorizos, dry salami, dry cervelat are slowly dried to a hard texture. (Jacobs.)

Sausage Casings. Natural casings are made from hog intestines for fresh frying sausages, and from sheep intestines for chipólatas and frankfurters. Skinless sausages are prepared in cellulose casing, which is then peeled off.

Sausage Factor. *See* Meat factor.

Sauté. Toss in hot fat without browning (sauté potatoes usually cooked first and browned).

Savarin, Brillat. Noted French gastronome (1755–1826) chiefly famous for his book "The Physiology of Taste".

Saveloy. Highly seasoned smoked sausage; the addition of saltpetre gives rise to the bright red colour. Originally a sausage made from pig's brains.

Savory. A plant with strongly flavoured leaves used as seasoning in sauces, soups, salad dishes. Summer savory is an annual, *Satureja hortensis*, winter savory is a perennial, *Satureja montana*. The plants are cut down at flowering time and dried for later use. (Merory.)

Saxin. Trade name (Burroughs, Wellcome Ltd.) for saccharine.

Scald. Defect occurring in stored apples consisting of formation of brown patches on the skin with browning and softening of the tissues underneath. Due to accumulation of gases given off during ripening.

Scampi. Norway Lobster or Dublin Bay Prawn. *See* Lobster.

Scenedesmus. *See* Algae.

Schardinger's Enzyme. The same as xanthine oxidase which oxidizes a whole range of aldehydes to acids, and also xanthine and hypoxanthine to uric acid.

Scleroproteins. *See* Albuminoids.

Scomberoid poisoning. Caused by products of microbial spoilage of one group of fish, scomberoid fish, including tunny, mackerel, sardines, pike-mackerel. Due to formation of relatively large amounts of histamine from the amino acid histidine by organism *Proteus morganii*.

Scone. A variety of tea cake originally made from oatmeal and sour milk, in Scone, Scotland.

SCP. Single Cell Protein.

Scrapple. Meat dish prepared from pork carcass trimmings, maize meal, flour, salt and spices—cooked to a thick consistency.

Scrod. Young cod.

Scuppernong. Name of the most widely cultivated of the muscadine grapes, used chiefly in wine rather than as a dessert grape.

Scurvy. *See* Vitamin C.

Scurvy Grass. *Cochlearia officinalis;* grows on the seashore and is a good source of vitamin C.

Scutellum. Area surrounding the embryo of the cereal grain; scutellum plus embryo is the germ. Rich in vitamins. (B. & R., KJ.)

S.D.A. *See* Specific dynamic action.

S.D.S. Sucrose disstearate. *See* Sucrose esters.

S.E. Starch equivalent.

Sea Slug. *See* Bêche-de-mer.

Seaweed. Used as a mineral supplement for cattle as it contains 15–20% ash on dry weight, including about 60 minerals. Also contains carotene, vitamin B_1, folic acid, vitamin E, and is said to be the only vegetable source of vitamin B_{12}.

Occasionally incorrectly claimed as a source of protein but most seaweeds are low in protein and of very low biological value.

Seaweed Extract. *See* Carageenan.

Secretin. A hormone, secreted by the intestinal mucosa, which travels via the bloodstream to the pancreas and stimulates this organ to secrete. Is a small, basic polypeptide, destroyed by pepsin and trypsin, and therefore ineffective when given by mouth. (Hawk, BDS.)

Sedoheptulose. A seven carbon sugar. Also called sedoheptose. *See* Hexosemonophosphate shunt.

Seitz Filter. Asbestos disc with pores so fine that they will not permit passage of bacteria, thus solutions filtered through a Seitz filter emerge sterile.

Selenium. Highly toxic element; High levels in the soil can accumulate in plants and render them toxic.

Acts synergistically with vitamin E (*See* Factor 3). (Gilbert, GMW.)

Self-raising Flour. *See* Flour, self-raising.

Semolina. The granular starchy product obtained from the endosperm of hard wheat; the fine floury part of the endosperm is semolina flour. Soft wheats give endosperm that does not hold together in granules during cooking.

Used for the preparation of alimentary pastes (macaroni, spaghetti, etc.) and as a milk pudding.

In U.S.A. farina (*which see*) is defined as the purified middling of hard wheat other than Durum wheat.

Sequestrants. Substances that combine with a metal ion or acid radicle and render it inactive, e.g. citrates, tartrates, phosphates, and various calcium salts. *See also* Ethylenediamine tetra-acetic acid.

Sequestrene. Trade name (Geigy Industrial Chemicals, U.S.A.) for ethylenediamine tetra-acetic acid, disodium and disodium calcium salts.

Serendipity Berry. *Dioscoreophyllum cumminsii.* West African fruit with an extremely sweet taste. Active principle called **monellin.**

Serine. A non-essential amino acid; amino hydroxypropionic acid. (BDS.)

Serosal. In reference to the intestine means the outer side of the intestinal wall as distinct from the inner or mucosal side.

Serum. Clear liquid left after the protein has been clotted; reference both to blood and to milk. The serum from milk, occasionally referred to as lacto-serum, is whey.

Serum, Blood. Blood plasma without the fibrinogen. When blood clots, the fibrinogen is converted to fibrin which is deposited in strands that trap the red cells and form the clot. The clear liquid that is exuded is the serum. (BDS.)

Serum Butter. *See* Butter, whey.

201

Sesame. *Sesamum indicum.* Tropical and sub-tropical plant, also known as **sim-sim** in East Africa and **benniseed** in West Africa. Seeds are small and in most varieties, white; used whole in sweetmeats, in stews and to decorate cakes and bread, and for extraction of the oil.

Composition per 100 g: 20 g protein, 50 g fat, 16 g carbohydrate, 5 g fibre, 592 kcal (2·5 MJ), 1 mg B_1, 0·25 mg B_2, 5 mg nicotinic acid. (OF, Platt.)

Seven Foods Plan. *See* Basic 7 Foods Plan.

Seville Orange. Spanish term for the bitter orange, *which see*, under Orange, bitter.

Sex Hormones. *See* Hormones, sex, *and* Oestrogens.

Sfumatrice. Machine for obtaining the oil from the peel of citrus fruit. Based on the principle that the natural turgor of the oil sacs forces out the oil when the peel is folded. (Brav.)

Shaddock. Alternative name for pomelo, *Citrus grandis*, from which grapefruit is descended (named after Captain Shaddock who introduced it into West Indies).

Sharples Centrifuge. Continuous high-speed centrifuge (15,000 to 30,000 revs. per min) consisting of vertical cylinder. Used to separate liquids of different densities or to clarify by sedimenting solids.

Sharps. *See* Wheatfeed.

Shashlik. Similar to shishkebab omitting steeping the meat in wine. According to some recipes the same as shishkebab.

Shea Butter. *See* Vegetable butters.

Shearling. Sheep 15–18 months old.

Shellfish, Edible. Include prawns, shrimps, lobsters, crayfish and crabs.

Zoologically they are of the Order Decapoda, Sub-order Macrura (prawns, shrimps, lobsters and crayfish) and Sub-order Brachyura (crabs).

See under separate entries.

Sherbet. A water ice, made from sugar, water and fruit flavouring, whipped with egg white to give a fluffy texture.

There is also milk sherbet containing a small amount of milk.

Shishkebab. Lamb (although beef sometimes used) cut into cubes steeped in onion, garlic and wine, for a few hours, impaled on a skewer; pieces of meat alternating with tomatoes, mushrooms, or pieces of eggplant, dusted with flour and then broiled.

Shortening. Soft fats that produce a crisp, flaky effect in baked products. Lard possesses the correct properties to a greater extent than any other single fat.

Unlike oils, shortenings are plastic and disperse as a film through the batter and prevent the formation of a hard, tough mass.

Shortenings are compounded from mixtures of fats or prepared by hydrogenation and are still called **lard compounds** or **lard substitutes.**

Shrimp. The pink shrimp commonly sold at fishmongers is *Pandalus montagui. See* Prawns.

Analysis without shell: protein 22·3%, fat 2·4%, carbohydrate 0; kcal 114 (0·48 MJ), Ca 320 mg, Fe 1·8 mg, vitamin B_1 0·03 mg, B_2 0·03 mg, nicotinic acid 3 mg —per 100 g. (M&W.)

202

Sialic Acid. Many tissues, body fluids and mucoproteins contain substances which give a purple colour with Ehrlich's reagent; they have been isolated and variously called **sialic** acid, **neuraminic** acid, **hemataminic** acid, **lactaminic** acid and **gynaminic** acid.

Their components have not been characterized but they may play an important rôle in the body.

Sialogogue. Substance that stimulates the flow of saliva.

Siderophilin. Or transferrin, an iron-carbonate-protein complex, the form in which iron is transported in the blood plasma.

Siderosis. Accumulation of haemosiderin, an iron-protein complex, in the liver, spleen and bone marrow, in cases of excessive blood destruction, and on poor diets relatively rich in iron. Said to be a common disorder among the Bantu people, who cook their maize in iron pots and consume up to 100 mg of iron per day. (DP.)

Sild. Young herring, *Clupea harengus*.

Silica Gel. Drying agent.

Silicones. Organic compounds of silicon; in the food field they are used as antifoaming agents, as semi-permanent glazes on baking tins and other metal containers, on non-sticking wrapping paper.

Silver. Not of interest in foods apart from its use in covering "nonpareils"—the silver beads used to decorate confectionery. Present in traces in all plant and animal tissues but has no function nor is enough ever absorbed to cause toxicity. *See also* Oligodynamic. (GMW.)

Simmer. *See* Cooking.

Simon's Metabolites. Name given to two compounds found (by Simon and co-workers) in the urine of rabbits as metabolites of vitamin E. Called Simon's metabolites in place of the long chemical names but now known by the trivial names of tocopheronic acid and tocopheronolactone.

Sim-sim. *See* Sesame.

Singharanut. *See* Chestnut, Water.

Single Cell Protein. Name given to bacteria, algae and yeasts grown in mass culture as a source of dietary proteins.

Sippet. A small piece of bread, fried or toasted, served as a garnish to a mince or hash.

Sippy Diet. For peptic ulcer patients; hourly feeds of small quantities, 150 ml., of milk, cream or other milky food. *See also* Lenhartz diet *and* Meulengracht diet. (DP.)

Sister Laura's Food. Trade name (Sister Laura Food Co.) for an infant food comprising wheat flour, sugar and salt. No vitamins are claimed.

Sitapophasis. Refusal to eat as expression of mental disorder.

Sitology. Science of foods (from the Greek *sitos*—food).

Sitomania. Mania for eating.

Sitophobia. Fear of food, also phagophobia.

Sitosterol. The main sterol found in vegetable oils, similar in structure to cholesterol with an extra ethyl group.

Skin Factor. Obsolete name for biotin.

Skyr. *See* Milks, fermented.

Sliwowitz. Plum brandy, originating in Yugoslavia. Some of the stones are included with the fruit and produce a characteristic bitter flavour from the hydrocyanic acid (0·008% HCN is present in the finished brandy).

Sloe. Wild sour plum of the blackthorn (*Prunus spinosa*), almost only use is for the manufacture of Sloe gin. (Merory.)

SLR Factor. *Streptococcus lactis* factor. *See* Folic acid.

SM. Protein-rich baby food (15% protein) made in Ethiopia from teff, peas, chick peas, lentils and skim-milk powder.

SMA. Trade name (John Wyeth Ltd.) for a milk preparation for infant feeding modified to resemble the composition of human milk. (AEB.)

Smell. *See* Organoleptic.

Smoke Point. A term used with reference to frying oils; the temperature at which the decomposition products become visible (bluish smoke). The temperature varies with different fats and ranges between 160 and 260°C.
See also Flash point *and* Fire point. (Bailey.)

Smoking. Meat and fish are often smoked after pickling to assist preservation and improve the flavour. Hard woods, oak, elm, and ash, produce a smoke containing aldehydes, phenols and acids with a preservative action, a surface dehydration also helps preservation. (Baum.)

Smörgäsbord. Scandinavian; table laden with delicacies such as fish, meat and cheese, as traditional gesture of hospitality.

Smörrebrod. Danish open sandwiches: literally means smeared bread.

SMS. Sucrose monostearate. *See* Sucrose esters.

Smut. A group of fungi that attack wheat; includes loose or common smut (*Ustilago triciti*) and stinking smut or bunt (*Tilletia triciti*). (KJ.)

S.N.F. *See* Solids-not-fat.

SO₂. *See* Sulphur dioxide.

Snibbing. Topping and tailing of gooseberries.

Soapstock. In the refining of crude edible oils the free fatty acids are removed by agitation with alkali. The fatty acids settle to the bottom as alkali soaps and are known as soapstock or "foots". (Bailey.)

Soda Bread. Made from flour and whey, or butter milk, using sodium bicarbonate and acid in place of yeast. Common in Ireland.

Sodium. A dietary essential which is almost invariably satisfied by the normal diet. The body contains about 100 g. of sodium, and the average diet contains 3–6 g, equivalent to 10 g · of sodium chloride. The intake varies enormously in different individuals and the excretion varies accordingly.
Vegetables are relatively poor in sodium and rich in potassium. Animal foods are rich in sodium. *See also* Water balance, Salt-free diets, *and* Sodium-potassium-ratio. (AEB.)

Sodium Bicarbonate. *See* Baking powder.

Sodium Chloride. Common salt —the commonest form in which sodium is consumed. *See* Sodium *and* Salt-free diets.

Sodium Glutamate. *See* Glutamate, sodium.

Sodium-Potassium Ratio. The body contains about three times as much potassium as sodium. Vegetables and fruits contain a great excess of potassium, e.g. potatoes 80:1; boiling with salt reduces this ratio to approx. 3:1.

Sodium Silicate. *See* Water-glass.

Soft Drinks. Legal standards for fruit content (ready-to-drink without dilution)—citrus-and-barley, lime juice and soda, 47 fl. oz per 10 gall; other types, 80 fl. oz per 10 gall.

Drinks requiring dilution, squash, crush, cordial or concentrate: citrus-and-barley, 1½ gall per 10 gall; citrus fruit, 2½ gall per 10 gall (25%); other fruits, 1 gall per 10 gall.

Comminuted whole orange: ready-to-drink, 5½ lb orange per 10 gall; for dilution, 27½ lb per 10 gall. (Bell.)

Sol. A colloidal solution, i.e. a suspension of particles intermediate in size between ordinary molecules (as in a solution) and coarse particles (as in a suspension). A jelly-like sol is a gel. (Hawk.)

Solanaceae. I.e. egg plant, peppers, potatoes and tomatoes.

Solanine. Toxic glycoside found in potato and especially the sprouts; consisting of glucose, galactose and rhamnose plus the alkaloid solanidine. A considerable portion is removed with the peel and some is leached out on cooking. (B. & R.)

Solids-not-fat. Refers to the solids of milk excluding the fat, i.e. protein, lactose and salts. S.N.F. serves as an index of milk quality and is determined by measuring the specific gravity in the lactometer.

Normal specific gravity is 1·032 at 60°F (15·5°C).

Per cent total solids $=0.25 \times$ S.G. $+ 1.2 \times$ percentage fat $+ 0.14$. (Davis.)

Solvents. For food additives—isopropyl alcohol, propylene glycol, diethylene glycol, monoethyl ether, hexylene glycol, monoacetin, diacetin, triacetin.

Sorbate. *See* Sorbic acid.

Sorbet. A semi-frozen water ice flavoured with liqueur. In a large-scale dinner sorbet is served before the roast to clear the palate.

Sorbic Acid. Formula $CH_3.CH:CH.CH:CH.COOH$. Used to inhibit selectively growth of yeasts and moulds (not bacteria). Metabolized in the same way as the naturally occurring caproic acid (of butter) and so generally held to be harmless.

Used in margarine (0·05%), fruit juice (0·02%), sauces, cheese, jam, flour confectionery (0·1%). Permitted in U.K. in flour confectionery and cheese.

Potassium sorbate is more soluble in water. Occurs in certain berries as the free acid and the delta-lactone; first claimed as antimycotic in 1945.

Is active as the undissociated acid and therefore the concentration for preservation is related to the acidity of the food. Effective at pH 5·0–7·0.

Sorbistat. Sorbistat K. Trade names (Pfizer) for sorbic acid, *which see*, and its potassium salt.

Sorbitol. A six-carbon sugar alcohol formed by the reduction of fructose. Although it is metabolized in the body it appears to be tolerated by diabetics and is therefore used to sweeten diabetic foods. 60% as sweet as sucrose.

Found in plum, apricot, cherry and apple but not in raspberry, blackcurrant, strawberry or currant. (AEB).

Sorcerer's Milk. *See* Witches' Milk.

Sorenson Titration. Method of titrating amino acids and ammonium salts by adding formaldehyde, which combines with the amino groups, and titrating the carboxyl groups (or acidic radical of the ammonium salt). (Hawk.)

Sorghum. *Sorghum vulgare.* A cereal that thrives in semi-arid regions; important human food in tropical Africa, central and north India and China. Sorghum produced in United States and Australia is used for animal feed. Also known as **kaffir corn** (in South Africa), **guinea corn** (in West Africa), **jowar** (in India) and **millo maize.** The white grain variety is eaten as meal, red grained has a bitter taste and is used for beer; sugar syrup is obtained from the crushed stems of the sweet sorghum.

Composition per 100 g: 10 g protein, 3 g fat, 70 g carbohydrate, 2 g fibre, 4·5 mg iron, 0·5 mg vitamin B_1, 0·12 mg B_2, 3·5 mg nicotinic acid. (OF, Platt.)

Sorghum Syrup. Juice of the sugar sorghum which is related to the sugar cane.

Souchong. *See* Tea.

Soursop. *See* Custard Apple.

Souse. A cooked meat product treated with vinegar.

Soxhlet. An apparatus for the extraction of solids, mostly used for the extraction of fat. The solid is contained in a "thimble" and is percolated by fresh solvent continuously. The fat-laden solvent siphons over into a flask from which it is boiled off to be repercolated, while the fat is left in the flask. (Hawk.)

Soya. A bean (*Glycine max*) of importance as a source of both oil and protein. The protein is of high biological value, higher than many other vegetable proteins and is of great value for animal and human food.

When raw it contains a trypsin inhibitor destroyed by heat.

Native of China where it has been cultivated for 5,000 years; grows 2–3 ft high with 2–3 beans per pod. The original variety was 20% protein with no fat but modern varieties contain 40% protein and 20% fat.

Soybean Curd. Precipitate from soybean milk: water 85%, protein 7%, fat 4%, carbohydrate 3%, fibre 0·1%; kcal 76 (0·32 MJ), Fe 1·8 mg, vitamin B_1 0·05 mg, B_2 0·04 mg, nicotinic acid 0·5 mg —per 100 g. (Platt.)

Soybean Flour. Dehulled, ground soya bean, The unheated material is a rich source of amylase and proteinase and is useful as a baking aid. The heated material has no enzymic activity but is a valuable food.

Full fat: Protein 39%, fat 21%; kcal 357 (1·5 MJ), Ca 197 mg, Fe 6·2 mg, vitamin A 42 μg, B_1 0·77 mg, B_2 0·28 mg, nicotinic acid 2 mg.—per 100 g.

Defatted: Protein 46%, fat 5%; kcal 261 (1·1 MJ), Ca 247 mg, Fe 7·4 mg, vitamin A 33 μg, B_1 0·7 mg, B_2 0·3 mg, nicotinic acid 2 mg.—per 100 g.

There is about 25% carbohydrate in the bean, of which 12% is polysaccharide (dextrins, galactans and pentosans) and 12·5% sugars (6% sucrose, 5% stachyose and 1·5% raffinose). (FAO.)

Soybean Milk. Extract of the bean: water 93%, protein 3·4%, fat 1·5%, carbohydrate 1%, fibre 0·4%; kcal 32 (0·13 MJ), Fe 0·6 mg, vitamin B_1 0·09 mg, B_2 0·04 mg, nicotinic acid 0·2 mg—per 100 g. (Platt.)

Soyolk. Trade name (Soya Foods Ltd.) for full fat soya flour.

Soy Sauce. The fermented soya bean commonly eaten in China and Japan. Traditionally the bean, often mixed with wheat, is fermented with *Aspergillus oryzae* over a period of one to three years. The modern process is carried out at a high temperature or in an autoclave for a short time.

Water 68%, protein 6%, fat 1%, carbohydrate 5%, kcal 53 (0·2 MJ), Ca 100 mg, Fe 5·5 mg, vitamin B_1 0·02 mg, B_2 0·06 mg, nicotinic acid 0·3 mg—per 100 g. (Platt.)

SO₂. *See* Sulphur dioxide.

Spaghetti. *See* Alimentary pastes.

Spans. Trade name (Atlas Co.) for a group of compounds made by reacting sorbitol with fatty acids; are surface active or emulsifying agents and have been used, for example, as crumb softeners in bread.

Specific Dynamic Action. This is the name given to the increase in metabolism that follows the ingestion of foods, normally amounting to 5–7% of the food intake.

The reason for specific dynamic action (SDA) is not known, but it is suggested that it is partly the result of flooding the cells with metabolites and partly the heat of deamination of amino acids. In practice it means that 5–7% should be added to calculated calorie requirements (called thermic effect). (DP.)

Specificity. In relation to enzymes refers to the ability of an enzyme to catalyse only a limited range of reactions, or, in some cases, a single reaction. Specificity is the main distinction between enzymes and catalysts, as the latter are non-specific.

Examples, arginase will hydrolyse L-arginine only, not even the D-isomer; esterase will hydrolyse the whole group of compounds containing the ester linkage, but no others. (WHSS.)

Specificity, Stereochemical. Used in reference to enzymes; those that will attack one stereochemical isomer but not the other. Thus there are distinct L- and D- amino acid oxidases that will attack only the corresponding isomer and leave the other untouched. (WHSS.)

Spectrophotometer. Optical instrument that measures the amount of light absorbed at any particular wavelength. Used extensively to measure substances that have specific absorption in the infra-red or ultra-violet range, or are coloured, or can react to form coloured derivatives. Similar in this way to the absorptiometer.

Spelt. Coarse type of wheat, mainly used as cattle feed.

Spent Wash. Liquor remaining in the whisky still after distilling the spirit. A source of unidentified growth factors detected by chick growth.

When dried is known as distillers' dried solubles.

Sphingomyelins. Complex phosphatides found in brain and nerve tissue and as part of cell structure; composed of the base sphingosine plus fatty acids, phosphoric acid and choline. (BDS.)

207

Spices. Distinguished from herbs only in that part instead of the whole of the aromatic plant is meant, such as root, stem, seeds.

Originally used to mask putrefactive flavours. Some have preservative effect because of their essential oils, e.g. cloves, cinnamon and mustard.

Consumed in too small a quantity to provide any nutrients except possibly for curry powder which contains 22 mg iron per ounce. (Baum, Merory.)

Spinach. Leaves of *Spinacia oleracea*. A rich source of carotene, and vitamin C; also contains oxalic acid, which renders calcium insoluble and non-available.

Protein 1·8%, fat 0·2%; kcal 17 (0·07 MJ), Ca 66 mg, Fe 2·4 mg, vitamin A 2·3 mg, B_1 0·9 mg, B_2 0·16 mg, nicotinic acid 0·5 mg, vitamin C 48 mg—per 100 g. (FAO.)

Spirits. *See* Alcoholic beverages *and* Proof spirit.

Spirit, Silent. Highly purified alcohol, or neutral spirit, distilled from any fermentable material.

Spirometer, or Respirometer. Apparatus used to determine energy produced by calculation from the oxygen consumed.

Spirulina. Blue-green alga which can make use of atmospheric nitrogen; eaten for centuries round Lake Chad in N. Africa and in Mexico. *See* Algae.

Spores. In relation to bacteria they are the resting state; thick-walled, highly resistant to damage by heat. Under suitable conditions they germinate to produce bacteria.

Not all bacteria can form spores; the so-called spore-bearers are a hazard in pasteurization and sterilization as the spores can remain undamaged in the processing and the material is consequently not sterile. (Baum.)

Sprat. *Sprattus sprattus (Clupea sprattus)* related to the herring; young is **brisling.**

Composition per 100 g (fried, weighed with head): 19·6 g protein, 33·4 g fat, 390 kcal (1·64 MJ), 620 mg calcium, 4 mg iron. (M&W.)

Spray Dryer. Equipment in which material to be dried is sprayed as a fine mist into a hot-air chamber and falls to the bottom as dry powder. Period of heating is very brief and so damage is avoided. Dried powder consists of hollow particles of low density. Widely applied to many foods (e.g. milk) and pharmaceuticals. (RJC.)

Spreading Factor. *See* Hyaluronidase.

Springers. *See* Swells.

Squalene. A hydrocarbon, $C_{30}H_{50}$, found in liver of shark and rat; suggested as a possible intermediate in the synthesis of cholesterol in the body.

Squash, Fruit. *See* Soft drinks.

Squash. *See* Gourds.

Stabilizers. (*See also* Emulsifying agents.) Substances that stabilize emulsions of fat and water, e.g. gums, agar, egg albumin, cellulose ethers; used to produce the texture of meringues and marshmallows, lecithin for crumb-softening in bread and confectionery, glyceryl monostearate and polyoxyethylene stearate for crumb-softening.

The legally permitted list includes also superglycerinated fats, propylene glycol alginate and stearate, methyl-, methylethyl-, and sodium carboxymethyl-celluloses, stearyl tartrate, sorbitan esters of fatty acids.

Bread may contain only super-glycerinated fats and stearyl tartrate.

Stachyase. Enzyme that hydro-lyses the tetrasaccharide stachyose to fructose and a mannosaccharide consisting of glucose and two mole-cules of galactose. Found in the digestive juices of crustaceans and molluscs.

Stachyose. A non-reducing tetra-saccharide composed of one unit of fructose, two of galactose and one of glucose. Hydrolysis yields fructose and manninotriose; be-lieved to be used to a limited extent by animals.

Present in many foods such as soya, beans, lupins, tubers of *Stachys tuberifera*, etc. Also called **mannotetrose** and **lupeose.**

Stackburn. Name given to heat retention within stack of cans when stored after sterilization without being cooled. A high temperature is maintained in the centre of the stack for long periods and causes deterioration of the contents and accelerates internal corrosion. (FM.)

Staling. As applied to baked pro-ducts such as bread, is thought to be due to the slow passage of water from the starch to other compon-ents of the bread. It is suggested that anti-staling agents (*see* Suc-rose esters) function by forming an insoluble coating round the starch granules, which slows down the passage of water. (KJ.)

St. Anthony's Fire. *See* Ergot.

Staphylococcal Poisoning. *See* Food poisoning.

Staple Food. The principal food, e.g. wheat, rice, maize, etc.

Starch. Complex polysaccharide composed of units of glucose; consists of about one quarter amylose and three-quarters amy-lopectin; the form in which car-bohydrate is stored in the plant and does not occur in animal tissue. (Glycogen is sometimes referred to as **animal starch.**)

All starches are broken down by acid hydrolysis, or during digestion, first to maltose and then glucose, but the various starches such as potato, maize, cereal, arrowroot, sago, etc., have different structures.

It is the principal carbohydrate of the diet and hence the major source of energy for man and animals. *See also* Amylopectin *and* Amylase. (BDS.)

Starch, Animal. *See* Glycogen.

Starch, Arum. From root of the arum lily; similar to sago.

Starch, Derivatized. *See* Starch, modified.

Starch Equivalent. A measure of the energy value of animal feedingstuffs; the number of parts of pure starch that would be equivalent to 100 parts of the ration as a source of energy.

Determined by direct feeding experiments or may be calculated from the formula: S.E. per 100 lb $=0.44 \times$ disgestible protein plus $2.41 \times$ digestible fat plus diges-tible carbohydrate plus fibre.

Protein has S.E. 0.94, crude fibre 1.0, ether extract of oilseeds 2.4. 1 lb starch equivalent has a net energy value of 1,071 kcal; 1 kg $\equiv 9.9$ MJ. (KJ, Abrams.)

Starches, Waxy. Those containing a high percentage of amylo-pectin; they do not form rigid gels when gelatinized but soft pastes. *See also* Maize, waxy. (Matz 2.)

Starch, Inhibited. *See* Starch, modified.

Starch, Modified. Starch altered by physical or chemical treatment to give special properties of value in food processing, e.g. change in gel strength, flow properties, colour, clarity, stability of the paste.

Acid-modified starch—acid treatment reduces the viscosity of the paste (used in sugar confectionery, e.g. gum drops, jelly beans.)

Oxidized starch—peroxide, permanganate, chlorine, etc., alter viscosity, clarity and stability of the paste (major use is outside the food industry).

Derivatized starch—chemical derivatives such as ethers and esters show properties such as reduced gelatinization in hot water and greater stability to acids and alkalies (**"inhibited" starch**)—useful where food has to withstand heat treatment as in canning or in acid foods. Further degrees of treatment can result in starch being unaffected by boiling water and losing its gel-forming properties.

See also Starch, pregelatinized. (Matz 2.)

Starch, Oxidized. *See* Starch, modified.

Starch, Pregelatinized. Raw starch does not form a paste with cold water and therefore requires cooking if it is to be used as a food thickening agent. Pregelatinized starch, mostly maize starch, has been cooked and dried.

Used in instant puddings, pie-fillings, soup mixes, salad dressings, sugar confectionery, as binder in meat products. Nutritional value the same as the original starch. (Matz 2.)

See also Starch, modified.

Starch Syrup. *See* Glucose Syrup.

Starter. Culture of bacteria used to inoculate or start growth in, e.g., milk for cheese production, or butter to develop the flavour, or any fermentation.

Steam Baking. In baking an even temperature is maintained in the oven by means of closed pipes through which steam circulates. This is sometimes erroneously believed to mean that the bread is baked in live steam.

Steaming. *See* Cooking.

Steapsin. Obsolete name for pancreatic lipase.

Stearic Acid. Long-chain fatty acid with a total of 18 carbon atoms (octadecanoic acid $CH_3(CH_2)_{16}COOH$); present in most animal and vegetable fats as the triglyceride. Used in pharmacy and cosmetics.

Steatorrhoea. Excess of fat in the stools. May be due to lack of bile, lack of lipase in the digestive juices, or defective absorption of fat. Treatment by feeding low-fat diet.

See also Coeliac disease.

Steer. Bull castrated when very young; if castrated after reaching maturity known as a stag.

Stercobilin. One of the brown pigments of the faeces; formed from the bile pigments, which, in turn, are formed as breakdown products of the haemoglobin of obsolete red blood cells. (BDS.)

Stereoisomerism. Occurs when compounds have the same molecular formula, and the same structural formula, but with the atoms arranged differently in space. There are two subdivisions, namely, optical isomerism (*see* Optical activity) and geometrical isomerism (*see* Cis-trans isomerism).

Sterile. Free from all micro-organisms—bacteria, moulds and yeasts.

When foods are sterilized, as in canning, they are preserved indefinitely as they are protected from recontamination in the can, and also from chemical and enzymic deterioration. (Baum.)

Sterilization, Cold. Applied to preservaion with sulphur dioxide, but more particularly to sterilization with radioactive materials. Very large doses of ionizing radiation are required to inhibit enzyme activity and the growth of micro-organisms, and some foods develop unpleasant flavours on such treatment. *See* Irradiation.

Sterilization, Radiation. *See* Irradiation.

Steroids. Compounds that contain the cyclopenteno-phenanthrene ring system

include vitamin D, male and female sex hormones, hormones of the adrenal cortex, sterols such as cholesterol, toad poisons, cardiac glycosides of the digitalis group, and some of the carcinogenic hydrocarbons.

The steroid alcohols, i.e. steroids carrying the —OH alcoholic grouping, are sterols. (BDS.)

Sterols. Alcohols derived from the steroids, *which see.* Include cho-lesterol, widely distributed in animal tissue including brain and egg yolk, coprosterol in faeces, ergosterol in yeast which is the precursor for the synthetic vitamin D_2, and sitosterol and stigmasterol in plants. (BDS.)

Stevioside. Naturally occurring, non-nutritive sweetening agent, 300 times as sweet as sucrose, thus the sweetest natural compound.

It is a glucoside of steviol, which has a steroid structure, and is present in the leaves of a Paraguayan shrub, *Stevia rebaudiana.*

Not accepted for use in foods.

Stewing. *See* Boiling.

Stickwater. The aqueous fraction from pressing cooked fish in the manufacture of fish meal. Contains amino acids, vitamins, and minerals and is added to animal feed or mixed back with the fish meal and dried.

Also known as fish solubles. (Tressler.)

Stilboestrol. Synthetic substance with potent activity as female sex hormone; widely used clinically and for food production (for chemical caponization of cockerels and to stimulate the growth of cattle).

Stiparogenic. Foods that tend to cause constipation.

Stiparolytic. Foods that tend to prevent or relieve constipation.

St. John's Bread. *See* Carob seed.

Stobb. Strawberry stalk.

Stockfish. Unsalted fish that has been dried naturally in air and sunshine; mostly prepared in Norway. Contains 12–15% water, and 1 lb is made from $4\frac{1}{2}$ lb of fresh fish.

Analysis after boiling, protein

211

32%, fat 0·9%, carbohydrate 0; kcal 140 (0·59 MJ), Ca 22 mg, Fe 1·8 mg—per 100 g.

Stock; Meat, Vegetable, Bone Stock. Liquid in which the meat or bone or vegetable, or a mixture of these, has been boiled until most of the water-soluble matter has been extracted.

Meat and bone contains collagen, which is converted into gelatin by prolonged boiling, hence the stock may set to a gel on cooling.

The main nutritive value of stock is the mineral content.

Storage, Gas. *See* Gas storage.

Stork Process. The name given to the process of ultra-high temperature sterilization of milk followed by sterilization again inside the bottle.

Stout. *See* Beer. So-called milk stout merely has added lactose (milk sugar).

Strandin. A substance isolated from brain tissue which dries in long strands; composed of fatty acid, sphingosine, carbohydrate and a small proportion of neuraminic acid.

Strawberry. Fruit of genus *Fragaria*. Protein 0·8%, fat 0·5%; kcal 35 (0·15 MJ), Ca 26 mg, Fe 0·8 mg; vitamin A 15 μg, B₁ 0·03 mg, B₂ 0·06 mg, nicotinic acid 0·3 mg, vitamin C 58 mg—per 100 g. (FAO.)

Strepogenin. Name given to a peptide-like fraction from natural sources, claimed to be essential for micro-organisms and higher animals. The need for special peptides for the latter has not been confirmed. (Sebrell.)

Streptococcal Poisoning. *See* Food poisoning.

Streptococcus Lactis Factor. A fermentation product of the mould *Rhizopus nigricans*, known as rhizopterin, which is essential to *S. lactis* R. Related to folic acid, *which see*.

Streptodornase. *See* Streptokinase.

Streptokinase. Proteolytic enzyme prepared from haemolytic streptococci. Used clinically to liquefy thick pus in empyemata and to remove the fibrin clot covering wounds. Streptodornase is a similar enzyme preparation that attacks pus cells.

Struvite. Small crystals of magnesium ammonium phosphate which occasionally form in canned fish—resemble broken glass. (Tressler.)

Substrate. In relation to enzymes refers to the substance on which the enzyme acts. Thus the substrate for the enzyme amylase is starch, which is hydrolysed to maltose.

Substrate can also mean the medium on which micro-organisms grow.

Subtilin. Antibiotic isolated from a strain of *B. subtilis* grown on a medium containing asparagine. Used as a food preservative (not permitted in Great Britain) as it reduces the thermal resistance of spores and is effective against thermophilic flat sours; thus subtilin permits a reduction in the processing time.

Sucaryl. Trade name (Abbott Laboratories) for sodium or calcium salt of cyclo hexyl sulphamate.

Succory. Another name for chicory.

Succotash. Stew of green maize and lima beans (butter beans), an American-Indian dish.

Succus Entericus. Intestinal juice, *which see*.

212

Suchar. Activated carbon, used to decolorize solutions.

Sucrase. *See* Invertase.

Sucrol. *See* Dulcin.

Sucron. Trade name (Accepted Foods Ltd.) for mixture of saccharine and sucrose, four times as sweet as sucrose alone.

Sucrose. Cane sugar or beet sugar. A disaccharide composed of a molecule of glucose linked to one of fructose; these two monosaccharides are formed by the hydrolysis of sucrose.

Crude brown sugar is 97% carbohydrate, and contains 1% water, 0·2% protein, 2 mg Fe, 0·02 mg vitamin B_1, 0·1 mg B_2, 0·3 mg nicotinic acid—per 100 g.

Refined white sugar is close to 100% pure and contains no minerals or vitamins. (BDS, Platt.)

Sucrose Distearate. *See* Sucrose esters.

Sucrose Esters. Di- and tri-laurates and mono- and di-stearates of sucrose. Used as emulsifiers, wetting agents and surface active agents, e.g. for washing fruits and vegetables, as anti-spattering agents, anti-foam agents and anti-staling or crumb-softening agents.

Sucrose Intolerance. *See* Disaccharide Intolerance.

Sucrose Mono Stearate. *See* Sucrose esters.

Suet. Fat prepared from the kidneys of oxen and sheep. (Hilditch.)

Sugar. Usually refers to sucrose or table sugar obtained from the sugar cane or sugar beet. May also refer to any of the sugars such as milk sugar (lactose) fruit sugar (fructose), grape sugar (glucose), malt sugar (maltose). The simplest carbohydrates are classified as sugars, subdivided into monosaccharides, disaccharides and polysaccharides.

Sugar Beet. *Beta vulgaris* subsp. *cicla,* the most important source of sugar (sucrose) in temperate countries; contains 15–20% sugar; biennial related to the garden beetroot but with white, conical roots. (OF.)

Sugar Cane. The plant, *Saccharum officinarum,* from the juice of which sugar is prepared.

Sugar, Caster. Ordinary sugar (sucrose) crystallized in small crystals.

Sugar Doctor. To prevent the crystallization or "graining" of sugar in sugar confectionery, a substance called the sugar doctor or candy doctor is added. This may be a weak acid, such as cream of tartar, which "inverts" part of the cane sugar during the boiling, or invert sugar or starch syrup. (Jacobs.)

Sugar Esters. *See* Sucrose esters.

Sugar, Icing. Powdered sucrose.

Sugaring—of Dried Fruits. A type of deterioration of dried fruit on storage, most frequently on prunes and figs. A sugary substance appears on the surface or under the skin, consisting of glucose and fructose with traces of citric and malic acids, lysine, asparagine and aspartic acid.

When occurring under the skin of prunes it is called "red sugar".

Sugar Maple. *Acer saccharum;* the sap is evaporated down to a syrup, maple syrup, and crystallized to sucrose, maple sugar. (OF.)

Sugar Palm. *Arenga saccharifera,* grows wild in Malaysia and Indonesia; sugar (sucrose) is obtained from the sap. (OF.)

213

Sugar Tolerance. *See* Glucose tolerance.

Sulpha Drugs. Group of synthetic drugs derived from sulphanilamide (or aminobenzenesulphonamide) used to combat bacterial infection.

Sulphanilamide itself functions as an antivitamin to bacteria, as it inhibits the uptake of para-amino benzoic acid, an essential nutrient. These drugs include sulphapyridine, sulphadiazine, sulphathiazole, etc. (Hawk.)

Sulphate. The mineral sulphur occurs in foods and in the body in two main forms, (1) as sulphate—salts of sulphuric acid, and (2) in the amino acids methionine and cystine. *See* Sulphur.

Sulphite, Fixed. A term used when referring to sulphite as a preservative. Sulphites can combine with aldehydes, ketones, simple sugars, and possibly other food constituents, and such combined or fixed sulphite has no preservative action, only the undissociated acid is effective.

Sulphur. An element that is part of the amino acids cystine and methionine and is therefore present in all proteins. It is also part of the molecules of vitamin B_1 and biotin.

Apart from its presence as part of these compounds there appears to be no dietary need for sulphur in any other form and no deficiency has ever been observed, although it is essential for plants.

The old-fashioned remedy of sulphur and molasses was not only quite unnecessary but elemental sulphur is probably not used by the body. (Gil.)

Sulphur Amino Acids. Two amino acids, cystine and methionine, contain sulphur. As they are partly interchangeable they are classed together as the sulphur amino acids.

(Cysteine is of less importance.)

Sulphur Dioxide. Used in solution (as sulphurous acid) as a preservative, for sausage meat, liquid glucose, fruit, fruit pulp and juices, etc. One major advantage is that it is driven off by boiling.

Campden tablets used for domestic preservation are sodium sulphite, which liberates SO_2 in the presence of the fruit acid. Permitted limits: jam 40 ppm; fruit pulp 1,000–1,500 ppm; fruit cordial 350 ppm.

Stabilizes vitamin C but damages vitamin B_1.

Sulphuring. Preservation by sulphur dioxide.

Sulphur in Urine. Three groups of sulphur compounds are excreted, inorganic sulphates (sodium, potassium, calcium, magnesium and ammonium), organic sulphates (sulphuric esters of phenolic compounds), neutral sulphur (thiosulphates, thiocyanates, mercapturic acids, urochrome). (Hawk.)

Sultanas. Made by drying the golden sultana grapes (Turkey, Greece, Australia, and S. Africa); the bunches are dipped in alkali, washed, sulphured and dried. Sultanas of the European type produced in the U.S.A. are termed seedless raisins.

For analysis *see* Fruit, dried; *see also* Raisins, Muscatels *and* Currants.

Sunflower. *Helianthus annuus.* Seed used as source of edible oil, rich in polyunsaturated fatty acids; residual oilcake used for animal feed. Seeds also eaten raw.

Composition per 100 g: 27 g protein, 36 g fat, 23 g carbohydrate, 540 kcal (2·2 MJ), 100 mg calcium, 7 mg iron, 1·9 mg B_1, 0·2 mg B_2, 5·8 mg nicotinic acid. (OF, Platt.)

Sunlight Flavour. Name given to unpleasant flavours developing in foods after exposure to sunlight. In milk it is said to be due to the breakdown of methionine in the presence of vitamin B_2; in beer due to a change in the bitter principles from the hops.

Superglycinerated Fats. Normal fats are triglycerides, i.e. three molecules of fatty acid to each molecule of glycerol. Mono and diglycerides are known as superglycerinated.

Glyceryl monostearate (GMS) is solid at room temperature, flexible and non-greasy; used as a protective coating for foods, as plasticizer for softening the crumb of bread, to reduce spattering in frying fats, as emulsifier and stabilizer.

Glyceryl mono-oleate (GMO) is semi-liquid at room temperature.

Suprarenal Glands. *See* Adrenal glands.

Supro. Protein-rich baby food (24% protein) made in East Africa from maize or barley flour with torula yeast, skim-milk powder and flavouring.

Surface Area. Heat loss from the body, and therefore basal metabolism, is related to surface area. Calculated by formula of Du Bois or Meeh.

Du Bois: Area (sq. cm.) = weight (kg) to power of 0·425 × height (cm) to power of 0·725 × 71·84.

Meeh: Area = 11·9 × weight to power of 2/3. (BDS.)

Surfactants. Basically the same as emulsifiers, i.e. substances that lower the surface tension. When this effect occurs between two liquids or between a liquid and a solid the surfactant aids emulsification and wetting of powders. Examples are mono and diglycerides, polyethylene derivatives, pectins, alginates, gums, gelatin, lecithin.

Also retard hardening rate of jellies, and reduce stickiness of caramels.

Suspensoids. *See* Colloids, lyophobic.

Sustagen. U.S. trade name (Mead Johnson Laboratories) of food concentrate in powder form, also usable for tube feeding; mixture of whole and skim milk, casein, maltose, dextrins and glucose.

Protein 24%, fat 8%, carbohydrate 68%; vitamins A, B_1, B_2, nicotinic acid, C, D, E, B_{12}, calcium pantothenate, pyridoxine plus choline, calcium and iron.

Sweat. Solution of salt (about 0·3%), urea 0·03%, lactate 0·07%. Varies in composition but hypotonic to blood plasma. (BDS.)

Swede. Root of *Brassica rutabaga* or Swedish turnip. Protein 1·1%, fat trace, carbohydrate 4·3%; kcal 21 (0·09 MJ), Ca 56 mg, Fe 0·4 mg, vitamin A 3 μg, B_1 0·5 mg, B_2 0·04 mg, nicotinic acid 0·8 mg, vitamin C 28 mg—per 100 g. (M&W, FAO.)

Sweetbread. *See* Pancreas.

Sweeteners, Non-Nutritive. Refers to sweetening agents which are not sugars and have no food value, such as saccharin and cyclamate. (AEB.)

215

Sweetening Agents. Three groups: (1) the sugars of which the commonest is sucrose. Fructose has 173% of the sweetness of sucrose, glucose, 74%, maltose, 33% and lactose, 16%; (2) synthetic non-nutritive sweeteners such as saccharine (550 times as sweet as sucrose), dulcin (250 times), sucaryl (30 times), P4000 (4,000 times)—*see under* individual headings. (3) various other chemicals such as glycerol and glycine (70% as sweet as sucrose), and certain peptides.

Sweetex. Trade name (Boots Ltd.) for saccharine.

Sweet sop. *See* Custard Apple.

Swells. Applied to infected canned foods when gases produced by fermentation inside the can cause the ends to swell.

A "hard swell" has permanently extended ends. If the ends can be moved under pressure, but not forced back to the original position, they are "soft swells". "Springers" can be forced back, but the opposite end bulges.

A "flipper" is a can of normal appearance in which the end flips out when the can is struck.

Hydrogen swells are harmless, and due to acid fruits attacking the can. (Baum.)

Swift Stability Test. *See* Active oxygen method.

Syllabub. Also sillabub. Elizabethan dish made of milk or cream, mixed with wine or brandy, sweetened and whipped. (GH.)

Syneresis. Oozing of liquid from a gel when cut and allowed to stand (e.g. jelly or baked custard).

Synsepalum. *See* Miracle Berry.

Synthalin. Decamethylene-diguanidine; lowers blood sugar and used experimentally in the treatment of diabetes, but is toxic.

Syntonin. Old name given to degradation products of proteins.

Syrup. A solution of sugar which may be from a variety of sources such as maple, corn, sorghum, and stages in refining such as top syrup, refiners syrup and sugar syrup.

The product of refining called golden syrup is 20% water, sugar 79%, protein 0·3%, fat nil; kcal 297 (1·25 MJ), Fe 1·5 mg— per 100 g; vitamins present only in traces.

The sugar solutions used for canning fruit are also syrups; light syrup—15° Brix, syrup— 20 or 30° Brix, heavy syrup—30 or 40° Brix, extra heavy syrup— 40 or 50° Brix. (Degrees Brix=per cent sugar.) (Jacobs.)

Syrup, Corn. *See* Glucose syrup.

T

Tachycardia. Rapid heart-beat; a symptom, among other causes, of certain vitamin deficiencies.

Tachyphagia. Rapid eating.

Tachyphylaxis. Decreased effects on repeated injections of a substance.

Tachysterol. One of the compounds produced (along with vitamin D_2 or calciferol) by ultraviolet irradiation of ergosterol. It has no anti-rachitic activity until it has been reduced to dihydrotachysterol, also called AT-10.

AT-10 is also used for the treatment of deficient thyroid function.

Taette. *See* Milks, fermented.

Tafia. Spirit similar to rum made from sugar cane.

Takadiastase. Or Koji, an enzyme preparation produced by growing the fungus, *Aspergillus oryzae,* on bran, leaching the culture mass with water and precipitating with alcohol.

Contains a mixture of enzymes, largely diastatic; used for the preparation of starch hydrolysates.

Tallow, Rendered. Beef or mutton fat prepared from parts other than the kidney, by heating with water in an autoclave; used for soap and candles. When pressed separates to a liquid fraction, oleo oil, used in margarine, and a solid fraction, oleostearin, used for soap and candles. (Hilditch.)

Tallow, Solid. *See* Premier jus.

Tamales. Mixture of meat, spices and maize meal wrapped in corn husks or special paper. (Loes.)

Tamarind. Leguminous tree, *Tamarindus indica,* with pods containing seeds embedded in brown pulp, eaten fresh and used in seasonings and curries.

Composition per 100 g: 2 g protein, 74 g carbohydrate, 2 g fibre, 300 kcal (1·25 MJ), 3 mg iron, 0·4 mg vitamin B_1, 0·15 mg B_2, 1·5 mg nicotinic acid, 10 mg C. (Platt.)

Tammy. A cookery term meaning to strain through a fine woollen cloth—a tammy cloth.

Tangelo. Cross between tangerine and grapefruit.

Tankage. Ground, dried residue from slaughter house excluding all the useful tissues.

Tannia (also tanier). Corm of *Xanthosoma sagittifolium*; known as **new cocoyam** in W. Africa and as **yautia**: same family as taro.

Composition per 100 g: 2 g protein, 0·3 g fat, 31 g carbohydrate, 133 kcal (0·56 MJ), 1 mg iron, 0·1 mg B_1, 0·03 mg B_2, 0·5 mg nicotinic acid, 10 mg C. (OF, Platt.)

Tannins. Complex phenolic compounds (including several hydroxy groups) found in cell sap of many plants and responsible for the astringent taste of some foods, e.g. in tea, coffee, cocoa, nuts, apples, pears. (Griswold.)

Tansy. *Tanacetum vulgare.* Leaves and young shoots used for flavouring puddings and ómelettes. Tansy cakes made with eggs and young leaves used to be eaten at Easter. Tansy tea made by infusing the herb formerly used as tonic and for intestinal worms. Root, preserved in honey or sugar, was used for gout. (OF.)

Tapioca. Starch prepared from the root of the cassava plant. The starch paste is heated to burst the granules then dried either in globules resembling sago or in flakes. The term is also used of starch in general as in manioc tapioca and potato flour tapioca.

Tapioca-macaroni. A mixture of 80–90 parts tapioca flour, with 10–12 parts of peanut flour, or tapioca, peanut, semolina, 60:15:25, baked into shapes resembling rice grains or macaroni shapes; developed in India. Also referred to as **synthetic rice.**

Tares. Traditional English name

217

for the vetches, which are pulses, *which see*.

Taro. Corm of *Colocasia esculenta* and *C. antiquorum;* called **eddo** or **dasheen** in W. Indies, **old cocoyam** in W. Africa.

Composition per 100 g: 2 g protein, 26 g carbohydrate, 113 kcal (0·48 MJ), 1 mg iron, 0·1 mg B_1, 0·03 mg B_2, 1 mg nicotinic acid, 5 mg C. (OF, Platt.)

Tarragon. Dried leaves and flowering tops of the bushy perennial plant, *Artemisia dracunculus*. Has an anise-like flavour and is used to flavour vinegar, and pickles, and is one of the ingredients of *fines herbes*.

Tarragon vinegar is made by steeping the fresh herb in white wine vinegar and is used in making sauce tartare and French mustard.

Tartar. Name given by the alchemists to animal and vegetable concretions, such as wine lees, stone, gravel and deposits on teeth, as they were all attributed to the same cause.

Tartar Emetic. Potassium antimonyl tartrate, produces inflammation of the gastro-intestinal mucosa and used to be used as an emetic. (Clark.)

Tartaric Acid. A dibasic acid, dihydroxysuccinic COOH.CHOH. CHOH.COOH. Occurs in fruits, the chief source is grapes; used in preparing lemonade, added to jams when the fruit is not sufficiently acidic (citric acid also used) and in baking powder.

Tartar emetic is the potassium antimonyl salt, and **Rochelle salt** is potassium sodium tartrate. *See also* Argol *and* Cream of tartar. (Cohen.)

Tartazine. Yellow colour permitted in food in most countries; trisodium salt of 5-hydroxy-1-p-sulphophenyl- 4-p-sulphophenyl-azopyrazole-3-carboxylic acid; called Yellow No. 5 in U.S.A.

Tartronate. Salt of tartronic (or hydroxymalonic) acid. Suggested as coenzyme in the decarboxylation of oxalo succinic acid in the citric acid cycle and also claimed as a dietary essential for the rat but not confirmed. (Cohen.)

Taste. *See* Organoleptic.

Taste Buds. Situated mostly on the tongue; about 9,000 elongated cells ending in minute hairlike processes, the gustatory hairs. (Merory.)

Taurocholic Acid. *See* Bile.

Tea. Introduced into England 1659. Prepared from the tender leaves, leaf buds and tender internodes of different varieties of *Thea sinensis*.

Black tea—leaves fermented (actually an oxidation) before drying.

Green tea — (unfermented) steamed and dried only; light in colour, more tannin than black tea.

Oolong tea—fermented only slightly; intermediate between the first two.

Of the black teas, Flowering Pekoes are made from the top leaf buds, Orange Pekoe from the first opened leaf, Pekoe from the third leaves, and Souchong from the next leaves. World consumption of coffee (1957) 2·7 million tons, tea 0·9 m tons, but as 1 lb of tea makes about four times the amount of beverage as coffee, more tea is drunk than is coffee. U.K. consumes ⅓ of total world tea consumption.

The infusion made from 100 g of tea contain 0·9 mg vitamin B2 and 6 mg nicotinic acid.

Tea, Black. *See* Tea.

Tea, Green. *See* Tea.

Teaseed Oil. Oil from the seed of *Thea sasangua*, cultivated in China; used as salad oil and for frying; similar in properties to olive oil.

Teeth, Mottled. *See* Mottled teeth.

Teff. Millet-like cereal grain; major protein of the diet of Ethiopia. *See* Millet.

Teg. Two-year-old sheep.

Tempeh. Soya bean fermented by a fungus; eaten in Indonesia.

Temptein. Trade name (Miles Lab. U.S.A.) for textured vegetable protein.

Tenderizer. Usually refers to the enzyme papain, when used to tenderize meat. Weak acids such as vinegar and lemon juice and 2% sodium chloride also tenderize meat. (Meat.)

Tenderometer. Instrument to measure the stage of maturity of peas to determine if they are ready for canning. Measures the force required to effect a shearing action.

Tenuate. *See* Anorectic drugs.

Tequila. Distilled liquor obtained from a fermented mash made from the cultivated cactus *Agave tequilana*; 90–100 degrees proof; common in Mexico.

Mescal is similar but made from the mescal Agave, which grows wild, and is much cheaper. (Jacobs.)

Terpeneless Oil. *See* Terpenes.

Terpenes. Components of the essential oils of citrus fruits; hydrocarbons of the general formula $C_{10}H_{16}$; also sesquiterpenes $C_{15}H_{24}$. Include limonene, alpha, beta, and gamma terpinene, alpha and beta phellandrene. Limonene is 90% of oil of orange.

Although terpenes constitute 90–95% of citrus oils they are not responsible for the characteristic flavour, and as they readily oxidize and polymerize to produce unpleasant flavours they are removed from citrus oils by distillation or solvent extraction leaving the so-called **terpeneless oils.** Further, the terpenes are not very soluble so that unless they are removed the oils cannot be used for flavouring beverages and clear jellies. (Brav.)

Terramycin. Antibiotic isolated 1950 from *Streptomyces rimosus*. Now known as oxytetracycline. *See* Tetracyclines.

Testa. In reference to cereal grains the test is a fibrous layer between the pericarp and the inner aleurone layer. (KJ.)

Test Meal. *See* Fractional test meal.

Tetany. Oversensitivity of motor nerves to stimuli, particularly affects face, hands and feet. Caused by reduction in the level of ionized calcium in the bloodstream and can accompany severe rickets. (DP.)

Tetracyclines. Group of closely related antibiotics, tetracycline, oxytetracycline (terramycin) and chlortetracycline (aureomycin). The last two are used in some countries for preserving food and, when added to animal feed at the rate of a few mg per ton, improve growth.

Of special use for eviscerated poultry; the bird is dipped in solution of 10 ppm, and, when stored at 34–37°F, shelf life is extended from 10–14 to 17–21 days. 2 ppm left in the poultry, much reduced on cooking.

Also of great value in extending the storage life of fresh fish by 2–3 days, by adding 5 ppm antibiotic to the ice or chilled water, or by dipping fillets into water containing 5–20 ppm. (Bell.)

Tetraenoic Acid. An acid with four double bonds, such as the essential fatty acid, arachidonic acid.

Tetraodontin poisoning. Caused by fish of *Tetraodontidae* family (puffer fish) and amphibia of *Salamandridae* family due to toxins in the entrails (Japan).

Tetra Pack. Tetrahedral cartons used to pack milk and other beverages. Used widely in U.S.A. where milk sold in self-service stores, but more expensive than re-usable glass bottles.

Tewfikose. A sugar once claimed as distinct from lactose obtained from the milk of the Egyptian buffalo. (Davis & Mac.)

Texgran. Trade name (Swift Edible Oil Co., U.S.A.) for textured vegetable protein. (FM.)

Texatrein. Trade name (Cargill, Inc., U.S.A.) for textured vegetable protein made by extrusion.

Texture. A physical quality of food determined principally by the feel in the mouth, excluding temperature and taste. Texture includes roughness, smoothness, graininess, chewiness, succulence, grittiness, and is a resultant of density, viscosity, surface tension, etc.

Some discussions of texture include visual appearance and in evaluating bakery products tactile methods are included. (Matz.)

Textured Vegetable Protein. Spun or extruded vegetable protein made to simulate meat. (FM.)

Theine. Alternative name for caffeine.

Thaumatin. See Katemfe.

Therapeutic Diets. Those formulated to treat disease or metabolic disorders. (AEB.)

Thermization. Heat treatment, less severe than pasteurization, e.g. heat treatment of milk for cheese-making whereby the number of organisms is diminished.

Thermoduric. Bacteria that are heat resistant but not thermophilic. Found in milk. They survive pasteurization temperatures but do not develop at them. Usually not pathogens but indicative of insanitary conditions. (Tanner.)

Thermopeeling. A method of peeling tough-skinned fruits in which the fruit is rapidly passed through an electric furnace at about 900°C then sprayed with water.

Thermophiles. Bacteria that prefer temperatures of 55°C (131°F) and above; can tolerate temperatures up to 75–80°C (167–176°F). Some strains reported to survive boiling 24 hours at pH 6·1.

Include the "flat sours" that produce acids from carbohydrates but no gas (*Bacillus stearothermophilus*), anaerobes not producing H_2S (*Clostridium thermosaccharolyticum*), and anaerobes producing H_2S (*Clostridium nigrificans*).

Thermophilic bacteria are responsible for spontaneous combustion in hay stacks. (Baum.)

Thiamin. Vitamin B_1.

Thiaminase. An enzyme present in many species of fish that hydrolyses thiamin and can therefore cause vitamin B_1 deficiency. *See* Chastek's paralysis.

Thiochrome. Compound to which vitamin B_1 can be oxidized (for example, by potassium ferricyanide) and which gives a strong blue fluorescence in ultra-violet light. This is used as an assay of the vitamin.

Thioctic Acid. Lipoic acid (1-2-dithiolane-3-valeric acid).

Thiopanic Acid. *See* Pantoyltaurine.

Thirst. *See* Water balance.

Threonine. An essential amino acid; the latest of the amino acids to be discovered, 1935; amino hydroxybutyric acid. (BDS.)

Thrombin. Plasma protein involved in coagulation of the blood, *which see*.

Thrombokinase. Or thromboplastin. Liberated from damaged tissue and blood platelets; converts prothrombin to thrombin in the coagulation of the blood, *which see*.

Thromboplastin. Or Thrombokinase. *See* Coagulation, blood.

Thunberg Tube. A test-tube carrying a curved hollow stopper that is used to hold one of the reactants; the whole tube can be evacuated through a side-arm. It is used to study oxidation reactions where it is necessary to keep the reactants separate until the oxygen has been removed from the system. (Hawk.)

Thuricide. Name given to a living culture of *Bacillus thuringiensis* which is harmless to man but kills off insect pests. Known as a microbial insecticide. Used to treat certain foods and fodder crops to destroy pests such as corn earworm, flour moth, tomato fruit worm, cabbage looper, etc. The bacillus is mass-produced and stored like a chemical.

Thyme. Dried leaves and flavouring tops of *Thymus vulgaris* used in sausage and as flavouring in soup, meat, fish and poultry dressing.

Thymine. *See* Pyrimidines *and* Nucleic Acid.

Thymonucleic Acid. Alternative name for deoxyribonucleic acid. *See* Nucleic acid.

Thyroglobulin. The protein-bound form in which thyroxine and triiodothyronine exist in the thyroid gland; it is broken down under the influence of the thyroid-stimulating hormone of the pituitary gland to liberate the free hormones which pass into the blood stream. Here they travel in combination with plasma protein as the so-called **protein-bound iodine** (PBI). The concentration of PBI in the blood is thus an index of thyroid activity. (BDS.)

Thyroid Gland. Endocrine gland situated in the neck; secretes four hormones, thyroxine (most abundant), diiodothyronine and two triiodothyronines.

Controls the basal metabolism of the body; when deficient (hypothyroidism) the metabolism is slowed down, when the activity of the gland is excessive (hyperthyroidism) there is an increased

221

metabolic rate. Hence the use of thyroid extract as an aid to slimming.

Cretinism is a thyroid deficiency starting in childhood. A deficiency of iodine in the diet causes hyperplasia of the thyroid gland which is **goitre** (*which see*). (BDS.)

Thyroxine. Hydroxyphenyl-tetra-iodotyrosine; hormone from the thyroid gland (*which see*), converted into the more active tri-iodothyronine in the tissues. (BDS.)

Tin. Of no known biological function. Its resistance to corrosion in the absence of oxygen permits its use as a lining to steel cans. Corrosion of tinned cans takes place through pinholes in the tin lining. (GMW.)

Tintometer. Instrument for measuring depth and shade of colour visually by comparison with a range of coloured glass slides. The Lovibond Tintometer is the best known.

Used for the chemical determination of substances that can be converted to coloured compounds, e.g. many minerals and vitamins.

Tisane. French term for a medicinal tea or infusion made from herbs (camomile, lime blossoms, fennel seeds, etc.).

Tobasco Sauce. Tobasco peppers are macerated, fermented and left to cure for periods up to three years, then bottled with vinegar. (Loes.)

Tocol. *See* Vitamin E.

Tocopherol. *See* Vitamin E.

Tocopheronic Acid. A water-soluble degradation product of alpha-tocopherol (vitamin E) isolated from the urine of animals fed tocopherol, together with tocopheronolactone, the lactone of tocopheronic acid, which is highly vitamin-E active.

Tocopheronic acid is 2-(3-hydroxy - 3 - methyl - 5 - carboxyl) - pentyl, 3, 5, 6-trimethyl benzoquinone.

Tocotrienol. *See* Vitamin E.

Toffee. A sweetmeat that is essentially a dispersion of minute globules of fat in a supersaturated sugar solution; made from fat, milk, sugar and confectioners' glucose. No real distinction between toffees and caramels except that toffees are boiled at a slightly higher temperature, 260–270°C compared with 250–255°C for caramels. Composition: water 4·8%, sugars 70%, protein 2%, fat 17%, kcal 435 (1·83 MJ), Ca 95 mg, Fe 1·5 mg. (M&W.)

Tofu. A Japanese product, soy bean curd. Contains 5–8% protein, 3–4% fat, 2–4% carbohydrate and 84–90% water.

Tomatine. An antifungal substance isolated from wilt-resistant tomatoes.

Tomato. Fruit of *Lycopersicon esculentum*. Protein 1·1%, fat 0·3%; kcal 19 (0·08 MJ), Ca 11 mg, Fe 0·6 mg, vitamin A 200 μg, B_1 0·06 mg, B_2 0·04 mg, nicotinic acid 0·5 mg, vitamin C 23 mg— per 100 g. (FAO.)

Tomato Ketchup, Catsup, Catchup or Sauce. Preparation of tomato purée, sugar, vinegar, salt and spices.

Legally in U.K. must contain not less than 6% by weight of tomato solids excluding seeds and other coarse substances. No fruit other than tomato may be used except onion, garlic and spices.

"Ketchup" or "catsup" derived from Chinese "koechiap" or "kitsiap" which is the brine of pickled fish, and now applied to a thick sauce made from pulp of fruits such as tomato or green walnuts.

Topfer's Reagent. Dimethylaminoazobenzene; an indicator with a pH range $2 \cdot 9$–$4 \cdot 0$, changing red to yellow. Often used in titration of the acidity of gastric contents as it changes colour only in the presence of free hydrochloric acid. (Hawk.)

Toppings. *See* Wheatfeed.

Torry Kiln. Machine developed by the Fisheries Research Station at Torry (U.K.) for the controlled smoking of fish. (FM.)

Tortillas. Eaten in Central America. Flat circular cakes made from whole maize that has been soaked in water containing lime, boiled, ground and cooked. The lime appears to add considerable amounts of calcium to the diet.

Torula. *See* Yeast.

Torularhodin. Carotenoid pigment in red yeast, *Torula rubra*, with vitamin A activity.

Torulin. Antibiotic produced during aerobic culture of *Torula utilis*.

Tous-les-mois. Queensland arrowroot, used as a source of starch.

Toxins. Generally means poisons produced by bacteria. They are antigenic and stimulate the body tissues to produce specific neutralizing substances (antibodies).

Exotoxins are liberated by bacteria, are unstable to heat, e.g. destroyed by heating at 60°C for 1 hour, and include toxins responsible for botulism, tetanus and diptheria.

Endotoxins, inside the cell, more stable to heat. (Baum.)

TPN. Triphosphopyridine nucleotide. *See* Nicotinamide adenine dinucleotide.

Trace Elements. Refers to mineral salts needed by the body in very small amounts—iodine, copper, manganese, magnesium, cobalt and zinc—as distinct from those required in relatively large amounts, such as sodium, potassium, calcium, phosphorus, sulphur and chlorine.

Of these trace elements only iodine is of importance in the diet as the others are almost always in adequate supply. This is not true of domestic animals amongst which various mineral deficiencies occur in certain areas.

Sixty minerals have been identified in plants, of which about one third have been shown to be essential to plant or animal nutrition. (Gilbert, GMW.)

Tragacanth. A gum obtained from shrubs of the genus *Astragalus*. Used as emulsifying agent in pharmaceutical preparations and as a thickener. (Jacobs.)

Trans-. *See* Cis-trans isomerism.

Transamination. Transfer of the amino group, —NH_2, from one compound to another, usually under the influence of an enzyme, transaminase. Thus glutamic acid under the influence of glutamic-alanine-transaminase conveys its amino group to pyruvic acid to form alanine, leaving keto-glutaric acid.

The prosthetic group of the enzyme is pyridoxal, vitamin B_6, which acts as an intermediate amino carrier. (WHSS.)

Transferrin. Or siderophilin, an iron-carbonate-protein complex, the form in which iron is transported in the blood plasma.

Trepang. Bêche-de-mer.

Tricarboxylic Acid Cycle. See Citric acid cycle.

Trichinosis (Trichiniasis). Disease due to infection with *Trichinella spiralis*, a worm that is a parasite in pork muscle. Destroyed by heat and by freezing. The infection is caused by eating undercooked pork or sausage meat. (Tanner.)

Triglycerides. See Glycerides.

Trigonelline. The betaine of nicotinic acid, the form in which nicotinic acid is excreted in the urine; formula $C_7H_7NO_2$; has no vitamin activity.

Also found in seeds of Fenugreek and in coffee.

Triiodothyronine. The active hormone of the thyroid gland into which thyroxine is converted in the tissues. It is synthesized in the body from the amino acid tyrosine and iodine. See Thyroid gland *and* Thyroglobulin. (BDS.)

Triotin. Unidentified urinary excretion product of biotin, together with miotin and rhiotin. (Sebrell.)

Tripe. Lining of the stomach of ruminant; usually the ox. There are various kinds such as blanket, honeycomb, book, monk's hood and reed according to which part of the stomach is used. Contains a large amount of connective tissue which is converted into gelatin on prolonged boiling.

Water 75%, protein 16%, fat 8·5% (Hutch.)

Tripeptide. See Polypeptide.

Triphosphopyridine Nucleotide. See Nicotinamide adenine dinucleotide phosphate.

Triticale. Cross between wheat and rye; under investigation as a potential crop; some lines rich in protein.

Tritium. See Hydrogen, heavy.

Truffle. Edible fungus that grows underground; the best varieties are found in France and Italy although some are found in Gt. Britain.

Black or Perigord truffle (*Tuber melanospermum*) and white truffle (*T. album* and *T. niveum*) which is held in lower regard. They contain about 75% water, 9% protein and 0·3% fat. Used as a savoury and for garnishing. (GH.)

Trusoy. Trade name (British Soya Products Ltd.) for full fat soya flour, heat-treated.

Trypsin. Proteolytic enzyme of the pancreatic juice that attacks parts of the protein molecule left unattacked by pepsin. Functions at alkaline pH, 8–11. Secreted as the inactive precursor, trypsinogen, liberated by enterokinase. (BDS.)

Tryptophan. Essential amino acid; rarely, if ever, limiting in any food. Chemically amino indole propionic acid. (BDS.)

TSP. Trade name (Spillers Ltd.) for textured soya protein in extruded form.

Tuberin. The protein of potato, a globulin.

Tuber. Underground storage organ of some plants, for example potato, Jerusalem artichoke, sweet potato, yam.

Tun. A vat containing 210 imperial gallons.

224

Tuna or Tunny. Fatty fish, species of *Thunnus* and *Neothunnus*. Also name for prickly pear.

Turbidity Test for Milk. *See* Milk, turbidity test.

Turkey X Disease. *See* Aflatoxins.

Turmeric. Dried rhizome of *Curcuma longa* (ginger family), grown in India and Southern Asia. Deep yellow and used both as condiment and (permitted) dye-stuff. Used in curry powder and in prepared mustard.

Its pigment is used as a dye under the name **curcumin.** (Jacobs, Merory.)

Turnip. Root of *Brassica campestris*. Protein 0·8%, fat trace, carbohydrate 3·8%; kcal 18 (0·8 MJ), Ca 59 mg, Fe 0·4 mg, vitamin A 10 i.u., B_1 0·05 mg, B_2 0·04 mg, nicotinic acid 0·8 mg, vitamin C 28 mg—per 100 g. (M&W, FAO.)

Tuxford's Index. A formula for relating height to weight in children; heavier than average have an index greater than 1, lighter, have an index below 1.

For boys $\dfrac{W}{H} \times \dfrac{336 - m}{270}$

For girls $\dfrac{W}{H} \times \dfrac{308 - m}{235}$

W is weight in pounds, H is height in inches, m is age in months. (DP.)

TVP. Textured Vegetable Protein.

Twaddell. Scale for measurement of density.

1% salt—1·4° Twaddell—1·007 sp. gr.

2% salt—2·8° Twaddell—1·014 sp. gr.

4% salt—5·6° Twaddell—1·028 sp. gr.

10% salt—14·6° Twaddell—1·073 sp. gr.

20% salt—30·2° Twaddell—1·151 sp. gr.

Only used for densities greater than 1; density $= 1 + \dfrac{\text{degrees}}{200}$ ·(FM.)

Tweens. Trade name (Atlas Co.) of a group of compounds formed by reaction between a sorbitan ester of a fatty acid and ethylene oxide; they are surface active or emulsifying agents. *See also* Spans *and* Polyoxyethylene monostearate.

Tyrosinase. Enzyme that oxidizes tyrosine and other phenolic compounds with the ultimate production of brown and black pigments. Absent in albinos, and from the white areas of piebald animals.

It is present in the potato and is responsible for the dark colour produced when raw potatoes or the juice are allowed to autoxidize in air. (BDS, B. & R.)

Tyrosine. A non-essential amino acid that has some sparing action on the essential amino acid phenylalanine. Very little soluble and crystallizes out of solutions of protein hydrolysates.

Tyrosine is the starting material for the formation of melanin, the pigment in the hair and skin, increased after sunburn. Chemically amino hydroxyphenyl propionic acid. (BDS.)

Tyrosinosis. Inborn error of metabolism in which the administration of the amino acid phenylalanine results in the excretion of tyrosine. (BDS.)

U

Ubi-chromenol. Cyclized form of ubiquinone, *which see*.

Ubiquinone. General name given to a group of pigments widely distributed in nature, and first found in the livers of rats deficient in vitamin A.

Not a dietary essential: chemically a derivative of benzoquinone with polyisoprene side chains which differ in length and are distinguished by the number of carbons in the chain, e.g. ubiquinone 50, 45, etc.

Identical with Coenzyme Q.

U.F.A. *See* Non-esterified fatty acids.

Ugli. Citrus fruit, cross between grapefruit and tangerine.

U.H.T.S. Ultra high temperature sterilization, *which see*.

Ullage. Liquid left in cask or bottle after some has been removed or lost through defective container.

Ultracentrifuge. Centrifuge operating at very high speeds; will separate particles of different size in a colloidal suspension. Used to separate the different fractions of cells.

Ultra-centrifuged milk has been treated for a few seconds at 15,000–16,000 revs. per min. when spore-forming bacteria are sedimented.

Ultra High Temperature Sterilization. Treatment of milk at a very high temperature but for a short time, so causing very little flavour or nutritive damage. It is equivalent to pasteurized milk in nutritive value, flavour, and colour and superior bacteriologically; it is sterile and must be bottled aseptically.

Ultrasonic Homogenizer. Super-high-speed vibrator giving a cavitation force of 60 tons per sq. in. in the liquid. Used to cream soups, disperse dried milk, disperse essential oils in soft drinks, to stabilize tomato purée, to prepare peanut butter, etc.

Ultra-violet Irradiation. Lethal to bacteria (wavelength 2,900 to 2,100 Ångstrom units) but of poor penetrating power and only of value for surface sterilization or sterilizing the air. Also used for tenderizing and aging of meat, curing of cheese, and prevention of mould growth on the surface of bakery products.

Umbles. Edible entrails of any animal (more particularly deer) which used to be made into pie—umble pie or humble pie.

Unesterified Fatty Acids. *See* Fatty acids.

U.N.I.C.E.F. The United Nations Children's Fund (UNCF) originally the United Nations International Children's Emergency Fund.

Unsaturated Fatty Acids. *See* Fatty acids.

Uperization. A method of sterilizing milk by injecting steam under pressure to raise the temperature to 150°C. The added water is evaporated off.

Uracil. *See* Pyrimidines *and* Nucleic Acids.

Urea. The waste nitrogen of most mammals is excreted in the urine as urea, $CO(NH_2)_2$. Formed in the liver by the urea cycle (*which see*) and excreted by the kidneys. (BDS.)

Urea Cycle. Sequence of reactions in which the amino group of unwanted amino acids is converted to urea, the nitrogenous excretion product. Formulated by Krebs, and known as the Krebs urea cycle (not to be confused with the Krebs tricarboxylic acid cycle).

The cycle is: ornithine + ammonia + CO_2 → citrulline; citrulline + ammonia → arginine; arginine, under the influence of arginase, → urea and ornithine.

The synthesis of urea takes place in the liver, and it is excreted by the kidneys. (BDS.)

Urease. Enzyme that hydrolyses urea to ammonia and carbon dioxide; appears to be absolutely specific for urea and used for the quantitative determination of urea in body fluids, etc.

Obtained from the jack bean and water-melon seed; the first enzyme to be crystallized. (WHSS, BDS.)

Ureotelic. Animals that excrete their waste nitrogen as urea, e.g. the mammals.

Uric Acid. End-product of nitrogen metabolism in birds and reptiles and of purine metabolism in man and the anthropoid apes. Other mammals possess the enzyme uricase, which converts the uric acid to allantoin. See also Purines. (BDS.)

Uricase. See Uric acid.

Uricotelic. Animals that excrete their waste nitrogen as uric acid, e.g. birds and reptiles.

Urobilinogen. Pigment in urine derived from the bile pigments, which, in turn, are formed from haemoglobin. When urine is left to stand, the urobilinogen is oxidized in air to urobilin. (BDS.)

Urogastrone. Hormone similar to gastrin found in urine; little known of its function. (BDS.)

Uropepsin. Proteolytic enzyme in urine; produced by acidification of uropepsinogen, which is identical with gastric pepsinogen. Urinary output serves as a measure of the amount of peptic glandular tissue.

V

Vac-ice Process. Alternative name for Freeze-drying.

Vacreation. Deodorization of cream by steam distillation under reduced pressure (see also Deodorization); developed in New Zealand. (Davis.)

Vacuum Contact Plate Process. Method of dehydrating food in a vacuum oven in which material is heated by hot plates both above and below. As the material shrinks due to water losses, continuous contact is maintained by closing of the plates. Has the advantage over a simple vacuum oven of supplying heat more effectively to the food. (Also known as V.C.D.—Vacuum contact dryer.)

Valine. An essential amino acid, rarely, if ever, limiting in foods. Chemically amino isovaleric acid. (BDS.)

Valzin. See Dulcin.

Vanadium. Element not shown to be essential but found in several animal tissues and believed to play a biological role.

Vanaspati. Purified, hydrogenated, vegetable oil, used in India and similar to margarine; fortified with vitamin A, 25 i.u. per gram, vitamin D optional.

Vanilla. Extract of the vanilla bean, fruit of the orchid, *Aracus aromaticus* (or *Vanilla aromaticus*) and related species. Fruits are allowed to ferment, when the beans become dark brown in colour; they are crushed and extracted with alcohol.

Chief flavouring principle is vanillin or methyl protocatechuic aldehyde, but other substances present aid the flavour, and synthetic vanillin has not the true flavour.

Discovered in Mexico in 1571 and could not be grown elsewhere because pollination could be effected only by a small Mexican bee, until artificial pollination was introduced in 1820. Main growing regions now Madagascar and Tahiti.

Vanilla sugar—ground bean mixed with sugar.

Ethyl vanillin—a synthetic substance, does not occur in the vanilla bean; incorrectly named —ethyl replaces methyl of vanillin; $3\frac{1}{2}$ times as strong in flavour, and more stable to storage than vanillin. (Jacobs, Merory.)

Vasoconstriction. Constriction of the blood vessels; the reverse of vasodilatation. (BDS.)

Vasodilatation. Dilation of the blood vessels; the reverse is vasoconstriction. Caused by a rise in body temperature and serves to lose heat from the body. (BDS.)

V.C.D. *See* Vacuum contact drying process.

Veal. Meat of the young calf, not less than three weeks old.

Protein 14·9%, fat 11%; 163 kcal (0·68 MJ), Fe 1·8 mg; vitamin A 7 μg, B_1 0·1 mg, B_2 0·2 mg, nicotinic acid 4·9 mg, —per 100 g. (FAO.)

Vegans. Those who consume no animal foods. (Vegetarians often consume milk and/or eggs.)

Vegetable Butters. Naturally occuring fats that melt rather sharply because they contain a preponderance of a single triglyceride.

Cocoa butter—from *Theobroma cacao*, cocoa bean, used in chocolate. Borneo tallow or green butter—from Malayan and E. Indian plant, *Shorea stenoptera*, resembles cocoa butter. Shea butter—from African plant, *Butyrospermum parkii*, softer than cocoa butter. Mowrah fat or illipé butter—from Indian plant, *Bassia longifolia*, used for soap and candles. (Bailey.)

Vegetable Casein. Name once used for wheat gluten.

Vegetables, Plants or parts of plants cultivated for food. Some foods that are botanically fruits, such as tomatoes and cucumbers, and seeds, such as peas and beans, are included with the vegetables.

As a source of nutrients most of the vegetables are useful sources of vitamin C and minerals, the root vegetables supply carbohydrate, but only the seeds are an important source of protein. (FB.)

Verdoflavin. Name given to a substance isolated from grass, later shown to be riboflavin.

Verjuice. Extracted juice of green or unripe fruit, usually applied to apple and grape which have a green tint when unripe; in earlier days used as a drink but now only for culinary purposes.

Vermicelli. *See* Alimentary pastes.

Vermouth. Wine to which has been added a mixture of aromatic and bitter herbs, such as angelica, cinchona, coriander, wormwood, angostura, etc.

Sweet or Italian vermouth, 15–17% alcohol (by vol.) and 12–20% sugar (by weight). Dry or French type 3–5% sugar, 18–20% alcohol. (Jacobs.)

Versene. Trade name for ethylenediamine tetra-acetic acid, *which see*.

Verv. Trade name (Patterson Co., U.S.A.) for calcium stearyl-2-lactate, used to reduce baking variations in flour. It produces a more extensible dough, more easily machined, and gives a loaf with better keeping properties and more uniform structure.

Vetches. Pulses, *which see*.

Vicilin. Globulin protein in pea and lentil.

Vienna Bread. A loaf with a very crisp, thin, highly glazed crust, with cuts on the upper surface, coarser than ordinary bread and with gas holes. It is baked in an oven which retains the steam.

Vieth's Ratio. With reference to milk is the ratio of anhydrous lactose: protein: ash which is normally 13:9:2.

Villi, Intestinal. Small, finger-like processes covering the surface of the small intestine in large numbers. They provide an enormous surface area for the absorption of digested food from the small intestine. (BDS.)

Vinasses. The residual liquors from sugar-beet molasses; contain appreciable quantities of betaine.

Vinegar. This term may lawfully be applied only to a product of double fermentation. (The term "non-brewed vinegar", usually a coloured solution of acetic acid, is not permitted.) It is made from malt, wine, cider or spirits.

The first fermentation produces alcohol; the second fermentation, for which the organism *Acetobacter* is added, converts the alcohol to acetic acid, and also produces the characteristic flavour due to esters and higher alcohols. The acetic acid content is 5%.

Acetobacter grows as a film on the surface—"mother of vinegar". (Tanner.)

Violet BNP. Sodium salt of 4:4'-di(dimethylamino)-4''-di-(p-sulphobenzylamino) triphenyl-methanol anhydride.

Viosterol. Irradiated ergosterol, i.e. vitamin D_2.

Virol. Trade name (Virol Ltd.) for a vitamin preparation composed of malt extract, starch syrup and egg with added vitamins.

Protein 3·4%, fat 12%, carbohydrate 60%; Ca 108 mg, Fe 27 mg, kcal 349 (1·46 MJ)—per 100 g. (M&W.)

Viscogen. Thickening agent for whipping cream. Two parts of lime (CaO) in six parts of water, added to five parts of sugar in ten parts of water; used at the rate of ½–1 oz. per gallon of cream. (Davis.)

Viscometer. Instrument for measuring the viscosity of liquids. (Matz.)

Viscosity. A term used of liquids to define their resistance to flow (i.e. the internal friction). (Matz.)

Visual Purple or Rhodopsin. Pigment in the retina of the eye,

229

consisting of retinol plus protein, which is necessary for vision in dim light. *See* Vitamin A.

Vitamers. Substances structurally related to vitamins, possessing some biological activity though often less than the true vitamin.

Vitamin. Naturally-occurring organic substance essential in very small amounts for the normal functioning of the living cell. Thus a factor essential for an animal or micro-organism and not essential for man is, nevertheless, termed a vitamin.

It is now questionable whether it is desirable to group together substances as varied in function as, for example, the B vitamins that function as coenzymes, and substances like vitamin D that appears to function as a hormone.

The confusion in vitamin nomenclature has been partly clarified by the recommendations of the International Union of Nutritional Sciences (Nutr. Abstr. Rev. 1970, **40**, 395) and the International Union of Pure and Applied Chemistry (Europ. J. Biochem. 1967, **2**, 1). There is still a difference as shown below.

	IUNS	IUPAC
1. Generic descriptor:	Folacin	Folic acid

Specific compounds:

(a)	Folic acid	Pteroyl glutamic acid
(b)	Folic acid glutamate (2)	Pteroyldiglutamic acid
(c)	Tetrahydrofolic acid	Tetrahydropteroyl glutamic acid

2. Generic descriptor: Menaquinone (vitamin K)

Specific compounds:

(a)	Phytylmenaquinone	Phylloquinone none
(b)	Multiprenylmenaquinones	Menaquinone-n
(c)	Prenylmenaquinone-6	Menaquinone-6

For other vitamins there is agreement between the two recommendations as follows:

A generic descriptor indicates a group of substances with the specific biological activity; thus "vitamin A" is used in terms of vitamin A deficiency; otherwise specific chemical names are used, as retinol (old name vitamin A alcohol), dehydroretinol (vitamin A2), carotene.

Riboflavin and thiamin spelled without the final "e". Niacin is a generic descriptor, specific terms are nicotinic acid and nicotinamide. Vitamin B_6 is the generic descriptor, specific chemical substances are pyridoxine, pyridoxal and pyridoxamine. (*See* individual vitamins).

Vitamin A. Includes both retinol (previously called preformed vitamin A) and carotene (previously termed vitamin A precursor). Essential for formation of glycoproteins of the mucous tissue by acting as a carrier for the monosaccharides involved; thus maintains normal condition of moist epithelial tissues lining mouth, respiratory and urinary tract; essential for growth. The aldehyde, retinal, is needed for vision in dim light in combination with protein to form visual purple.

Deficiency leads to **night blindness, xerophthalmia** (drying of tear ducts) and **keratomalacia** (ulceration of the cornea), blindness and stunting of growth.

Occurs as retinol in fish liver oils (cod and halibut), milk and butter, and as carotene in green vegetables, carrots and palm oil.

Daily recommended intake 750 μg for adult (2,500 i.u.). Vitamin A content of foods expressed as retinol equivalents: 1 μg retinol = 6 μg beta-carotene = 12 μg other active carotenoids = 3·3 i.u. retinol = 10 i.u. beta-carotene. (Sebrell, FB.)

Vitamin A₂. Old name for dehydroretinol, the form found in livers of freshwater fish; has 40% of biological activity of retinol.

Vitamin B_c. *See* Folic Acid.

Vitamin B Complex. *See under* individual B vitamins. These vitamins occur together in cereal germ, liver and yeast; are all coenzymes; and historically were discovered by separation from what was known originally as "vitamin B": hence they are grouped together as the B complex. The vitamin B₂ complex is of purely historical origin and includes all except B₁.

Vitamin B_p. Called the antiperosis factor for chicks, but can be replaced by manganese and choline.

Vitamin B_T. An essential dietary factor for the mealworm, *Tenebrio molitor*, and certain related species; now known to be identical with carnitine. In higher animals carnitine plays a part in fat synthesis by transferring acetyl across the mitochondrial membrane but it is not a dietary essential.

Vitamin B_w. Or Factor W; probably identical with biotin.

Vitamin B_x. Obsolete name for para-amino benzoic acid.

Vitamin B₁. Thiamin. Thiamin pyrophosphate is the coenzyme, cocarboxylase, needed in oxidative decarboxylation, e.g. the conversion of ketoglutarate to succinate and of pyruvic acid to acetyl. A deficiency of the vitamin leads to impaired metabolism of carbohydrate and clinically results in the disease beriberi in which pyruvate accumulates in the blood.

The daily requirement is related to the amount of carbohydrate oxidized (the non-fat calories)— 0·6 mg per 1,000 non-fat calories or 0·4 mg per 1,000 total Cals. (daily total approx. 1 mg). Thiamin is water-soluble and there is little storage in the body.

Occurs in cereal grains (little in white flour and white rice but these are enriched with added thiamin in many countries), in yeast, meat, especially pork, pulses, egg.

Obsolete name aneurine.

It is one of the more labile of the vitamins and is destroyed by heat under alkaline conditions, by sulphur dioxide, and is lost by leaching into the cooking water. The baking of bread can lead to 15–30% loss; up to half can be lost in cooked meat and fish, depending on the conditions. (Sebrell, FB.)

Vitamin B₂. Riboflavin. In combination with a number of different proteins it forms a group of coenzymes called flavoproteins, essential for the oxidation of carbohydrates. Flavoproteins act as intermediary hydrogen carriers and include flavin mononucleotide, flavin adenine dinucleotide, cytochrome c reductase, etc.

A deficiency of riboflavin impairs cell oxidation and results clinically in a set of symptoms known as ariboflavinosis. These include cracking of the skin at the corners of the mouth (angular stomatitis) fissuring of the lips (cheilosis) and tongue changes (glossitis); seborrhoeic accumulations appear around the nose and eyes.

Recommended intake—$0 \cdot 55$ mg per 1,000 kcal or an average of $1 \cdot 5$ mg per day. It occurs in yeast, liver, milk, eggs, cheese and pulses.

Processing losses are partly due to leaching into the water and partly to exposure to light. 50% of the riboflavin of milk can be destroyed in 2 hours by exposure to bright sunlight, and even on a dull day the losses can be 20%. The products of photoxidation of the vitamin B_2 destroy the vitamin C. (Sebrell, FB.)

Vitamin B_3. Name given to substance that was probably pantothenic acid.

Vitamin B_4. Name given to what was later identified as a mixture of arginine, glycine and cystine.

Vitamin B_5. Name given to a substance later presumed to be identical with vitamin B_6 or possibly nicotinic acid.

Vitamin B_6. Generic descriptor for three derivatives of 2-methylpyridine, namely the hydroxy compound, pyridoxine (previously known as adermin and pyridoxol),

the aldehyde, pyridoxal, and the amine, pyridoxamine; all equally active.

Deficiency causes convulsions and acrodynia (skin disorder) in rats, abnormal red cells in dairy cattle, anaemia in dogs and epileptiform seizures in human babies.

Functions as coenzyme for specific amino acid decarboxylases and deaminases, transaminases and transmethylases.

Rarely deficient in human diets; recommended intake thought to be about 2 mg per day; occurs in nuts, meat, fish, whole grain.

Obsolete names adermin, yeast eluate factor, factor I and factor Y. *See also* Transamination. (Sebrell.)

Vitamin B_7. When a new factor was discovered that was claimed to be essential for chick growth and feathering, the claimant stated that as nine factors were known the new factors should be called vitamins B_{10} and B_{11}. In fact the B vitamins had been numbered only up to B_6, hence B_7, B_8 and B_9 have never existed.

Vitamin B_8. *See* Vitamin B_7.

Vitamin B_9. *See* Vitamin B_7.

Vitamin B_{10}. The names B_{10} and B_{11} were given to two factors claimed to be essential for chick growth and feathering, they were later shown to be a mixture of vitamin B_{12} and folic acid.

Vitamin B_{11}. *See* Vitamin B_{10}.

Vitamin B_{12}. Essential for nucleic acid synthesis and so essential for formation of red blood cells. Deficiency gives rise to **pernicious anaemia.**

Although a dietary essential, cases of dietary deficiency have been observed in very rare instances only, in individuals living solely on fruits and vegetables, i.e. Vegans, since it is found, apart from some seaweeds, only in animal foods. Pernicious anaemia is usually due to an inability to absorb the vitamin through lack of the "**intrinsic factor**" normally present in the gastric mucosa.

Richest sources meat, liver and kidney; recommended intake not given in U.K. tables but 5 μg in U.S.A. tables.

Vitamin B_{12} is the generic descriptor; specific compounds are cyanocobalamin (formerly B_{12}a), hydroxocobalamin (formerly B_{12}b) and nitritocobalamin.

Essential growth factors for animals were variously termed **Animal Protein Factor** (APF), **Cow Manure Factor** and **Zoopherin** before they were shown to be identical with vitamin B_{12}. (Sebrell, AEB.)

Vitamin B_{13}. See Orotic acid; not an established vitamin.

Vitamin B_{14}. Not an established vitamin; a substance found in human urine which increases the rate of cell-proliferation in bone-marrow culture.

Vitamin B_{15}. Pangamic acid, which see; no evidence that it is a dietary essential.

Vitamin C. L-xylo-ascorbic acid (The isomer, D-araboascorbic acid, or isoascorbic acid or erythorbic acid has only slight biological activity, 1/20th, but is used as an antioxidant in foods). Controls production of intercellular cementing substances because it is essential for the hydroxylation of proline to hydroxyproline, a step in the synthesis of collagen. Breakdown of this matrix allows seepage of blood from capillaries, subcutaneous bleeding, weakness of muscles, soft, spongy gums leading to loss of teeth—in other words scurvy.

Easily oxidized, especially in foods kept hot, and leached into cooking water. Recommended intake 30 mg per day according to United Kingdom and FAO authorities; 45 mg according to U.S.A. authorities.

Occurs in fruits and vegetables; used as antioxidant and bread improver.

D-xyloascorbic acid, L-araboascorbic have zero biological activity; L-rhamno- has 1/5th of activity of vitamin C; D-arabo- has 1/20th. (DP, FB.)

Vitamin D. Formed in the skin under the action of ultraviolet light which converts 7-dehydrocholesterol into vitamin D_3 or cholecalciferol. Also synthesized as D_2 or ergocalciferol by irradiation of ergosterol.

Term D_1 was given originally to an impure mixture and is not used now.

Converted into 25-hydroxy derivative in liver and then into 1,25-dihydroxy derivative in kidney. This is 300–1,000 times more potent than vitamin D and stimulates absorption of dietary calcium from intestine and calcium turnover in bone.

Deficiency causes rickets in young children, osteomalacia in adults. Not widely distributed in foods—egg yolk, butter, fatty fish and enriched margarine.

Recommended intakes 10 μg (400 i.u.) for infants and children and 2·5 μg (100 i.u.) for adults.

Excess can be harmful. (Sebrell, AEB.)

Vitamin E. Generic descriptor for group of fat-soluble compounds essential for reproduction in animals. Essential for man (not for reproduction so far as is known) but rarely, if ever, deficient in the diet. Deficiency symptoms vary considerably in different animal species—sterility in mouse, rat, rabbit, sheep and turkey; muscular dystrophy in several species; capillary permeability in chick and turkey; anaemia in monkey. Many substances have vitamin E-like activity, eight in particular, (old names in brackets): 5,7,8-trimethyl tocol (alpha tocopherol); 5,8-dimethyl tocol (beta); 7,8-dimethyl tocol (gamma); 8-methyl tocol (delta-tocopherol); 5,7,8-trimethyl tocotrienol (alpha tocotrienol); 5,8-dimethyl tocotrienol (beta); 7,8-dimethyl tocotrienol (gamma) and 8-methyl tocotrienol (delta). All expressed as alpha-tocopherol equivalents.

These compounds are antioxidants with varying potencies and their natural occurrence in vegetable oils protects the latter against rancidity. (AEB.)

Vitamin F. *See* Essential fatty acids.

Vitamin G. Obsolete name for vitamin B_2.

Vitamin H. *See* Biotin.

Vitamin K. Fat-soluble vitamin essential for the production by the liver of prothrombin and several other factors involved in the blood clotting system. Hence called the antihaemorrhagic vitamin.

There is a discrepancy between the nomenclature of the International Union of Pure and Applied Chemistry and that of the International Union of Nutritional Sciences (given in brackets). Generic descriptor: Menaquinone, 2-methyl-1,4-naphthoquinone. Specific compounds phylloquinone (phytylmenaquinone), the 3-phytyl derivative, formerly called vitamin K1—used therapeutically. Compounds with prenyl side chains are menaquinone-n (multiprenylquinones) such as menaquinone-6 (prenylmenaquinone-6). Potency expressed as phylloquinone (phytylmenaquinone) equivalents.

The old designation vitamin K2 (naturally-occurring) was given to 2-methyl-difarnesyl-1,4-naphthoquinone. Synthetic analogues were termed K3 (menaquinone); K4 or menadiol, the hydroquinone form; K5, 4-amino-2-methyl-1-naphthol (used as a food preservative); K6, 2-methyl-1,4-naphthalene diamine (toxic); K7, 4-amino-3-methyl-1-naphthol.

Widely distributed in greenstuffs and synthesized by bacteria in the intestine but not known how much is absorbed; dietary deficiency is not encountered (except in newborn infants with a sterile intestine) only failure of absorption. (Sebrell, AEB.)

Vitamin L. Vitamins L_1 and L_2 are factors in yeast said to be essential for lactation; they have not become established.

Vitamin M. *See* Folic acid.

Vitamin P. Name formerly given to a group of plant flavonoid substances that affect the strength of the walls of the blood capillaries, namely, rutin (in buckwheat), hesperidin, eriodictin and citrin (in the pith of citrus fruits).

234

(Citrin is a mixture of hesperidin and eriodictin.) Now considered that the effect is pharmacological and that they are not dietary essentials; sometimes called "bioflavonoids".

Called vitamin P from "permeabilitäts vitamin". Once claimed as a cure for the common cold. *See also* Flavonoids, *and* Capillary fragility. (Brav.)

Vitamin PP. *See* Nicotinic acid.

Vitamin—pronunciation. According to Fowler's Modern English Usage (Oxford University Press) vitamin is the better pronunciation, in conformity with other words derived from *vita*, but seems unlikely to hold its own against the more popular vītamin.

Vitamins (Content of Foods). According to the Code of Practice no claims for the presence of a vitamin or mineral in a food should be made unless the amount ordinarily consumed in a day contains one-sixth of the daily requirements.

No claim should be made that the food is a rich or excellent source unless half of the daily requirement is present; no reference to the prevention of disease unless the full day's requirement is present.

For this purpose the requirements are taken to be: vitamin A 900 μg, B_1 0·9 mg, B_2 1·8 mg; nicotinic acid 12 mg; vitamin C 30 mg; D 12 μg; calcium 0·75 g, iron 10 mg; iodine 0·1 mg; phosphate 0·75 g. (Bell.)

Vitamins, Fat-soluble. *See* Fat-soluble vitamins.

Vitamins, Water-soluble. *See* Water-soluble vitamins.

Vitamin T. A factor found in insect cuticle, mould mycelia and yeast fermentation liquor, claimed to accelerate maturation and promote protein synthesis. Also known as **torulitine.** Said to be a mixture of folic acid, vitamin B_{12} and desoxyribosides and not a new factor.

Vita-Wheat. Trade name (Peak Frean Ltd.) for a crispbread, *which see.* Composition: protein 8·6%, fat 10·3%, carbohydrate 77·8%; Ca 44 mg, Fe 3·4 mg, kcal 423 (1·8 MJ)—per 100 g. Phytic acid phosphorus 59% of total phosphorus (372 mg per 100 g). (M&W.)

Vitellin. One of the proteins of egg yolk; approximately four-fifths of the total protein; is a phosphoprotein and accounts for one-third of the phosphorus of egg yolk. (B. & R.)

Vodka. Made from neutral spirit, i.e. alcohol distillate (in Russia mainly from potatoes), with little or no acid present so that there is no ester formation and hence no flavour.

Vol. Trade name for commercial ammonium carbonate, a mixture of ammonium bicarbonate and carbamate. Used as aerating agent in baking as it breaks down when heated to give carbon dioxide, ammonia and steam, without leaving any residue.

Votator. Machine used for the continuous manufacture of margarine; the fat and water are emulsified, and the subsequent conditioning process carried out in the same machine.

W

Warburg and Christian's Coenzyme. Nicotinamide adenine dinucleotide phosphate.

Warburg Apparatus. Small vessel attached to a manometer in which reactions that involve gas exchange can be followed. The vessel is immersed in a constant-temperature bath and shaken continually to equilibrate the gas in solution, where the reactions are taking place, with the gas in the gas phase, where it is being measured.

Living tissues as slices, minces, homogenates, and micro-organisms are examined in this way. (Hawk.)

Warburg's Respiratory Enzyme. Enzyme postulated by Warburg as part of the cell oxidation system; later shown to be cytochrome oxidase. (WHSS.)

Warburg's Yellow Enzyme. A flavoprotein that is part of the cell oxidation chain; passes on the hydrogen from reduced Coenzyme I to cytochrome. (WHSS.)

Water Balance. The balance between intake and excretion. Intake as drinks averages 1–1·5 litres per day, as aqueous part of food, 0·5-litres, and formed in the body by oxidation of foodstuffs, 300–500 ml, total 2–3 litres.

Losses as water from the lungs, 400–500 ml, through the skin 400–500 ml, in faeces 80–100 ml, in urine 1–1·8 litre.

Total body water 40–44 litres (80 pints) as blood plasma (2–3 litres), extracellular water (10 litres) and intracellular water (27–30 litres).

The kidney controls the volume of extracellular water by excreting water. Ingestion of sodium chloride raised the osmotic pressure of the extracellular water causing thirst.

Watercress. Leaves of *Nasturtium officinale*; recommended 1597 in John Gerarde's Herball as cure for scurvy; not cultivated commercially until early 19th century.

Composition per 100 g: 2·9 g protein, 0·7 g carbohydrate, 15 kcal (0·06 MJ), 220 mg calcium, 1·6 mg iron, 1,700 μg vitamin A, 0·1 mg B_1, 0·6 mg nicotinic acid, 60 mg C. (OF, M&W.)

Water, Demineralized. Water that has been purified by passage through a bed of ion-exchange resin which removes mineral salts. Demineralized or deionized water is as pure as, and can be purer than, distilled water.

Water, Extracellular. *See* Water balance.

Water-glass. Sodium silicate; used to preserve eggs, as a layer of insoluble calcium silicate is formed around the shell which seals the pores.

Water Hardness. Soap-precipitating power of water due to the formation of insoluble calcium and magnesium salts of the soap. Temporary hardness is removed by boiling, permanent hardness is not.

May be measured in degrees Clarke; one degree = 1 part of calcium carbonate per 100,000 parts of water.

Water, Intracellular. *See* Water balance.

Water, Metabolic. *See* Metabolic water.

Waters, Natural. *See* Mineral waters, natural.

Water-soluble Vitamins. All the members of the B complex (thiamin, riboflavin, nicotinic acid, pantothenic acid, pyridoxine, biotin, folic acid, para-amino benzoic acid, choline, inositol and B_{12}) and vitamin C.

Unlike the storage of vitamins A and D in the liver, there is no specific site for storage of the water-soluble vitamins, they are merely dispersed in solution through the blood and tissues. *See also* Fat-soluble vitamins.

Wax, Apple. Peel wax contains triacontane, heptaconsanol and malol.

Waxes. Esters of fatty acids with long-chain monohydric alcohols (fats are esters of fatty acids with the three-carbon trihydric alcohol, glycerol). E.g. beeswax, ester of palmitic acid with myricyl alcohol; spermaceti, cetyl palmitate.

Animal waxes are often esters of the steroid alcohol, cholesterol. (BDS.)

Weatings. *See* Wheatfeed.

Weende Analysis. The same as proximate analysis, named from the Weende Experimental Station in Germany which laid down, in 1865, methods of determining crude fibre, ether extract, ash, nitrogen, and soluble carbohydrate by the difference of the sum of these from the total.

Weetabix. Trade name (Weetabix Ltd.) for a breakfast cereal prepared from wheat flakes.

Protein 10·9%, fat 1·9%, carbohydrate 77·0%; Ca 36 mg, Fe 4 mg, vitamin B_1 0·6 mg, B_2 1·0 mg, nicotinic acid 7 mg, Calories 351—per 100 g. (M&W.)

Weighting Oils. *See* Brominated oils.

Wetzel Grid. Children are grouped by physique into five groups, ranging from tall and thin to short and thick-set. A healthy child will grow, as measured by height and weight, along one of these channels at a standard rate, if he deviates from the channel malnutrition is suspected. (DP.)

Wey. 48 bushels of oats or 40 bushels of salt or "corn".

Whalemeat. (Edible portion only.) Protein 20%, fat 4%; kcal 125 (0·53 MJ), Fe 2·4 mg, vitamin A 80 i.u., B_1 0·03 mg, B_2 0·1 mg, nicotinic acid 4·4 mg—per 100 g. (FAO.)

Whale Oil. Used, after hardening by hydrogenation, for lower-quality margarines; also in soap making.

Wheat. The most important of the cereals and one of the most widely grown crops. Many thousand varieties are known but there are three main types: *Tricitum vulgare*—used mainly for bread, *Tricitum durum* (Durum wheat)—largely used for macaroni, and *Tricitum compactum* (Club wheat) too soft for ordinary bread.

The berry is composed of the outer branny husk, 13% of the grain, the germ or embryo (rich in nutrients) 2%, and the central endosperm (mainly starch) 85%.

Composition (FAO figures) hard wheat: protein 12·2%, fat 2%; calcium 37 mg, iron 4 mg, calories 332, vitamin B_1 0·45 mg, B_2 0·13 mg, nicotinic acid 5·4 mg—per 100 g.

Soft wheat: protein 10·5%, fat 1·9%; vitamin B_1 0·38 mg, B_2 0·08 mg, nicotinic acid 4·3 mg —per 100 g, other values the same as hard wheat.

See also Extraction rate, Flour and Wheatfeed. (KJ, OF.)

Wheatfeed. Residue from the milling of wheat to produce flour, also known as **millers' offal** and **wheat offals.**

Bran itself consists of the husk of the grain with some adhering endosperm. Particles with less husk and more endosperm are variously known as middlings, sharps, toppings. Very coarse middlings are known as pollards. These various designations have been dropped and the two categories weatings and superfine weatings used.

Weatings—middlings or sharps containing not more than $5 \cdot 75\%$ fibre; **superfine weatings**—richer type of middlings containing not more than $4 \cdot 5\%$ fibre. Coarse bran contains about 10% fibre. All three fractions contain about 15% protein, 3–4% fat and 60–70% carbohydrate. (KJ.)

Wheat Germ. *See* Germ.

Wheatmeal, National. Name given to the 85% extraction flour when introduced in U.K. in February 1941 (as distinct from wholemeal which is 100% extraction). Later called National flour. It was milled to contain as much of the germ and aleurone layer as possible, having most of the nutritional properties of wholemeal flour with higher digestibility and a more attractive loaf.

A loaf described as wheatmeal must contain not less than $0 \cdot 6\%$ fibre calculated on dry weight.

Wheat, Puffed. Trade name of a breakfast cereal prepared by heating wheat grains under pressure and then rapidly releasing the pressure when the superheated steam in the grain suddenly expands so puffing or "exploding" the grain.

Protein $13 \cdot 9\%$, fat $2 \cdot 0\%$, carbohydrate $75 \cdot 3\%$; Fe $3 \cdot 3$ mg, vitamin B_1 $1 \cdot 2$ mg, kcal 358 ($1 \cdot 5$ MJ)—per 100 g. (M&W.)

Wheat, Shredded. Trade name (Nabisco, Ltd.) of a breakfast cereal prepared from wheat grains.

Protein $9 \cdot 7\%$, fat $2 \cdot 8\%$, carbohydrate 79%; Fe $4 \cdot 5$ mg, kcal 362 ($1 \cdot 5$ MJ)—per 100 g. Phytic acid phosphorus 80% of total P (287 mg/100 g). (M&W.)

Whey. The residue from milk after removal of the casein and most of the fat (as in cheese-making); also known as **lacto-serum.**

Contains about $\cdot 1\%$ protein (lactalbumin and lactoglobulin) together with all the lactose, water-soluble vitamins and minerals and therefore has some food value although it is 92% water.

Whey cheese can be made by heat coagulation of the protein, and whey butter from the small amount ($0 \cdot 25\%$) fat.

Dried whey is added to processed cheese; most whey is fed in liquid form to pigs.

Whey Butter. *See* Butter, whey.

Whiskey, Whisky. A grain spirit distilled from barley, rye or other cereal which has first been malted and then fermented. Most brands of whisky are a blend of pure malt whisky with spirit distilled from grain.

Oxford Dictionary permits both spellings; the Trade regard whisky as the Scotch variety and whiskey as the Irish and American varieties. The name is derived

238

from the Gaelic uisgebeatha—water of life.

White Blood Cells. *See* Leucocytes.

White Cell Count. *See* Leucocytes.

White Rice. *See* Rice.

Whole-wheat Meal. Flour or meal prepared by milling the whole wheat grain, i.e. 100% extraction rate.

Whortleberry. *See* Bilberry.

Wills' Factor. A factor in autolysed yeast effective in promoting red blood cell formation, probably folic acid.

Wilson's Formula. *See* Blood volume.

Windberry. *See* Bilberry.

Wine. Essentially a fermentation of sugar by yeast to produce alcohol, together with flavouring agent supplied by the fruit or vegetable.

Table wines are produced from grapes with sugar content such that the alcohol produced is 11–14% by volume, dessert wines from grapes with higher sugar content and fortified by the addition of brandy distilled from grape wine, to 17–21% alcohol. *See also* Alcoholic beverages.

Wineberry. *Rubus phoenicolasius*; similar to raspberry, orange coloured.

Winterization. Applied to edible oils, meaning the removal of the more saturated glycerides so that the oil remains bright and clear at low temperatures. The oil is simply chilled and the solidified palmitates and stearates filtered off.

Witches' Milk. Secretion of the mammary gland of the newborn of both sexes; due to the presence of the hormone prolactin that travels from the blood of the mother into the foetus. Also known as **sorcerers' milk**. (Hawk.)

Wood Alcohol. Methyl alcohol, CH_3OH; highly toxic. Its presence in methylated spirits accounts for the toxicity of the latter.

Worcester Sauce. Characterized by spicy flavour, sediment and thin supernatant liquid. Recipes usually secret but basically soya, tamarinds, anchovies, garlic and spices, plus sugar, salt and vinegar, matured six months in oak casks.

Work. *See* Energy.

World Food Programme. Part of Food and Agriculture Organisation of the United Nations; intended to give international aid in the form of food from countries with a surplus.

Wort. *See* Beer.

X

Xanthine. *See* Purines *and* Nucleic acids.

Xanthine Oxidase. An enzyme present in milk and in liver; specific for the two purines, xanthine and hypoxanthine (which it oxidizes to uric acid), and will also oxidize a range of aldehydes to the corresponding

acids. It is identical with **Schardinger's enzyme** of milk. (WHSS.)

Xanthophyll. Yellow, hydroxy carotene derivative; occurs in all green leaves together with the chlorophyll and carotene, also present in egg yolk. Has no vitamin A activity.

Also known as **lutein** and **luteol.**

Xanthophylls. Collective term for hydroxylated carotenoids or carotenols.

Xanthoproteic Test. For proteins (actually for the benzene nucleus of tyrosine and tryptophan which occur in nearly all proteins). Yellow colour on boiling with nitric acid, turns orange on adding ammonia. (Hawk.)

Xerophthalmia. Occurs in advanced vitamin A deficiency. Epithelium of the cornea and conjunctiva of the eye deteriorates because of impairment of the tear glands, resulting in dryness then ulceration.

Xyloascorbic Acid. *See* Ascorbic Acid.

Xylose. Pentose sugar found in plant tissues as complex polysaccharide; 40% sweetness of sucrose. (Hawk.)

Y

Yams. Tubers of perennial climbing plants of a number of species of *Dioscorea*. The wild species contain toxins (saponins and alkaloids) and these can appear in cultivated varieties under poor conditions of growth.

Largely carbohydrate 25%, only 2% protein, iron 1 mg, vitamin B_1 0·05 mg, B_2 0·06 mg, nicotinic acid 0·4 mg, vitamin C 15 mg—per 100 g. (TND.)

Yarmouth Bloater. *See* Red herring.

Yautia. *See* Tannia.

Yeast. Fungi; consist of cell wall enclosing cytoplasm and nucleus, some can spore ("true yeasts"), others reproduce only by cell division ("false yeasts").

Saccharomyces cerevisiae used in brewing and baking; *S. cerevisiae* var. *ellipsoideus* used in wine making (occurs on grapes). Other species of this genus used in production of fermented milk liquors, like Koumiss, Kefir, etc.

Sub-genus *Zygosaccharomyces* can ferment highly concentrated sugar products like jam, honey and sugar confectionery, and therefore important to the food technologist.

Also in the Tribe Saccharomyceteae are *Pichia* and *Hansenula*, contaminants in brewing that form esters instead of alcohol from sugar. Also grow as films on pickle brines—film yeasts.

Varieties such as *Candida utilis* called Food Yeast (formerly *Torula utilis*) are grown on waste carbohydrate sources and petroleum residues, as a potential supplement to animal feed. Composition varies with growing conditions, approx. 50% protein of NPU about 50, and relatively high concentrations of most of the B vitamins, 5% fat (*Rhodotorula gracilis* can produce 50% fat.) (Baum. FM.)

Yeast Adenylic Acid. Adenosine-3-phosphoric acid. Muscle adenylic acid is adenosine-5-phosphoric acid. (BDS.)

Yeast Eluate Factor. Obsolete name for vitamin B_6.

Yeast Extract. A preparation of the water-soluble fraction of autolysed yeast, valuable both as a rich source of the B vitamins and for its strong savoury flavour. Yeast (commercially brewers' yeast) is allowed to autolyse, extracted with hot water and concentrated by evaporation. Commercial preparations are Marmite and Yeastrel, *which see*.

Yeast Fermentation, Bottom. Fermentation during the manufacture of beer with a yeast that sinks to the bottom of the tank. Most beers are produced this way; ale, porter and stout being the principal beers produced by **top fermentation**. (Matz.)

Yeast Filtrate Factor. Obsolete name for pantothenic acid.

Yeastrel. Trade name (Brewers Foods Supply Co.) for a yeast extract; contains 4·2 mg vitamin B_2 and 40 mg nicotinic acid—per 100 g.

Yeatex. Trade name (English Grains Ltd.) for yeast extract—autolysed brewers' yeast—used as a flavouring ingredient. Composition 41% protein, 10% carbohydrate; 1 mg thiamin, 2 mg riboflavin, 40 mg nicotinic acid, 5 mg pantothenic acid, 2·5 mg pyridoxine, 1 mg folic acid per 100 g.

Yellow Colours. Oil yellow GG—mixture of 4-phenylazoresorcinol and 4:6-di(phenylazo)resorcinol.

Yellow 2G—disodium salt of 1-(2:5-dichloro-4-sulphophenyl)-5-hydroxy-3-methyl-4-p-sulphophenylazopyrazole.

Yellow RFS—disodium salt of 4-sulpho-4-(sulphomethylamino)-azobenzene.

Yellow RY—disodium salt of 6-p-sulphophenylazoresorcinol-4-sulphonic acid.

Sunset yellow FCF—disodium salt of 1-p-sulphophenylazo-2-napnthol-6-sulphonic acid; yellow-orange colour used to simulate the colour of eggs or orange, called Yellow No. 6 in U.S.A.

Oil yellow XP—3-methyl-1-phenyl-4-(2:4-xylylazo)-5-pyrazolone.

Naphthol yellow S—disodium or potassium salt of 2:4:dinitro-1-naphthol-7-sulphonic acid.

Yellow Enzyme. *See* Warburg's yellow enzyme.

Yerba Maté. *See* Maté.

Yestamin. Trade name (English Grains Ltd.) for a variety of preparations of dried Saccharomyces yeast (debittered brewers' yeast) used to enrich foods. Composition 45% protein, 1-2% fat, 36% carbohydrate; 4·5-27 mg thiamin, 3-6·5 mg riboflavin, 20-60 mg nicotinic acid, 1·8-6 mg pantothenic acid, 2-3 mg pyridoxine, 2 mg folic acid per 100 g.

Yoghurt. *See* Milks, fermented.

Yolk Index. Index of freshness of an egg; ratio of height to diameter of yolk under defined conditions. As the egg deteriorates the yolk index decreases. (Griswold.)

Yuksov disease. Another name for Haff disease, *which see*.

Z

Zeaxanthin. One of the carotenoid pigments in maize, egg yolk and *Physalis* (Chinese lantern); has no vitamin A activity; used as a colouring.

Zedoary Root. Of *Curcuma zedoaria*, an Indian plant of the ginger family. Used in the manufacture of flavours and bitters.

Zein. Protein obtained from maize (*Zea mais*), soluble in alcohol but not water or dilute alkali. Of poor nutritive value as it completely lacks lysine and is poor in tryptophan. (B. & R.)

Z-enzyme. Enzyme found associated with amylases, that attacks the few 1:3-beta-links present in amylose. Pure, crystalline beta-amylase will convert only 70% of amylose to maltose, it requires the presence of the Z-enzyme for complete conversion. (WHSS.)

Zest. Outer skin of citrus fruits. *See* Flavedo.

Zinc. Essential for plant growth, and a dietary essential for man and animals. Deficiency results in hypogonadism. Present as part of enzymes carbonic anhydrase and uricase, and in crystalline insulin.

Found in traces in most foods; excess is harmful. Oysters concentrate zinc from seawater and can contain up to $0 \cdot 3\%$. *See also* Parakeratosis. (Gilbert, GMW.)

Zitoni. *See* Alimentary Pastes.

Zizanie. *See* Rice, wild.

Zomotherapy. Treatment by raw meat or raw meat-juice. Used for anaemia, neurasthenia, in convalescence. (Hutch.)

Zoopherin. Vitamin B_{12}.

Zwieback. German term for twice-baked bread. Ordinary dough plus eggs and butter, baked, sliced, baked again to a rusk and sometimes sugar coated.

Zymase. Name given to the mixture of enzymes in yeast that is responsible for fermentation.

Zymogens. The inactive form in which some enzymes exist before being liberated by the action of a kinase. E.g. trypsinogen and pepsinogen are secreted in the intestine and converted into their active forms trypsin and pepsin. (BDS.)

Zymotachygraph. An instrument that measures the gas produced in a fermenting dough and the amount escaping from the dough. (KJ.)

242

RECOMMENDED INTAKES—FOOD AND AGRICULTURE ORGANISATION

Subject	Age (years)	kcal	MJ	Protein (g/kg)	Calcium (g)	Iron* (mg)	Vitamin A (i.u.)	Vitamin A (µg)	Thiamin (mg)	Riboflavin (mg)	Niacin (mg)
Children	0–1	110 per kg	0·47 per kg	1–3	0·5–0·6	7	1000	300	0·4	0·6	6·6
	1–3	1360	5·7	1·19	0·4–0·5	7	800	240	0·5	0·7	8·6
	4–6	1830	7·6	1·01	0·4–0·5	7	1000	300	0·7	0·9	11·2
	7–9	2190	9·2	0·88	0·4–0·5	7	1300	390	0·8	1·2	13·9
Boys	10–12	2600	10·9	0·81	0·6–0·7	7	1900	570	1·0	1·4	16·5
	13–15	2900	12·1	0·72	0·6–0·7	12	2400	720	1·2	1·7	20·4
	16–19	3100	13·0	0·60	0·5–0·6	6	1500	750	1·4	2·0	23·8
Adults		3000	12·6	0·57	0·4–0·5	6	2500	750	1·3	1·8	21·1
Girls	10–12	2350	9·8	0·76	0·6–0·7	18	2400	720	1·0	1·4	17·2
	13–15	2500	10·5	0·63	0·6–0·7	18	2400	720	1·0	1·4	17·2
	16–19	2300	9·6	0·55	0·5–0·6	19	2500	750	1·0	1·3	15·8
Adult		2200	9·2	0·52	0·4–0·5	19	2500	750	0·9	1·3	15·2
Pregnancy		+350	+1·5	+9	1·0–1·2	19	2500	750	0·4/1000 kcal	0·55/1000 kcal	6·6/1000 kcal
Lactation		+550	+2·3	+17	1·0–1·2	19	4000	1200	0·4/1000 kcal	0·55/1000 kcal	6·6/1000 kcal

* If animal foods comprise 10–25% of energy intake.
From "Requirements of Vitamin A, Thiamin, Riboflavin and Niacin", WHO Rpt. No. 362 (1967) and "Energy and Protein Requirements", WHO Rpt. No. 522 (1973).

243

RECOMMENDED INTAKES—FOOD AND AGRICULTURE
ORGANISATION (*continued*)

Subject	Age (years)	Vitamin C (mg)	Vitamin D (μg)	Vitamin B_{12} (μg)	Folate (μg)
Children	0–1	20	10	0·3	50
	1–3	20	10	0·9	100
	4–6	20	10	1·5	100
	7–9	20	2·5	1·5	100
Boys	10–12	20	2·5	2·0	100
	13–15	30	2·5	2·0	200
	16–19	30	2·5	2·0	200
Adults		30	2·5	2·0	200
Girls	10–12	20	2·5	2·0	100
	13–15	30	2·5	2·0	200
	16–19	30	2·5	2·0	200
Adult		30	2·5	2·0	200
Pregnancy		50	10	3·0	400
Lactation		50	10	2·5	300

From "Requirements of Ascorbic Acid, Vitamin D, Vitamin B_{12}, Folate and Iron", WHO Rpt. No. 452 (1970).

RECOMMENDED INTAKES OF NUTRIENTS FOR THE UNITED KINGDOM

Age range	Occupational category	Body weight kg	Energy kcal	Energy MJ	Protein g	Thiamin mg	Riboflavin mg	Nicotinic Acid mg equivalent	Ascorbic Acid mg	Vitamin A µg	Vitamin D µg cholecalciferol	Calcium mg	Iron mg
BOYS AND GIRLS													
0 up to 1 year		7·3	800	3·3	20	0·3	0·4	5	15	450	10	600	6
1 up to 2 years		11·5	1200	5·0	30	0·5	0·6	7	20	300	10	500	7
2 up to 3 years		13·5	1400	5·9	35	0·6	0·7	8	20	300	10	500	7
3 up to 5 years		16·5	1600	6·7	40	0·6	0·8	9	20	300	10	500	8
5 up to 7 years		20·5	1800	7·5	45	0·7	0·9	10	20	300	2·5	500	8
7 up to 9 years		25·1	2100	8·8	53	0·8	1·0	11	20	400	2·5	500	10
BOYS													
9 up to 12 years		31·9	2500	10·5	63	1·0	1·2	14	25	575	2·5	700	13
12 up to 15 years		45·5	2800	11·7	70	1·1	1·4	16	25	725	2·5	700	14
15 up to 18 years		61·0	3000	12·6	75	1·2	1·7	19	30	750	2·5	600	15
GIRLS													
9 up to 12 years		33·0	2300	9·6	58	0·9	1·2	13	25	575	2·5	700	13
12 up to 15 years		48·6	2300	9·6	58	0·9	1·4	16	25	725	2·5	700	14
15 up to 18 years		56·1	2300	9·6	58	0·9	1·4	16	30	750	2·5	600	15
MEN													
18 up to 35 years	Sedentary	65	2700	11·3	68	1·1	1·7	18	30	750	2·5	500	10
	Moderately active		3000	12·6	75	1·2	1·7	18	30	750	2·5	500	10
	Very active		3600	15·1	90	1·4	1·7	18	30	750	2·5	500	10
35 up to 65 years	Sedentary	65	2600	10·9	65	1·0	1·7	18	30	750	2·5	500	10
	Moderately active		2900	12·1	73	1·2	1·7	18	30	750	2·5	500	10
	Very active		3600	15·1	90	1·4	1·7	18	30	750	2·5	500	10
65 up to 75 years }	Assuming a sedentary life	63	2350	9·8	59	0·9	1·7	18	30	750	2·5	500	10
75 and over		63	2100	8·8	53	0·8	1·7	18	30	750	2·5	500	10
WOMEN													
18 up to 55 years	Most occupations	55	2200	9·2	55	0·9	1·3	15	30	750	2·5	500	12
	Very active		2500	10·5	63	1·0	1·3	15	30	750	2·5	500	12
55 up to 75 years }	Assuming a sedentary life	53	2050	8·6	51	0·8	1·3	15	30	750	2·5	500	10
75 and over		53	1900	8·0	48	0·7	1·3	15	30	750	2·5	500	10
Pregnancy, 2nd and 3rd trimester			2400	10·0	60	1·0	1·6	18	60	750	10	1200	15
Lactation			2700	11·3	68	1·1	1·8	21	60	1200	10	1200	15

U.S. RECOMMENDED DAILY DIETARY ALLOWANCES*

	Years	Weight (kg)	Weight (lb)	Height (cm)	Height (in)	Energy (kcal)	Protein (g)	Vitamin A activity (u.g.)	Vitamin A activity (i.u.)	Vitamin D (i.u.)	Vitamin E activity (i.u.)
Infants	0·0–0·5	6	14	60	24	kg × 117	kg × 2·2	420	1400	400	4
	0·6–1·0	9	20	71	28	kg × 108	kg × 2·0	400	1000	400	5
Children	1–3	13	28	86	34	1000	23	400	2000	400	7
	4–6	20	44	110	44	1800	30	500	2500	400	8
	7–10	30	56	135	54	2400	36	700	3300	400	10
Males	11–14	44	97	158	63	2800	44	1000	5000	400	12
	15–18	61	134	172	69	3000	54	1000	5000	400	15
	19–22	67	147	172	69	3000	52	1000	5000	400	15
	23–50	70	154	172	69	2700	56	1000	5000		15
	51+	70	154	172	69	2400	56	1000	5000		15
Females	11–14	44	97	155	62	2400	44	800	4000	400	10
	15–18	54	119	162	65	2100	48	800	4000	400	11
	19–22	58	126	162	65	2100	46	800	4000	400	12
	23–50	58	128	162	65	2000	46	800	4000		12
	51+	58	125	162	65	1800	46	800	4000		12
Pregnant						+300	+10	1000	5000	400	15
Lactating						+500	+20	1200	6000	400	15

* Food and Nutrition Board, National Academy of Sciences—National Research Council.

U.S. RECOMMENDED DAILY DIETARY ALLOWANCES (continued)

	Years	Weight (kg)	Weight (lb)	Height (cm)	Height (in)	Water-soluble vitamins Ascorbic acid (mg)	Folacin (mg)	Niacin (mg)	Riboflavin (mg)	Thiamin (mg)	Vitamin B_6 (mg)	Vitamin B_{12} (mg)
Infants	0·0–0·5	6	14	60	24	35	50	5	0·4	0·3	0·3	0·3
	0·6–1·0	9	20	71	28	35	50	8	0·6	0·5	0·4	0·3
Children	1–3	13	28	86	34	40	100	9	0·8	0·7	0·6	1·0
	4–6	20	44	110	44	40	200	12	1·1	0·9	0·9	1·5
	7–10	30	56	135	54	40	300	15	1·2	1·2	1·2	2·0
Males	11–14	44	97	158	63	45	400	18	1·5	1·4	1·6	3·0
	15–18	61	134	172	69	45	400	20	1·8	1·8	1·8	3·0
	19–22	67	147	172	69	45	400	20	1·8	1·5	2·0	3·0
	23–50	70	154	172	69	45	400	18	1·6	1·4	2·0	3·0
	51+	70	154	172	69	45	400	16	1·5	1·2	2·0	3·0
Females	11–14	44	97	155	52	45	400	16	1·2	1·2	1·6	3·0
	15–18	54	119	162	65	45	400	14	1·4	1·1	2·0	3·0
	19–22	58	126	162	65	45	400	14	1·4	1·1	2·0	3·0
	23–50	58	128	162	65	45	400	13	1·2	1·0	2·0	3·0
	51+	58	125	162	65	45	400	12	1·1	1·0	2·0	3·0
Pregnant						60	800	+2	+0·3	+0·3	2·5	4·0
Lactating						60	600	+4	+0·5	+0·3	2·5	4·0

U.S. RECOMMENDED DAILY DIETARY ALLOWANCES (continued)

	Years	Weight (kg)	Weight (lb)	Height (cm)	Height (in)	Minerals Calcium (mg)	Phosphorus (mg)	Iodine (mg)	Iron (mg)	Magnesium (mg)	Zinc (mg)
Infants	0.0–0.5	6	14	60	24	360	240	35	10	60	3
	0.6–1.0	9	20	71	28	540	400	45	15	70	5
Children	1–3	13	28	86	34	800	800	60	15	150	10
	4–6	20	44	110	44	800	800	80	10	200	10
	7–10	30	56	135	54	800	800	110	10	250	10
Males	11–14	44	97	158	63	1200	1200	110	18	350	15
	15–18	61	134	172	69	1200	1200	150	18	400	15
	19–22	67	147	172	69	800	800	140	10	350	15
	23–50	70	154	172	69	800	800	130	10	350	15
	51+	70	154	172	69	800	800	110	10	350	15
Females	11–14	44	97	155	62	1300	1200	115	18	300	15
	15–10	54	110	162	65	1200	1200	115	18	300	15
	19–22	58	126	162	65	800	800	100	18	300	15
	33–50	58	128	162	65	800	800	100	18	300	15
	51+	53	125	182	65	800	800	80	10	300	15
Pregnant						1200	1200	125	18+	450	20
Lactating						1200	1200	150	18	450	25

248

AVERAGE PORTIONS OF FOOD

Energy and protein content of edible portions

Food	Size of average portion (oz)	Energy per average portion (kcal)	(MJ)	Protein (g)
Apple	4	50	0·21	0·4
Apple pudding	4	280	1·1	3
Bacon, gammon	2	250	1·4	18
Banana	4	80	0·33	1
Beans, baked	4	100	0·42	7
Beans, butter	2	50	0·21	4
Beans, French	2	4	0·02	0·4
Beef, lean only	4	250	1·04	30
Beetroot	2	30	0·13	1
Blancmange	2	70	0·29	2
Bread	3 slices	280	1·17	9·6
Bread with butter		390	1·63	9·6
Butter	1	230	0·96	0
Cabbage	4	10	0·04	0·8
Cakes	2	240	1·00	4
Cake, cherry	2	260	1·09	5
Carrots	2	10	0·04	0·4
Cauliflower	2	6	0·03	0·8
Breakfast cereal	1	100	0·42	1·9
Cheese	1	120	0·50	7·2
Chicken, boiled or roast	4	220	9·20	33
Cod, fried	6	240	1·00	30
Egg	2	90	0·38	7
Fish cakes	4	240	1·00	14
Ham, boiled	4	490	2·05	18
Jelly	4	90	0·38	2·4
Kidney, stewed	4	180	0·75	29
Lettuce, raw	2	5	0·02	0·6
Luncheon meat, canned	4	380	1·6	13
Margarine	1	230	0·96	0
Marrow, boiled	2	4	0·02	0·2
Milk	1 glass	130	0·54	6·3
Mince-pie	2	220	0·92	7
Nuts, Brazil, Barcelona	2	360	1·50	16
Nuts, pea	2	340	1·40	16
Orange	4	40	0·17	0·8
Peas, fresh, boiled	2	30	0·13	3
Pineapple, canned in syrup	4	70	0·29	0·4
Plaice, fried	6	390	1·63	30
Plaice, steamed	6	150	0·63	30
Potatoes, boiled	6	140	0·59	2·4
Potatoes, chipped	6	410	1·71	7
Potatoes, roast	6	210	0·88	5
Salmon	4	160	0·67	22
Salmon, canned	6	240	0·96	22
Sardines in oil	1	85	0·35	6
Sardines in tomato	1	50		

Food	Size of average portion (oz)	Energy per average portion (kcal)	(MJ)	Protein (g)
Sausages, fried, pork	2	360	1·50	13
Sausage roll	2	260	1·09	4·6
Spaghetti, macaroni	4	130	0·54	4
Sprouts	4	20	0·08	3
Stew, Irish	4	170	0·71	4·4
Suet pudding	4	420	1·69	6
Tomato, raw	2	10	0·04	0·6
Trifle	4	160	0·67	4

94915